SEXUALITY IN ADOLESCENCE AND EMERGING ADULTHOOD

Sexuality in Adolescence and Emerging Adulthood

Raymond Montemayor

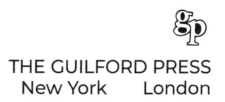

THE GUILFORD PRESS
New York   London

Library of Congress Cataloging-in-Publication Data

Names: Montemayor, Raymond, author.
Title: Sexuality in adolescence and emerging adulthood / Raymond Montemayor.
Description: New York, NY: Guilford Press, [2019] | Includes bibliographical
   references and index.
Identifiers: LCCN 2018035464 | ISBN 9781462537174 (hardcover : alk. paper) |
   ISBN 9781462537167 (pbk. : alk. paper)
Subjects: LCSH: Teenagers—Sexual behavior. | Adolescence.
Classification: LCC HQ27 .M628 2019 | DDC 306.70835—dc23
LC record available at *https://lccn.loc.gov/2018035464*

Preface

The idea for this book arose from an advanced undergraduate psychology course entitled Adolescent Sexuality that I taught for many years in the Department of Psychology at The Ohio State University. The course emerged from my interest in adolescent sexuality and from the desire of students for a course on that topic. Student demand for the course has been high, and the class is offered twice each year to 60–80 students per semester. In looking for an appropriate text for the course, I discovered that a book that surveyed the field of adolescent sexuality as I envisioned it did not exist. This is that book. It is an extensive, empirical survey of research on adolescent and emerging adult sexuality and is ideal for a course on that subject.

The book is interdisciplinary, not only drawing on research from psychology but also including findings from sociology, biology, medicine, anthropology, and newer disciplines, such as media studies and sexuality studies. This mix of disciplines reflects the diversity of questions and methods that characterize the vigorous area of research on adolescent sexuality.

The text emphasizes recent empirical research on adolescent sexuality. It is not possible to cover the vast literatures on each of the topic areas in the book, so the chapters are selective, highlighting contemporary research but covering older research where appropriate. Each chapter also includes "A Focus on Research" sidebar that is an examination of a research issue related to the chapter topic.

Where possible, research is reported in a developmental context, beginning in childhood, moving into adolescence, where most of the research is found, and ending in emerging adulthood. The book begins with an examination of sex play during childhood, moving to the unfolding of early sexual behavior during the middle school years, and to the growing expression of sexuality during the high school years into emerging adulthood. Sexuality does not suddenly appear at puberty, but has earlier childhood antecedents and includes precoital behaviors.

While the book is data driven, relying extensively on social science and biological research on adolescent sexuality, it may not be as theoretical as some might wish. This is because with some exceptions, most of the research on the sexual behavior of young people is the result of attempts to answer specific research or applied questions rather than to test theoretical ideas. Where theory is linked to research it is usually as an attempt to integrate or explain research findings, and those theories are presented where they seem useful.

■ ORGANIZATION

The book is organized in a question-and-answer format designed to pose interesting and important questions about adolescent sexuality, and to answer each question or at least present the best available evidence that addresses that question. This format is meant to engage the reader and to draw the reader into the particular issue under examination. This approach also highlights the manner in which science often proceeds, starting with an important question and attempting to supply an answer, or at least a provisional answer, to that question.

Each chapter can stand alone. There are some cross-references and interconnections among the chapters and those connections are presented in the text. There is something to be gained from reading all the chapters in the order given, but there is no need to follow that order. An instructor also may assign only particular chapters from the book.

One unique feature of the book is the extensive use of stories written by students about their sexuality, called "In Their Own Words." All the stories are written by undergraduate students taking my course on adolescent sexuality, each of whom wrote two papers about some aspect of their sexual lives. Students were instructed to write in a casual, colloquial style as if they were telling a story about themselves to a friend. Over the years, I collected hundreds of these stories, and 75 were selected to illustrate various ideas in the book. Students gave me permission to reprint each of their stories. I have retained the original language, spelling, punctuation, and grammar, only editing some of the stories to eliminate extraneous material or information that would compromise the anonymity of the writer. The stories bring to life and make human many of the research findings, putting a personal imprint on abstract ideas. The number of stories varies from chapter to chapter. Some topics do not include stories because students did not write on those topics.

■ AUDIENCE

The primary audience for this book includes undergraduate and graduate students taking courses in psychology, sociology, family science, education, health, nursing, public health, and social work or other fields with a focus on adolescence or human sexuality. The book is written for readers with little or no knowledge about research on adolescent sexuality. In addition to students, the book is written for teachers, clinicians, counselors, nurses, social workers, other practitioners, and policymakers who work with adolescents. The book is also appropriate for scholars and researchers looking for a broad-based survey of research on adolescent sexuality.

Practitioners, educators, and policymakers who work with adolescents may find the book especially useful as background material on sexual development and on the sexual activity of adolescents. Information on sexual development; lesbian, gay, bisexual, transgender, and questioning (LGBTQ) youth; and risky sexual behavior should be particularly valuable for clinicians and counselors who work directly with adolescents. Professionals involved in the legal system, from social workers to judges and policymakers, may benefit from an examination of research on the legal ramifications of adolescent sexual behavior. Educators may find the material on sex education, teen pregnancy, romantic relations, and peer influences germane to their interest in the behavior of middle school and high school students. Research on biology, sexually transmitted infections, and teen pregnancy may be especially useful for physicians and nurses in the field of adolescent medicine.

This book is a comprehensive synthesis and examination of empirical research on adolescent sexuality. It is an attempt to convey some of the important questions that have driven research in this area and to provide current answers to those questions. Much is known about this important topic, but much more remains to be discovered—perhaps, by you.

Acknowledgments

I am enormously grateful to the many colleagues, friends, and students who freely gave of their time and generously provided feedback during the lengthy period I spent conducting research for this book and the longer period of time writing it. There were times when I thought I would never finish, and their support and encouragement kept me on task and moving forward.

The book owes its life to C. Deborah Laughton, my enthusiastic editor at The Guilford Press, who sponsored it and saw it through to completion. Without C. Deborah's belief in me and in the book, there would be no book. She not only encouraged me to write the book but contributed to it in substantial ways by suggesting that I follow a question-and-answer format for the book and that I include "A Focus on Research" section in each chapter.

Two people were especially important in the process of writing this book: my friend and colleague John Gibbs, in the Department of Psychology at The Ohio State University, and my long-time friend Chet Cortellesi were tremendously helpful and I am particularly grateful to both of them. John helped me clarify and sharpen my ideas about adolescent sexuality during the many hours he and I spent together at our weekly lunches over the past several years. John was an inspiration and guide from start to finish, offering practical suggestions about writing, feedback on ideas for the book, and helpful advice about the arduous process of getting a book published. Chet has been a long-time and constant source of support and encouragement, and we spoke almost every day about my writing progress, or sometimes lack of progress. Chet cheered me on and held me accountable for my time, keeping me on track and moving ahead even on days when I did not much feel like writing.

My colleague and friend Jerry Winer generously read and extensively commented on several chapters, offering constructive criticism and advice, especially about the importance of tying research findings to intervention where possible. Five students provided valuable editorial assistance: Emily Corturillo, Shelby Kretz, and Alex Wasserman read and incisively commented on several chapters, and Edwin Szeto and Justyn Harvey collected valuable reference material for the LGBTQ chapter. I would also like to thank Guilford's reviewers of the manuscript, initially anonymous, whose thoughtful comments were very helpful in shaping the book: Terri D. Fisher, Professor Emeritus of Psychology, The Ohio State University at Mansfield; Wendy Hadley, Division of Psychiatry and Human Behavior, Brown University; Michael Kimmel, Department of Sociology, Stony Brook University; Toni Serafini, Department of Sexuality, Marriage, and Family Studies, St. Jerome's University/University of Waterloo; and Devon Hensel, Department of Pediatrics, Indiana University.

Friends from my movie group, including Denise Bronson, Charlie Flowers, and Pat Flowers, listened to my stories and offered valuable advice and feedback. My friend and colleague David Huron was on a writing journey himself—his progress and comments about my writing inspired me to stay on task.

I had many conversations with friends and relatives about my writing progress, including my neighbors Mark and Kathy Blanchard, close friends Paul Croshaw and Zina Brown, and my cousin Anthony Galindo, and I thank all of them for their interest and contributions.

Three people offered valuable personal and professional support and guidance. My dear friend and colleague Charles Wenar, who died too soon in 2008, encouraged me to teach a course on adolescent sexuality, which was the genesis of this book. Douglas Kramer has been and continues to be a guide through troubled waters and he taught me valuable life lessons that went far beyond writing this book. Radu Saveanu was a source of comfort and aid during an especially difficult time in my life when I did not think I was capable of finishing this book.

My loving wife, Kathleen Montemayor, gave me the freedom and time to obsessively devote myself to what at times seemed like an insurmountable and monumental task. Kathy provided reassurance, emotional support, and constant encouragement, often expressing confidence in me and in my ability to complete this daunting project. Thank you, Kathy, for everything, including your suggestions for improving the manuscript, and for your backing from the beginning to the end of this enormous undertaking.

Last, I want to gratefully thank all the students in my course on adolescent sexuality who over the years gave me permission to reprint their personal stories, bringing to life many of the ideas in this book. I removed any identifying information from the stories in order to protect the anonymity of the students. I am grateful to all the students who generously contributed to the book by sharing stories of their very personal sexual experiences.

Brief Contents

Extended Contents

Overview

The study of adolescent sexuality is an ongoing vigorous area of research as revealed by a recent search performed on PsycINFO with the search terms *adol** and *sexual** that turned up 34,036 English-language hits, 38% of which were studies published since 2010. The vitality of this field is due to the importance of sexuality to adolescents and to their development, and to the social and economic consequences adolescent sexual behavior has on us all.

The book includes 12 chapters, each of which is a summary and interpretation of research and theory on an area of study on adolescent sexual activity. The book presents some of the most important findings on adolescent sexuality to a wide range of nontechnical readers. The material is accessible to individuals with a variety of backgrounds. Research is described in nontechnical language except where technical terms are useful, in which case the terms are clearly defined.

Chapter 1 explores the idea that sexuality does not suddenly emerge with the onset of puberty. Sexuality is a developmental phenomenon, and the focus of this chapter is on some precoital activities, including sex play in childhood, masturbation, and oral sex, followed by an examination of sexual intercourse and the transition from virginity to nonvirginity. Historical trends in adolescent sexual behavior are then presented. The last section focuses on sexuality and gender issues, especially female sexual development.

Chapter 2 examines some of the important biological changes that occur during puberty, and the impact of biology on adolescent sexuality. Biology may not fully determine adolescent sexual behavior, but biology has an influence on sexual behavior, although the association between biological factors and adolescent sexuality is complex. The impact of gonadal hormones on the sexual behavior of young people is explored, followed by an investigation of the relationship between physical maturation and teen sexuality. Next is an examination of the impact of family stress on pubertal timing and adolescent sexual behavior. A presentation of recent research on the effect of teen brain development on adolescent sexuality follows. Next is a presentation of recent research on the effect of teen brain development on adolescent sexuality. The chapter ends with a consideration of genetic effects on the sexual behavior of adolescents.

Chapter 3 examines the impact of parents on adolescent sexual behavior. Research is presented on the relationship between family structure and adolescent sexuality, followed by the influence of fathers on teen sexuality. The next section is on the relationship between parental divorce and adolescent risky sexual behavior. The chapter ends with a discussion of the relationship between adolescent sexuality and four parenting attributes: parental support, control, monitoring, and attitudes about sexuality.

Chapter 4 focuses on parent–adolescent communication about sex. In the first section, differences between mother–adolescent and father–adolescent discussions about sex are examined. Next is a comparison of parent conversations about sex with their daughters and sons. The final sections focus on the possible impact of parent–teen communication about sex on adolescent sexual behavior, followed by an examination of interventions designed to improve the ability of parents to talk effectively to their teens about sex.

There is a strong association between the sexual activity of adolescents and the sexual activity of their peers. Chapter 5 examines the reasons for that association, focusing on peer socialization and peer selection. The chapter also explores the relationship between popularity and sexual activity followed by an examination of the sexual double standard and whether it still exists. Last, research on the relationship between membership in a deviant peer group and adolescent risky sexual behavior is presented.

Chapter 6 examines dating, romantic relations, and casual sex in adolescence and emerging adulthood. The relationship between dating and sexual behavior is explored, and dating and romantic relations among lesbian, gay, bisexual, transgender, and questioning (LGBTQ) adolescents are discussed. A hookup is defined and research on hookups is presented, especially on the extent of hookup behavior. Last, the antecedents of hooking up are examined along with studies on the psychological consequences of hooking up.

Chapter 7 reviews research on the relationship between sex in the media and adolescent sexual attitudes and behavior. The difficulty of establishing a causal relationship between sex in the media and sexual behavior is discussed. Research on sex on the Internet, on television, in movies, and in music is presented. The association between exposure to sex in the media and permissive sexual attitudes and behavior is examined, and the relationship between exposure to sex in the media and adolescent sexual risk-taking is explored. Issues related to sexting are discussed. Last is an examination of the association between viewing pornography and adolescent sexual attitudes and behavior.

Chapter 8 examines LGBTQ adolescents and emerging adults. An important focus of the chapter is on theory and research on the development of a sexual identity. There is a discussion of the victimization of LGBTQ adolescents and an examination of mental health problems among LGBTQ adolescents and emerging adults, especially depression, suicide, and substance use and abuse. Research on transgender adolescents is presented, and gender dysphoria (GD) is defined and examined. The chapter ends with a discussion of the mental health and substance use problems among transgender adolescents.

Teen pregnancy is explored in Chapter 9, which focuses not only on the causes of teen pregnancy but also on its consequences to young mothers, their children, and the fathers. The point is made that teens are disadvantaged as a result of an early pregnancy, but some of that disadvantage is present even before the pregnancy and birth. Next is an examination of the children born to teen mothers, focusing on their physical health, psychological and cognitive development, and social relations throughout childhood into adolescence. Research on the fathers of children born to teen mothers is presented, along with an examination of the consequences of being a teen father. Last is an overview of interventions designed to help teen families and improve the lives of family members.

In Chapter 10, the point is made that a substantial number of adolescents and emerging adults have a sexually transmitted infection (STI), and the incidence of STIs among the young is increasing. A discussion of condom usage is included as well as an examination of the psychological, social, and behavioral risk factors associated with acquiring an STI. The focus of the chapter is on understanding the risky sexual behavior of adolescents that may lead to an STI. A social-ecological perspective is used to examine the individual, interpersonal, and neighborhood influences on risky adolescent sexual behavior.

Chapter 11 evaluates the effectiveness of school-based sex education programs to influence adolescent sexual behavior, focusing specifically on comprehensive sex education and abstinence sex education. Results reveal that comprehensive sex education reduces risky teen sexual activity, but effects are modest and short term. Abstinence sex education is less effective in general, but a few programs have had some limited successes. The chapter ends with an examination of other attempts to reduce risky sexual behavior, including virginity pledges, parent education programs, peer-led sexuality courses, media interventions, and school-based health clinics.

Adolescent sexuality typically is presented as dangerous, risky behavior. In Chapter 12, a new perspective is examined that portrays sexual behavior as an unfolding of a normal developmental interest during adolescence and emerging adulthood. Research on the relationship between sexual activity and adolescent physical, psychological, and behavior problems is described and evaluated. Research is presented that reveals that adolescent sexuality is far from a negative experience for many, if not most, adolescents. The point is made that sexual activity can be a positive experience for some adolescents in some circumstances. Last is a presentation of a nonproblem-oriented approach to the study of adolescent sexuality that may lead to a more complete understanding of this important aspect of adolescent development.

CHAPTER 1

Sexuality from Childhood through Adolescence

Human sexuality is more than sexual intercourse and it does not begin in adolescence with the onset of puberty. Instead, sexuality is a developmental process, some aspects of which appear in infancy, are elaborated on in childhood, and fundamentally altered with the onset of puberty. Sexuality—broadly conceived to include sexual curiosity and exploration—antedates puberty by many years, first appearing early in life. Puberty brings with it the initiation of sexual desire and the capacity for sexual response, but the precursors of adult sexuality are present long before the emergence of genital sexuality during early adolescence.

Children are sexual beings, as Sigmund Freud long ago famously argued, an idea on which he built an elaborate theory of psychosexual development. The basic theory is that children are inherently sexual beings, whose sexuality unfolds through various sexual stages. Although most of Freud's principal contentions about early sexuality have been discredited, his basic insight that children have an interest in sexuality and engage in behaviors that appear to be sexual is an important observation about the development of sexuality. The low level of sex steroids present in a child's body prevent a child from having and experiencing a true adult sexual response, but children do engage in behaviors that are sexual in appearance and which give them pleasure.

■ SEX PLAY IN CHILDHOOD

What Is Sex Play in Childhood?

Childhood sex play is difficult to define, but it is important to provide some definition of the concept in order to distinguish it from child sexual abuse. There is no generally agreed-upon definition of *childhood sex play* (de Graaf &

The following story told by a female college student is an example of childhood sex play. Note the negative reaction of the father to the incident, a common reaction by parents.

IN THEIR OWN WORDS

When I was a younger child I experienced my first and only (as far as I can remember) childhood sex play experience. I was 3 years old at the time, as well as the boy who I experienced it with, my cousin, B. Every Sunday my family would go to church together and then go to my grandparents to spend time together. My grandparents had an extra room that they had converted basically into a playroom filled with toys for the grandchildren. B. and I were the only grandchildren there in the playroom at the time. I had just gotten a play doctor set for my birthday, which included a fake stethoscope and Band-Aids. We both thought it was the coolest thing ever, and we took turns playing doctor and patient. I don't exactly remember how, but eventually it got to the point that we each took turns pulling down our own pants and exposing our genitals, especially our butts. I have absolutely no idea why, but at the time we thought butts were the funniest things ever. It was all a very innocent thing. Mostly I would say that it stemmed from curiosity. There was absolutely nothing sexual about it at all. It seemed like it was part of being a doctor to us at the time. It was just play. But, unfortunately for us, my father walked in on us when I was showing my butt off. That put an end to that. My dad was furious, and I can't remember exactly what our punishment was, but I do remember both my cousin and I getting spanked pretty good. What had been a very innocent thing at the time from then after seemed very negative.

Rademakers, 2006), but the term includes prepubescent children's interest in and exploration of their own genitals or the genitals of others. When childhood sex play includes another child, the children are approximately the same age, perhaps no more than 2 years apart. Childhood sex play is not coercive and does not involve forced participation. In addition, childhood sex play may include children of the opposite sex or the same sex.

Sex play is a common activity during childhood, perhaps more common than many adults realize. Anthropologists report that what they refer to as "sexual rehearsal play" is common among nonhuman primates and among children in many nonindustrial societies (Josephs, 2015). It is a troubling activity for many contemporary Western parents, who often have two questions about it when they discover its occurrence in their own children: Is it normal? and What should I do about it (Moser, Kleinplatz, Zuccarini, & Reiner, 2004)?

What Are the Most Common Sex Play Behaviors among Young Children?

Studying sex play in childhood is difficult for reasons that are both practical and ethical. First, it is challenging, if not impossible, to question young children, especially those under the age of 6 years, about sex play because of the problem of defining and describing those behaviors to the children. Second, even if children could report on their own sex play, there are ethical reasons for not asking them to report on behaviors and feelings that could be embarrassing or upsetting. For these reasons, the study of sex play in childhood relies on the retrospective reports of adults, usually college students, about their behavior when they were young, or on parent reports, usually mothers, on the behaviors they have observed in their children. Occasionally, reports about childhood sexual behavior are obtained from early childhood educators in learning settings (Balter, van Rhijn, & Davies, 2016). There are limitations to all these methods that include the unreliability of memory and adults' lack of knowledge about child behavior when the adult is not present. Data collected using these techniques are not invalid, but their true validity is unknown and we should interpret these findings cautiously.

One study of Swedish adolescents found that sex play before the age of 13 was common (Larsson & Svedin, 2002). About 80% of older adolescents reported that they had engaged in solitary or mutual sexual play before they were 13 years old. The most common solitary activity was exploration of the self including genitals, and the most common mutual sexual play was kissing and hugging.

Friedrich and colleagues (1992) developed a child sexual behavior inventory that relies on mothers' reports of 38 behaviors assessing sexual behavior of children between 2 and 12 years of age. The five most common childhood sex play behaviors based on a sample of over 1,000 U.S. children who had not been sexually abused include the following: touches sex (private) parts when at home, touches or tries to touch their mother's or other women's breasts, stands too close to people, tries to look at people when they are nude or undressing, and is very interested in the opposite sex. The three least common behaviors are tries to have sexual intercourse with another child or adult, puts mouth on another child's/adult's sex parts, and asks others to engage in sexual acts with him or her (Friedrich, Fisher, Broughton, Houston, & Shafran, 1998). The findings reveal that sex play involving touching and looking is common among prepubescent children, but other behaviors, especially those involving attempted intercourse and oral sex, are uncommon and may be indicative of sexual abuse or other behavioral problems (Friedrich et al., 2001).

The most common feelings young adults remember having when they engaged in sex play during childhood are feeling excited (but not sexually excited), being silly/giggly, having pleasant body sensations, and feeling good/fine (Larsson & Svedin, 2002). Feelings of guilt are uncommon, although more females than males remember feeling guilty. Most young adults, especially males, remember positive feelings about their sex play (de Graaf & Rademakers, 2006).

Who Is Likely to Engage in Sex Play?

Young children under the age of 5 years are more likely to engage in sex play than older children. Several explanations are possible for the decrease in sex play as children get older. First, gonadal hormones decrease after about age 5 years, and remain low until puberty, perhaps leading to a declining interest in sex play in middle childhood (Udry & Campbell, 1994). Second, the decrease may reflect an increase in socialization as children get older and learn that sex play is inappropriate, especially in public. Third, children may become more secretive and cautious about their sex play as they get older, so mothers are less likely to observe this type of play among older children even though it does occur (Kellogg, 2009).

Boys are more likely to engage in sex play than girls. Some kinds of sex play that are more common among boys than girls include self-stimulation, looking at sexually explicit pictures, and sexual teasing (Larsson & Svedin, 2002). These early gender differences in sex play may be due to differences in socialization in which boys are given more freedom to express their sexual interests than girls. These differences are present even among children as young as 2 years old, however, which suggests the possibility of biological differences between genders in interest in sexuality.

Two family factors related to sex play include maternal education and parents' attitudes about childhood sex play (Friedrich et al., 1998). Mothers with more education report more sex play among their children than mothers with less education, which could be due to more lenient attitudes about sex play among educated mothers, or to more awareness of childhood sex play among educated mothers. Further, parents who think it is normal for children to be sexually curious report more sex play among their children than parents who do not think this is normal.

Differences in childhood sex play vary across cultures and ethnicities. For example, Dutch children engage in more sex play than U.S. children (Friedrich, Sandfort, Oostveen, & Cohen-Kettenis, 2000). These differences are undoubtedly due to differences in sexual socialization that begin at an early age. Dutch adults have more liberal attitudes about sexuality than U.S. adults, which may include more liberal attitudes about sex play in childhood. U.S. parents are less tolerant of childhood sex play than Dutch parents and may be more likely to punish it when it occurs. Other research on U.S. Latinos found that mothers reported more childhood sex play, especially interpersonal sex play, in comparison to white mothers, a difference that may reflect more tolerance of sex play among Latino parents (Kenny & Wurtele, 2013). Together, these studies reveal cultural differences in parental attitudes about childhood sex play and in differences in the frequency of childhood sex play.

What about Sibling Sex Play?

Sex play in childhood is a troubling occurrence for many parents who worry that it indicates psychological disturbance or may lead to sexual and other problems later in life. Of even greater concern is sibling sex play, not only for the same reasons about sex play among friends but, in addition, because it suggests a violation of the incest taboo. How common is sibling sex play and what effect does it have on later sexual development? About 15% of college students with a

The following example illustrates a typical sibling sex play experience that includes looking and touching.

IN THEIR OWN WORDS

... I do remember when I was between the ages of 5 and 9. My parents had a massage wand back massager that I was fascinated with (they still have it). My brother had showed me what to do with it. We would take turns putting this massage wand on each other's genitals. I continued to use this massage wand until my mom caught me with it. I remember telling her I put it on my belly but obviously, she knew I was lying. I was so embarrassed when she told me not to put it on my private parts. The words *private parts* still make me uncomfortable when she uses the phrase on my 5-year-old niece.

Along with the back massager wand, my brother showed me his penis when we were younger. He had me touch it a few times. I remember feeling a little embarrassed and that it felt really weird. He never touched me like that nor did I ever show him my "private parts."

sibling report that they engaged in some type of sibling sexual play when they were young (Finkelhor, 1980; Greenwald & Leitenberg, 1989). The median age of sibling sexual activity is about 10 years, a little older than typical sex play among friends. Sibling sexual activity often includes exhibiting genitals and touching genitals, in addition to a small percentage of young adolescents who have intercourse or attempt intercourse with a sibling. Force or the threat of force is uncommon when the sexual activity is between siblings who are close in age, but more common between siblings with a wider age gap.

Is Sex Play in Childhood Related to Sexual Behavior in Emerging Adulthood?

In general, nonaggressive sex play in childhood is unrelated to sexual behavior during emerging adulthood (Leitenberg, Greenwald, & Tarran, 1989; Okami, Olmstead, & Abramson, 1997). The absence of a relationship between childhood sex play and later sexual behavior suggests that these two types of behaviors are unrelated, although they have a surface similarity. Perhaps sex play in childhood has more to do with curiosity than with sexuality, while emerging adult sexuality is more strongly influenced by biological and psychosocial factors directly related to a sexual response.

There is no association between nonaggressive sibling sex play and later sexual behavior among young men, but some young females who engaged in sibling sex play are more sexually active in college than females who did not engage in sibling sex play (Finkelhor, 1980). Sibling sex play can be related to psychological difficulties in adolescence if the sex play involves force or the threat of force (Hardy, 2001; Krienert & Walsh, 2011).

There is one qualification to the general conclusion of no association between childhood sex play and emerging adult sexual behavior. If the sex play in childhood involves genital contact, even if it does not include intercourse, then emerging adults are more likely to engage in premarital sexual intercourse and have more intercourse partners than emerging adults who's sex play during childhood does not involve genital contact (Leitenberg et al., 1989). We need to be cautious about attributing an increase in emerging adult sexual behavior to genital contact during childhood, since there are many reasons why these behaviors might be related. Nevertheless, sex play involving genital contact may be different in some important ways from more typical sex play and indicate an early interest in sexuality that goes beyond typical sex play and persists into emerging adulthood.

■ MASTURBATION

The story of the idea that masturbation is a moral failure and a dangerous disease is well-known (Laqueur, 2003). Based on Judeo-Christian beliefs that masturbation is a sin against nature and God, medical practitioners in the United States and in the West in the 18th and 19th centuries provided health-related descriptions of the medical ills that could befall someone as a result of "self-abuse." Dr. R. V. Pierce's (1875) book *The People's Common Sense Medical Adviser in Plain English* provides an example of this concern, and includes an impassioned description of what the doctor terms *spermatorrhea,* or *seminal weakness,* that results from excessive masturbation. According to Pierce, masturbation "saps the vigor, undermines and ruins the constitution, and, if the victim marries and has not by such indulgences rendered himself entirely impotent, he becomes the father of puny offspring; or, more frequently, being entirely impotent, it renders both his own life and that of his companion most wretched" (p. 816). Pierce pays less attention to female masturbation, but it too is presented as a serious assault on one's physical and mental health.

We live in more enlightened times, but the stigma surrounding masturbation continues to exist, although to a considerably lesser degree and expressed in a much less impassioned language. The subject of masturbation remains a sensitive and dangerous topic of discussion, however, that has even cost people their careers. One famous case occurred in 1994, when U.S. surgeon general Joycelyn Elders was forced to resign her post after giving a speech in which she suggested that masturbation should be a topic taught in sex education courses (Greenberg, 1994).

What Percentage of Adolescents Have Masturbated?

Two conclusions emerge from several recent studies of the prevalence of masturbation among adolescents in the United States, Britain, and Australia: first, masturbation is common in adolescence and throughout the lifespan; and second, more males than females report that they have masturbated. In one study of U.S. adolescents between 14 and 17 years of age, about 75% of males and about 50% of females reported that they had masturbated (Robbins et al., 2011). The percentage of adolescents who have masturbated increases during adolescence, dramatically for males. Further, males of all ages masturbate more frequently than females. For example, 20% of males report that they masturbate four or more times per week, while only 7% of females report masturbating that often. These findings are representative of results from other studies of adolescents and adults in the United States (Das, 2007), Britain (Gerressu, Mercer, Graham, Wellings, & Johnson, 2008), and Australia (Smith, Rosenthal, & Reichler, 1996). One additional finding is that lesbian and gay adolescents are more likely to report masturbating than heterosexual adolescents, perhaps revealing a stronger sex drive among lesbian and gay adolescents (Gerressu et al., 2008).

Why Is Masturbation More Common among Males Than Females?

The findings that more males than females report they masturbate and masturbate more often are among the largest and most consistent differences between males and females for any aspect of sexuality (Petersen & Hyde, 2010). Why these gender differences exist is not well understood, but at least three explanations are possible. One is that there are no real differences in male and female masturbation, only gender differences in a willingness to report masturbation. The assumption underlying this explanation is that males are less ashamed about masturbating than are females, and so are more willing to report on an anonymous survey that they masturbate.

A second explanation for gender differences in masturbation is based on the existence of the sexual double standard that allows males more sexual freedom than females. According to this idea, masturbation is more acceptable for males than for females, a belief that when internalized leads females to suppress their sexuality, including their desire to masturbate.

A third explanation is that gender differences in masturbation may have a biological basis and are rooted in differences in those aspects of brain functioning that control sexual arousal. In addition, some have argued that gender differences in gonadal hormones, especially level of testosterone, lead to a heightened sexual drive among males. In line with the idea that gonadal hormones released during puberty have a stronger effect on male than female masturbation, consider Figure 1.1, based on data collected by Alfred Kinsey in the late 1940s and early 1950s on the prevalence of masturbation in males and females of different ages. The graph reveals two important findings. First, after puberty, significantly more males than females report that they have masturbated. Second, of more relevance for the biological explanation for gender differences in masturbation, note the shape of the two graphs. For males, the prevalence of masturbation increases dramatically after the onset of puberty

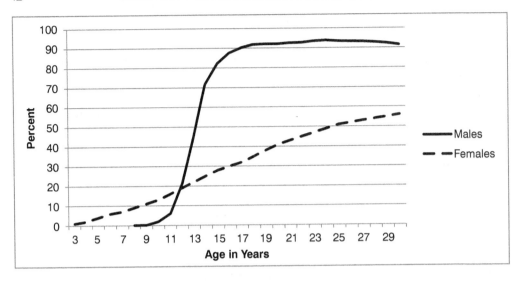

FIGURE 1.1. Percentage of males and females who have masturbated at least once. Adapted from Kinsey, Pomeroy, and Martin (1948) and Kinsey, Pomeroy, Martin, and Gebhard (1953).

during early adolescence. The percentage of males who have masturbated at age 15 is 13 times higher than the percentage of males who have masturbated at age 11, suggesting that male masturbation is highly related to the occurrence of biological changes that begin during puberty. In contrast, there is no evidence of a puberty effect for females. For females, the prevalence of masturbation gradually increases year by year between childhood and emerging adulthood.

Why Are Some Adolescents More Likely to Masturbate Than Others?

More adolescents and emerging adults report masturbating in the 1990s and 2000s than in the 1960s and 1970s, a generational shift found in the United States (Herbenick et al., 2010; Laumann, Gagnon, Michael, & Michaels, 1994), Germany (Dekker & Schmidt, 2003), Finland, Sweden, and Russia (Kontula & Haavio-Mannila, 2002). More adolescents today report that they masturbate more frequently, and that they begin to masturbate at an earlier age than adolescents in the past. It is possible that adolescents today simply are more comfortable reporting that they masturbate, but another possibility is that a real change in behavior has occurred as ideas about masturbation have become more liberal and masturbation has become more acceptable (Day, 2013).

Masturbation varies by race and ethnicity. Hispanic adolescents report the highest rate of masturbation, followed by white adolescents, and Asian American males and females, while African American youth, especially females, report the lowest rate (Das, 2007; Laumann et al., 1994; Okazaki, 2002; Robbins et al., 2011). These group differences highlight the impact of culture on

A FOCUS ON RESEARCH

Survey research is built on the idea that what people think, believe, or have done is accurately reflected in their answers to survey questions. Answers to survey questions are thought to have high *validity*, which is the degree to which a question measures what it is designed to measure. Studies of adolescent sexual behavior, including masturbation, are not based on actual observations of behavior or on biological markers of sexual activity, but on self-reports. The assumption is that the validity of self-reports of sexual behavior is high, because it is thought that adolescents generally tell the truth when they participate in anonymous studies of sexuality. It is not known to what extent this assumption is true since some adolescents may underreport their behavior and indicate they did not engage in a behavior when they did, while others may overreport their behavior and report they did engage in a behavior when in fact they did not. There are many reasons for these inconsistencies, such as misremembering a behavior that took place in the past, or bragging about sexual conquests that did not occur. One study of masturbation during adolescence reveals that reports of masturbation may not be perfectly valid.

Young males reported twice on whether they had masturbated during adolescence, the first time when they were adolescents and the second time several years later when they were young adults (Halpern, Udry, Suchindran, & Campbell, 2000). The results indicated that male adolescents reported less masturbation during adolescence than they did when they were young adults, suggesting that some adolescents are reluctant to admit that they masturbate. In other research, female college students reported they had intercourse with a fewer number of partners when they thought their answers would be anonymous and a higher number of partners when they thought the researcher could detect dishonesty. The results suggest that under standard testing conditions adolescents may be influenced by social desirability and answer questions in a way they think they should answer the questions, even if it means distorting the truth (Alexander & Fisher, 2003). The finding that some adolescents may not always tell the truth does not invalidate results of studies of sexual behavior, but it does suggest that the actual percentages may be somewhat different from what is reported.

sexual behavior and reveal the effect cultural ideas about sexuality can have on masturbation.

Reports of masturbation and frequency of masturbation increase with more education. High school graduates are more likely to masturbate than young men and women who did not graduate from high school, and college graduates are more likely to masturbate than young adults who did not graduate from college (Laumann et al., 1994). Further, more education is associated with reports of more pleasure from masturbation. Education appears to decrease the taboo about masturbating, leading to more masturbation and to experiencing more pleasure from masturbation.

Religion is another factor related to reports of masturbation. Young women who are religious report less masturbation than women who are not religious, a relationship that is not as strong for men (Gerressu et al., 2008). Apparently, religious beliefs inhibit female masturbation more than male masturbation.

In the following story, a young man describes the first time he masturbated. Note that religion did not seem to have an impact on whether he masturbated, but his religious beliefs had an impact on his reactions to masturbation. He first felt ashamed about what he was doing, and later unburdened when he was told that masturbation was not a sin.

IN THEIR OWN WORDS

It was the evening in the year 2000; I remember it for the movie that I had seen that evening. It was early on in the television debut of the film *Austin Powers.* After 90 minutes I was introduced to the notions of penis enlargement pumps, orgasms, and sex toys, as well as getting a healthy eyeful of half-naked women. It must have been the combination of psychedelic '60s free love and nonstop sex jokes that made me connect the idea of sex with pleasure. I guess I didn't know before then what an orgasm was, but after hearing Powers's pleasured moans, I figured it out. And what's more is that the penis pump reference made me realize that the penis was the center of the male orgasm. That evening I was in the bath when I began to figure out how the general act is done. In mimicking the idea of a penis pump, I used a plastic cup and the water to form a seal so that I could induce a certain amount of pressure around my penis. Though it did not work as a penis pump, the activity at least led to an erection,

and through trial and error I made it all the way to discovering masturbation. I remember thinking that night that I had never done this before, and was surprised that I had not figured it out before then. I continued the practice semiregularly.

I was nine at this time. . . . I was raised Roman Catholic, but the odd thing is that no one had informed me at that point that masturbation was a sin. The shame was soon to follow. Though masturbation was already something that I kept a secret because it seemed like something private, it now was something to be ashamed of and hidden. . . . I decided I must stop. And I did, I stopped masturbating for an entire year (I believe when I was 13). Though the abstinence didn't last, being religious . . . did have a drastic effect on my masturbatory habits. It was a few years later that I confessed this particular sin to a priest, and he informed me that it was not a sin. That was good enough for me to stop feeling ashamed.

What Is the Relationship between Masturbation and Interpersonal Sexual Behavior?

Findings on the relationship between masturbation and interpersonal sexual behavior are inconsistent. In one study of adolescents, masturbation was positively related to partnered sexual behavior for males and females (Robbins et al., 2011). In another study, masturbation was positively related to sexual intercourse for females, but not for males (Gerressu et al., 2008), while in two other studies, masturbation and intercourse were unrelated (Leitenberg, Detzer, & Srebnik, 1993; Smith et al., 1996). It is not clear what accounts for these inconsistencies, but it does not appear that a simple relationship exists between masturbation and partnered sexual activity.

■ ORAL SEX

Parental panic about oral sex among preteenage children reached a crescendo in the early 2000s. Newspapers broke stories with headlines such as "Parents Are Alarmed by an Unsettling New Fad in Middle Schools: Oral Sex" (Stepp, 1999), which breathlessly reported on a new fad sweeping the country—middle school oral sex parties. The parties even had a name—Rainbow Parties—at which girls supposedly wore different-colored lipstick and boys competed to acquire as many different colors of lipstick on their penises as they could (Ruditis, 2005). Oprah Winfrey devoted an entire show to the "oral sex epidemic." What was going on? Was it true then, or true now, that large numbers of adolescents as young as 11- and 12-year-olds were engaging in casual oral sex? Had oral sex become cool? In this section, the scholarly literature on oral sex during adolescence is examined to assess the extent of oral sex, and to identify what personal characteristics are related to oral sex behavior.

How Prevalent Is Oral Sex among Teens?

The most recent estimates of the prevalence of oral sex reveal that it is common among emerging adults, somewhat less common among teens, and rare among middle school students. In the mid-2000s, about 80% of emerging adults ages 20–24 years had heterosexual oral sex, while about half of all U.S. teens ages 15–19 years had oral sex with members of the opposite sex (Copen, Chandra, & Martinez, 2012). Estimates of the prevalence of oral sex in Canada and the United Kingdom also reveal that about half of older teens have had oral sex (Sexuality and U, 2016; Stone, Hatherall, Ingham, & McEachran, 2006), indicating that adolescent involvement in oral sex does not uniquely arise from aspects of U.S. culture.

Good estimates of the national prevalence of oral sex among U.S. middle school students do not exist, but one extensive study of the sexual behavior of middle school students in the Los Angeles school district reveals that about 4% of 6th graders, 6% of 7th graders, and 13% of 8th graders reported that they had heterosexual oral sex (DeRosa et al., 2010). About twice as many boys as girls reported oral sex, 11% versus 5%, a discrepancy that could be due to reporting irregularities or to a pattern of boys having sex with older girls who were not in middle school.

The finding that many adolescents engage in oral sex has implications for sex education. It is important to discuss some of the dangers associated with oral sex, especially the possibility of transmission of sexually transmitted infections (STIs) and HIV/AIDS, in order to disavow adolescents of the widely held notion that oral sex is risk-free (Hoffman, 2016).

Has the Prevalence of Teenage Oral Sex Increased over the Past Several Years?

Survey researchers have not been tracking the prevalence of oral sex among U.S. teens over a long period of time, so it is not possible to ascertain whether the sudden concern about teen oral sex in the early 2000s represented a real increase in oral sex at that time or simply an increase in awareness and media attention. What data do exist does suggest that a real increase in oral sex among U.S. adolescents occurred between the mid-1970s and 2010, but there is no evidence of a sudden rise in oral sex behavior during the early 2000s (Child Trends, 2015a; Newcomer & Udry, 1985). Data on oral sex among Canadian 9th and 11th graders reveal about a 5% increase in oral sex between 1994 and 2002–2003 (Sexuality and U, 2016), indicating a general increase in oral sex among Canadian adolescents but no sharp increase in it in the early 2000s.

Are There Gender Differences in Oral Sex?

There are no strong gender differences in reports of oral sex among heterosexual adolescents, which one would expect since it takes two to have oral sex, but there are differences in reports of giving and receiving oral sex that are difficult to explain. About the same number of males and females report giving oral sex, but more males than females report receiving oral sex (Child Trends, 2015a; Jozkowski & Satinsky, 2013), although this pattern is not always found (Lindberg, Jones, & Santelli, 2008). Since the percentage of males who report receiving heterosexual oral sex should equal the percentage of females who report giving oral sex, it is difficult to explain how more males could report receiving oral sex than females report giving oral sex. Several possibilities might explain this puzzle: some females may have oral sex with more than one male, females may underreport giving oral sex, or males may overreport receiving oral sex. As we saw when we examined masturbation, reports of oral sex tell us something about the actual occurrence of oral sex, but we must not take those reports at face value since we need to be cautious about accepting self-reports of sensitive sexual behavior.

Another gender difference exists in the relationship between how pleasurable oral sex is and how often it is performed. Most young men report that giving oral sex is rewarding, but they are *less* likely to actually give oral sex, while young women report that giving oral sex is less pleasurable, but they are *more* likely to give oral sex (Lewis & Marston, 2016; Wood, McKay, Komarnicky, & Milhausen, 2016). How to explain this gender inconsistency? One answer is that females are more oriented to giving than to receiving sexual pleasure. Another answer is that more females than males are ambivalent about receiving oral sex and so do not ask for it even though they enjoy it and males are willing to do it, while males usually do not perform oral sex unless a female indicates she wants it. Further research is needed to better understand the complicated issue of gender differences in oral sex.

In the following story, a young woman describes her feelings about performing oral sex on her boyfriend, which eventually was reciprocated. Note that oral sex precedes vaginal intercourse.

IN THEIR OWN WORDS

Now, I hadn't had many boyfriends in high school. Two, to be exact. A., my first boyfriend, was a great friend, but not exactly the best boyfriend material. Our dating relationship got about as far as holding hands, hugging, and kisses on the cheek. It wasn't so much as a bad relationship; he and I just didn't really know how to move past being best friends. My second boyfriend, M., although he was also one of my best friends, was completely different and yet very similar. He knew what to do in a relationship. He was experienced in the whole dating thing, but he was still a virgin when I started dating him. We grew together in our relationship, both in maturity and eventually, sexually. We took things slowly. M. waited for me to allow certain things, like touching and petting, slowly taking things further and further. If I said no, he apologized and said we would wait until I was ready.

M. and I didn't start to move closer to oral sex and sexual intercourse until the summer after we started dating, roughly 8 months. We were both still virgins when we started with oral sex. It started with me giving and him receiving for a while, but then, as I grew more comfortable with the idea, slowly it transitioned to both of us giving and both receiving. At first, with me giving and M. receiving, I felt a little bad about what I was doing, especially if it turned out that he wasn't going to be the guy I married, but then I came to be OK with it. When we both started giving and receiving, I didn't feel bad at all, I felt good about it. I knew that I was sharing something very intimate with someone I really cared about.

Nearly a year after we started dating was when we finally moved on to having sex. I was just shy of 18 by about 2½ months.

Young men and women have different motivations for engaging in oral sex. Although both young men and women report physical pleasure as a reason for engaging in oral sex, young women also emphasize the importance of interpersonal and emotional reasons for giving oral sex (Vannier & O'Sullivan, 2012). Giving and receiving physical pleasure matter, but sexual desire, attraction, and emotional connection also matter, especially when it comes to giving oral sex by females. Thus, females are more likely to give oral sex if they are emotionally involved with their partner, while males focus on their own physical pleasure.

Why Do Adolescents Engage in Oral Sex?

There are many reasons for engaging in oral sex. The most common reasons among college students are giving pleasure, receiving pleasure, and avoiding sexual intercourse (Chambers, 2007). Other reasons include fostering intimacy, feelings of obligation, and foreplay. Students report that they are most comfortable engaging in oral sex in a committed relationship in contrast to a noncommitted or primarily sexual relationship. Together, these findings suggest that the primary motivation for engaging in oral sex is mutual pleasure between individuals in a committed relationship. Oral sex is about pleasure, but college students report that the pleasure is greater when oral sex occurs in a close romantic relationship (Vannier & Byers, 2013).

Other reasons for engaging in oral sex include avoiding the risks associated with vaginal sex, including a pregnancy and contracting an STI (Cornell & Halpern-Felsher, 2006). In addition, many adolescents indicate that teens have oral sex because their friends are doing it, or because they feel pressured to do it. Adolescents also report that engaging in oral sex increases their popularity.

Are Teens Who Have Oral Sex More Popular Than Teens Who Do Not?

Adolescents who engage in oral sex are rated by peers as more popular than adolescents who do not engage in oral sex (Prinstein, Meade, & Cohen, 2003). However, popularity decreases as the number of oral sex partners increases. There are no gender differences in these findings, a pattern many will find surprising, given the stereotype that having many sexual partners enhances the social status of males but lowers the status of females. This study is not the last word on the relationship between oral sex and social status for males and females, but the results indicate that the interplay of oral sex with gender and social status is complicated.

Who Engages in Oral Sex?

Age, gender, and race/ethnicity are all related to engaging in oral sex. Older adolescents and emerging adults are more likely to engage in oral sex than younger adolescents, and the difference is substantial (Brewster & Tillman, 2008). Part of the reason for this age effect is that all forms of sexual activity—including oral sex, vaginal sex, and anal sex—increase with age, suggesting that oral sex is part of a general pattern of sexual development that begins in early adolescence and continues on into emerging adulthood and beyond. Even an activity as personal and private as oral sex is influenced by age norms about when it is appropriate (Holway, 2015).

Teens who engage in oral sex during early adolescence are risk takers. Young adolescents who engage in oral sex also are likely to drink alcohol, use other drugs, have little interest in school, and receive poor grades (Bersamin, Walker, Fisher, & Grube, 2006; Ompad et al., 2006). In addition, young adolescents who engage in oral sex are high-sensation seekers who enjoy taking sexual risks and who are more likely to have unprotected sex (Ronis & O'Sullivan, 2011; Salazar et al., 2011).

Among white, African American, and Hispanic youth, white youth are most likely to give and receive oral sex, and this is especially true for white males (Child Trends, 2015a). African American youth are least likely to participate in oral sex, especially to give oral sex, and this is particularly true for

African American females (Brewster & Tillman, 2008). Further, when African American females do engage in oral sex, they tend to engage in it at an older age, after they have had sexual intercourse for the first time, while white females are more likely to engage in it either before or around the same age as first sexual intercourse (Auslander, Biro, Succop, Short, & Rosenthal, 2009). Clearly, cultural differences exist in the meaning of oral sex, which lead to racial and ethnic differences in oral sex engagement and timing (Auslander et al., 2009; Wilson, 1986).

Adolescents who have liberal attitudes about oral sex are more likely to eventually engage in it than adolescents with more conservative sexual attitudes (Lyons, Manning, Giordano, & Longmore, 2013). One consequence of having liberal attitudes about sex is a willingness to engage in sexual activities other than traditional sexual intercourse, such as oral sex.

Is Oral Sex Really Sex According to Adolescents?

In 1998, President Bill Clinton was roundly criticized and almost impeached for infamously declaring at a press conference that he "did not have sexual relations" with Monica Lewinsky, a White House intern, when, in fact, Lewinsky had performed oral sex on Clinton. The president interpreted the phrase *have sexual relations* narrowly to mean sexual intercourse, excluding oral sex, an interpretation some Americans shared, but others did not. Adolescents also differ in their interpretation of what it means to have sex, especially when it comes to oral sex.

One poll of U.S. teens ages 13–16 years found that about three-quarters of teens classify oral sex as a sexual act (NBC News/People Magazine, 2005). Based on results from one study of undergraduates enrolled in a human sexuality course, only about 20% of college students consider oral contact with genitals to be sex (Hans, Gillen, & Akande, 2010). The percent of college students who consider oral–genital contact to be sex decreased from about 40% in 1991 to 20% in 2007, suggesting that among university students a shift has occurred in the meaning of oral sex. It is not clear what might account for this shift, but one possibility is that the focus on penile–vaginal intercourse in sex education classes and the emphasis on sexual abstinence in abstinence sex education courses may have led students who engage in oral–genital contact to declassify it as sex in order to maintain a conception of themselves as sexually chaste.

Is Oral Sex a Substitute for Sexual Intercourse?

Do adolescents have oral sex in place of sexual intercourse or in addition to sexual intercourse? Some have suggested that many adolescents have oral sex instead of intercourse as a way of remaining a virgin, since many do not define oral sex as sex (Uecker, Angotti, & Regnerus, 2008). Substituting oral sex for vaginal intercourse is one way to maintain what has been called "technical virginity," an idea based on considerable media speculation, but little empirical evidence. The evidence that does exist does not support the idea that oral sex is a substitute for sexual intercourse. Instead, most adolescents who engage in oral sex also have sexual intercourse (Haydon, Herring, Prinstein, & Halpern, 2012; Holway, 2015; Song & Halpern-Felsher, 2011).

Oral sex and sexual intercourse do not appear to follow one sequence. For some adolescents, oral sex precedes sexual intercourse (Song & Halpern-Felsher, 2011), while for others, it follows (Haydon et al., 2012). What is more true than not is that adolescents who engage in one of these behaviors most likely will engage in the other within a year (Halpern & Haydon, 2012).

Where Does Oral Sex Fit into the Sex Lives of Lesbian, Gay, Bisexual, and Transgender Adolescents?

Oral sex starts earlier, is more common, more frequent, and involves more partners than either mutual masturbation or anal sex among gay and bisexual young men (Dodge et al., 2016). Virtually all gay and bisexual men between ages 18 and 25 years report that they have engaged in oral sex with a male partner at some point in their lives, and about half report that it was within the past 30 days (Dodge et al., 2016). Oral sex is considerably more common than insertive or receptive anal intercourse (Outlaw et al., 2011). Young men who have sex with men (YMSM) first engage in oral sex when they are in their mid- to late teens, and do not engage in anal sex until they are in their early 20s (Dyer, Regan, Pacek, Acheampong, & Khan, 2015). A general pattern of progression from oral sex to both receptive and insertive anal sex with men is typical among YMSM (Bruce, Harper, Fernández, & Jamil, 2012). It is common for YMSM to have oral and anal sex without a condom (Kapadia, Bub, Barton, Stults, & Halkitis, 2015), which raises concerns about the transmission of STIs, including HIV/AIDS.

Virtually all of the research on lesbian, gay, bisexual, and transgender (LGBT) oral sex has centered on gay and bisexual males, focusing on issues of safe and unsafe sex, and on the spread of STIs, especially HIV/AIDS. Less is known about oral sex among lesbians and bisexual females.

■ VIRGINITY AND SEXUAL ABSTINENCE

Self-reported virginity varies as a function of grade in school; about 76% of U.S. 9th graders indicate that they have not had sexual intercourse, a figure that steadily decreases to about 42% of 12th graders (Kann, Olsen, et al., 2016). We do not know what percentage of these virgin adolescents chose virginity and what percentage were virgin because of a lack of opportunity. Whatever the reason for their abstinence, the majority of virgin students have positive feelings about not having sex (Heywood, Patrick, Pitts, & Mitchell, 2016). Further, there is school variation in the percentage of adolescents who have not had sexual intercourse, meaning that in some schools virginity is the norm, while in other schools sexual activity is the norm, differences that inhibit or accelerate the typical increase in sexual experience that occurs as students get older (Coley, Lombardi, Lynch, Mahalik, & Sims, 2013; White & Warner, 2015).

Virginity is widely valued across cultures, especially for the young and for girls (Espinosa-Hernández, Bissell-Havran, & Nunn, 2015). In many cultures, female virginity is a cultural ideal, and virgins are coveted and pursued by desiring males (Bhana, 2016; Eltahawy, 2016). Virginity conveys status and respectability, and is rooted in traditional values about the desirability of female chastity. Further, female virginity often reflects positively on the family of origin in addition to securing more "bride wealth," which is payment and remuneration paid by the parents of the future husband to the parents of a virgin daughter.

Virginity, more specifically, losing one's virginity, is a theme of many popular teen movies. Consider just three examples: *American Pie* is the story of four teenage boys who form a pact to lose their virginity before prom night; the comedy *Superbad* is about two best friends who try to lose their virginity before they go off to college; in *Blockers* three girls make a plan to lose their virginity at their high school prom. These and other movies for teens, along with many episodes of TV shows about teens, all focus on the desire of teens, usually boys, to lose their virginity or on the struggle of adolescents, usually girls, to hold on to their virginity. These themes resonate with many teens who are at the stage in life when issues about virginity and sexual behavior loom large.

What Are the Attitudes of Adolescents and Emerging Adults about Virginity?

Despite the great interest in abstinence by sex educators and others, little is known about abstinence in general or the reasons why adolescents and emerging adults choose sexual abstinence. In one qualitative study of a group of U.S. 15- to 19-year-old females, researchers uncovered five motivations for abstinence (Long-Middleton et al., 2013). The most frequently occurring theme is *personal readiness,* which includes the feeling that one is simply not ready to have sex. *Fear* is the second most common theme related to the potential negative consequences of sex, including pregnancy and STIs. Third is *beliefs and values,* which reflect a moral standard, often based on religious teaching. *Partner worthiness* is a fourth theme reflecting the idea that the teen has not yet found the right partner and does not want to have sex with just anyone. The fifth theme is *lack of opportunity,* reflecting a lack of time, place, or person with whom to have a sexual relationship.

Sprecher and Regan (1996) surveyed college students at one U.S. midwestern university regarding their attitudes and feelings about being a virgin and discovered some important gender similarities and differences. According to the emerging adults in this study, the most important reasons for remaining a virgin are not being in love or not being in a relationship long enough to have sex. Students also indicated that they were virgins because they had not yet met the right person. Other reasons included fear of pregnancy and worries about AIDS and other STIs. College virgins do not abstain from sex because of low sexual desire, dispelling the idea that virginity is not a choice but an outcome of a low sex drive. Both male and female virgins indicate that they want sex and are looking forward to having sexual intercourse, but with the right person at the appropriate time. Young women focus more on interpersonal reasons for their virginity, while young men mention feelings of shyness and social awkwardness. Further, young women have a greater sense of pride and happiness about their virginity, while young men feel more embarrassment and guilt. More recent research essentially replicates these findings from the 1990s (Sprecher & Treger, 2015).

The attitudes of college students about their virginity are not much different from the feelings of high school students about their virgin status (Heywood et al., 2016). Girls say they feel good, happy, and fantastic about being a virgin, while boys are embarrassed, upset, and regretful. Girls give several reasons why they are virgins, including that they are proud to say no, do not feel ready to have sexual intercourse, and are not in love. Boys who are virgins also are proud to say no, and feel that they have not been in a relationship long enough to have sex, but also admit that they have an unwilling current partner. Both girls and boys report that they feel pressure from parents to remain a virgin, but boys, more than girls, indicate that they feel pressure from friends to have sex.

Why Are Some Adolescents Sexually Abstinent?

The values of parents and peers figure prominently in the decision to remain a virgin (Abbott & Dalla, 2008). Abstinent youth indicate that their values about premarital sex are strongly influenced by their parents, who stress the importance of remaining abstinent until marriage. Abstinent youth also choose friends who support those values and avoid associations with adolescents who approve of premarital sex. What the abstinent adolescents do is construct a social environment for themselves that includes like-minded peers who support their decision to remain abstinent.

One study of the relationship between sexual abstinence and alcohol abstinence among a large sample of Finnish adolescents and emerging adults found that sexual abstinence is correlated with alcohol abstinence and religiosity, suggesting that sexual abstinence is not a value separate from other values, but is embedded in a constellation of values and beliefs associated with a more conservative and traditional lifestyle (Winter, Karvonen, & Rose, 2014). Sexually abstinent adolescents are not like other adolescents in every way except that they are abstinent—instead, their lifestyle reflects some deeply held values that fundamentally differentiate the abstainers from those who are sexually active.

How Do Adolescents and Emerging Adults Think about Virginity Loss?

Losing your virginity is widely perceived by adolescents and emerging adults as an important event in the process of growing up (Carpenter, 2002). It is not a neutral experience for most young people. Happiness is the most common emotional reaction to having sexual intercourse for the first time, a reaction that is especially true for males (Vasilenko, Maas, & Lefkowitz, 2015). Virginity loss does not have a single meaning for all adolescents, but has multiple meanings for different adolescents. Carpenter (2005) has uncovered three broad themes that capture the ways young adults characterize their transition from virginity to nonvirginity. One theme is that virginity is a *gift* to someone you love with whom you are in a committed relationship. A second theme is that virginity is a *stigma* that needs to be shed at the first available opportunity to someone who may be a friend or a casual partner, a theme especially common among young men who describe their virginity status as unmasculine (Caron & Hinman, 2013). The third theme is that one's virginity and the loss of one's virginity is a positive transitional *process* into adulthood that should be physically and emotionally pleasurable.

One study of Canadian college students found that about 50% of the students describe their virginity loss as a process, 40% see the loss of their virginity as a gift, and about 10% view their virginity loss as a stigma (Humphreys, 2013). Young women are more gift oriented and young men are more likely to view their virginity as a stigma. Love is more important for individuals who are gift oriented, and these gift-oriented students are more involved with the person with whom they had sex.

What Does It Mean to Be a Lesbian, Gay, Bisexual, Transgender, Questioning Virgin?

According to Wikipedia, virginity is generally understood to mean "the state of a person who has never engaged in sexual intercourse," with sexual intercourse defined as when "a man puts his penis into the vagina of a woman." Now this is a perfectly acceptable definition for heterosexuals, but it is problematic when describing the sexual status of lesbian, gay, bisexual, transgender, questioning (LGBTQ) youth, many of whom have not had sexual intercourse, but who are sexually active and do not consider themselves to be virgins. What does it mean to be an LGBTQ virgin? Both gay males and lesbians are more likely to talk about the "first time" they have a particular sexual experience with someone of the same sex (Averett, Moore, & Price, 2014). Among gay males virginity loss can describe the first experience of oral sex, or the first experience of anal intercourse.

■ SEXUAL INTERCOURSE

What Percentage of U.S. Adolescents Have Had Sexual Intercourse?

As can be seen in Figure 1.2, there is a steady increase in the percentage of U.S. high school students in each grade who report that they have had sexual intercourse, from about 24% of 9th graders to about 58% of 12th graders (Kann,

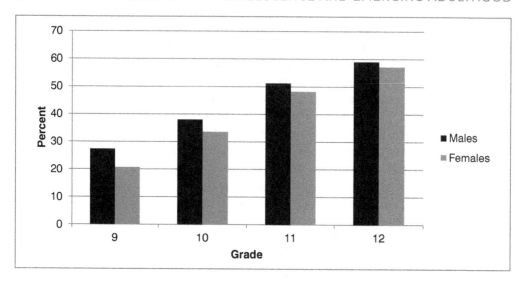

FIGURE 1.2. Percentage of U.S. high school students who have ever had sexual intercourse by grade, 2015. Adapted from Kann, McManus, et al. (2016).

Olsen, et al., 2016). About the same percentage of males and females in high school report sexual activity in each grade, but there are significant racial/ethnic differences in the percentage of students who have ever had sexual intercourse: 44% of white students, 49% of Hispanic students, and 61% of African American students.

Why Are Older Adolescents More Sexually Active Than Younger Adolescents?

As adolescents get older, they are more likely to have sexual intercourse. Why should age make a difference? Several important processes occur during adolescence that are related to an age increase in sexual intercourse. First, in the United States and in most Western countries, the period of adolescence and emerging adulthood is the time when it is expected that most individuals will form close relationships that have the potential of becoming sexual. The age when it is appropriate for an individual to become sexually active is a contested issue in the United States, but the period of adolescence increasingly is seen by adolescents and adults as the time when sexual debut will occur. It is not surprising then, that most adolescents expect to become sexually active sometime between middle adolescence and emerging adulthood.

Second, there are changing psychological and interpersonal factors during adolescence that are catalysts for sexual activity. Adolescence is a time for the development of autonomy. It is a time when teens begin to disengage from their parents and form their own values, apart from parental values.

Adolescents spend an increasing amount of time with peers and begin to show a natural interest in romantic relationships (Sales et al., 2012). Coupled with these interpersonal developments, most adolescents begin to develop more liberal views about sex than their parents.

Third, biology plays some role in the combination of forces that propel adolescents in the direction of sexual activity. Pubertal processes, especially an increase in sex steroids, are related to an increase in sexual cognitions and sexual drive, which also make it more likely that older adolescents will become sexually active (Halpern, Udry, & Suchindran, 1997, 1998). Thus, a combination of factors all converge during adolescence to make that period the time of life when more and more adolescents make the transition from virginity to nonvirginity.

Has There Been a Change in the Percentage of U.S. High School Students Who Have Had Sexual Intercourse over the Past Several Years?

Between 1991 and 2013, the percentage of U.S. high school students who have ever had sexual intercourse decreased from about 54% in 1991 to about 47% in 2013, which can be seen in Figure 1.3. Note that historical changes in the sexual behavior of high school students reveals two distinct periods: a period of decline from 1991 to 2001, and a period of stability from 2001 to 2013. The reasons for the shape of this graph are not well understood. Perhaps the pattern reflects a cultural emphasis on abstinence in the 1990s followed by a more

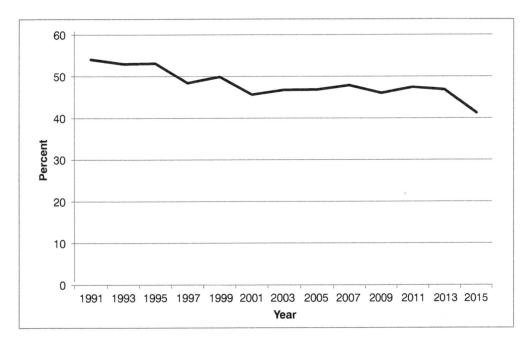

FIGURE 1.3. Percentage of U.S. high school students who have ever had sexual intercourse, 1991–2015. Adapted from Kann, McManus, et al. (2016).

recent emphasis on safer sex in the 2000s. Whatever the reasons, adolescents today are somewhat less likely to have sexual intercourse than adolescents in the 1990s.

■ GENDER AND ADOLESCENT SEXUALITY

In the past, gender differences in sexual behavior were large and common for many behaviors. These differences have narrowed over the past several decades for adolescents and adults, reflecting two important changes: first, more females are sexually active than ever before, closing the gender gap in sexual behavior; and second, more females are willing to report that they are sexually active than before, reducing the number of females who underreport their sexual activity.

How Do Young Men and Women Differ in Their Sexual Behavior and Sexual Expectations?

Men continue to report more sexual experiences and hold more permissive sexual attitudes than women (Petersen & Hyde, 2010). Most gender differences in sexuality are small, however. The largest differences are found for the following: men report that they are more likely to masturbate, view pornography, engage in casual sex, and have more liberal attitudes about casual sex than women. The magnitude of these differences decline between adolescence and adulthood.

Examinations of the relationship between gender and sexual behavior are complicated by the need to consider race and ethnicity in these comparisons. For example, the average age of first sexual intercourse is somewhat lower for males than for females. When race and ethnicity are taken into account a more complex picture emerges. For example, the average age of onset of sexual intercourse is lowest for African American males; similar for white, African American females, and Hispanic adolescents; and highest for Asian American adolescents (R-Almendarez & Wilson, 2013; Zimmer-Gembeck & Helfand, 2008). Explanations for these racial and ethnic differences in sexuality, especially for the young age and high number of sexual partners among African American males, focus on the social environment of African American youth, an environment that emphasizes traditional definitions of manliness, coupled with strong peer pressure to be sexually active.

The gendered nature of adolescent sexuality is especially evident in the perceptions youth have about gender differences in sexual behavior. Gender role expectations about sexuality held by youth across cultures show some common themes (Marston & King, 2006). Around the world, youth perceive males to have a higher sex drive than females. Males are viewed as motivated for sex by a desire for physical pleasure, while female sexual desire is linked to romantic love. Males are allowed and even expected to be sexually active before marriage. Males are perceived to be untrustworthy partners who may deceive females about their emotions in order to acquire sexual favors. Youth perceive males with many sexual partners to have higher social status than males with no or few sexual partners. In contrast, female virginity has higher social value than male virginity. Youth perceive females with no or few sexual partners to have higher social status than females with many sexual partners. Youth believe that having many sexual partners can damage a girl's reputation. The gender gap created by these differing perceptions and expectations is closing, however, especially in North America and Western Europe. For example, the expectation that females must remain virgins until they marry or risk social dishonor is no longer true for most people in the Western world.

What Accounts for Gender Differences in Sexual Behavior?

There is widespread agreement among researchers about the existence of gender differences in sexual behavior and in the messages and expectations young men and women receive about their sexuality, but there is much controversy about why these differences exist. Some argue that gender differences in sexual activity have their origins in hard-wired biological variations between males and females that have evolved over millennia (Buss, 2016). Even the most ardent proponents of biological explanations for gender-related sexuality typically do not propose that these differences are entirely the result of biological factors alone. The expression of male and female sexuality is also attributed to strong social-psychological forces that emerge from the cultural context in which males and females develop.

What about Sexual Desire?

More is known about what teens do than about why they engage in sexual activity, even though examining the whys of sexuality is important for understanding the what of adolescent sexuality. Further, an examination of why adolescents have sex reveals strong gender differences in sexual desire that illuminate the specific pressures and conflicted messages females receive about their sexuality. Although the gender gap in sexual behavior is narrowing, gender differences persist in sexual desire, and in how young men and women experience and understand their sexuality.

According to some feminists, female sexual desire is stifled by cultural and social constraints that hamper and suppress the expression of female sexuality (Dawson & Chivers, 2014). One illustration of this repression of female sexual desire is revealed in an investigation of girls' explanations for their sexual behavior (O'Sullivan & Meyer-Bahlburg, 2003). Most of the Latina and African American girls in this study are reluctant to admit that they are interested in sex and desire it. Few of these girls speak about sexual desire but, instead, interpret their sexual interests and activities as expressions of romantic motives that reflect their attraction to and love of their boyfriends. The girls go so far as to condemn sexual behavior that is purely motivated by sexual pleasure, but accept sexual activity when it occurs in a romantic relationship.

What Are Some of the Sexual Pressures Young Women Face?

Girls are bombarded by images of female sexuality that promote the idea that looking sexy is the pathway to high self-esteem, social status, and popularity (Tolman, 2012). In contrast to the message that girls need to develop an image of sexual availability if they want to be popular, girls are also taught the opposite message, which is that they should suppress their sexuality. Girls receive the mixed message that they should look sexy, but not be sexual, while sexual activity is an accepted part of the male gender role (Kiefer & Sanchez, 2007). These opposing forces create tension and apprehension in heterosexual romantic relations, with males pressuring females to have sex and females resisting. One consequence of this asymmetry is that girls who do not desire sex but are coerced into having it are likely to feel guilt, shame, and depression (Burrington, Kreager, & Haynie, 2011). Thus, the well-documented finding that sexual activity and depression are linked for some girls is partly explained by the fact that many sexually active girls are reluctant participants who are pressured into having sex by their persistent partners. In contrast, girls who are motivated to have sex by their own sexual desire report that they enjoyed their sexual experience and do not regret it (Impett & Tolman, 2006).

Feminist writers are especially interested in how gender norms affect adolescent sexuality, particularly female sexuality. One general theoretical point feminists make about female sexual development is that traditional gender role expectations continue to have a powerful impact on the sexual behavior and sexual desires of females. Deborah Tolman at the City University of New York has been a prolific writer and articulate spokesperson for this idea (Tolman, 2005). According to Tolman, traditional gender role expectations emphasize the need for girls to make themselves attractive to boys. As a result of this emphasis on making oneself attractive, girls learn to use their bodies in an attempt to make themselves objects of desire, while boys learn to treat girls as sexual objects (Fine & McClelland, 2006).

An important outcome of this sexual objectification is that girls are more focused on the impact they have on others, especially boys, than on their own sexual desires. Females are expected to emphasize the sexual pleasure of their partners over their own sexual pleasure. Most young females focus more on giving sexual pleasure than on receiving it, one consequence of which is that males receive more pleasure from sex than do females (Saliares, Wilkerson, Sieving, & Brady, 2017). Many females are unhappy about this imbalance, but they report that it is difficult to communicate with their partners about what they find pleasurable not only because they feel embarrassed and awkward talking about their own sexual preferences but also because they are reluctant to ask for what they want.

SUMMARY

■ SEX PLAY IN CHILDHOOD

Human sexuality does not suddenly appear with the onset of puberty. Sexuality is a developmental process that initially emerges in an early form in early childhood, is elaborated on in middle adolescence with the appearance of precoital activities, finally emerging in an adult form sometime in adolescence and emerging adulthood for an increasing number of individuals.

Sex play in childhood is a common expression of sexual curiosity among children. Typical activities include such behaviors as looking at naked other children, exposing oneself to other children, touching another child's genitals, kissing, and hugging. Not all children engage in sex play and several factors have been identified that are associated with sex play. Age and gender are especially important, and boys between ages 2 and 5 years are most likely to participate in sex play. Sex play is also related to higher parental education and to liberal parent attitudes about sex play. In general, childhood sex play is not related to adolescent or emerging adult sexual behavior, which suggests that sex play in childhood is not true sexual behavior but instead, is based on other nonsexual motivations—most likely, curiosity.

■ MASTURBATION

Masturbation has a long history of being condemned as a psychological and physical illness, despite the fact that large numbers of individuals engage in it. Masturbation is common throughout the lifespan and is considerably more common among males than females. Several explanations have been offered to account for this strong gender difference, which include the sexual double standard, biological differences in sex steroids, and methodological problems with the assessment of masturbation. More adolescents masturbate today than in times past. Other factors related to masturbation include race/ethnicity, education, and religion. Masturbation during adolescence does not appear to be strongly related to interpersonal sexual activity during adolescence or later during emerging adulthood.

■ ORAL SEX

Oral sex is uncommon in middle school, but considerably more common in adolescence and emerging adulthood. There is little evidence of a sudden increase in oral sex in the early 2000s. One perplexing gender difference is that more males report receiving heterosexual oral sex than females report giving it. Other gender differences include who gives oral sex and why. There are many motivations for engaging in oral sex, with the primary one being giving and receiving pleasure. Some factors related to who engages in heterosexual oral sex include age, gender, race/ethnicity, having liberal attitudes about sex, and being a risk taker. Many adolescents do not consider oral sex to be sex. Oral sex does not seem to be a substitute for sexual intercourse, but often occurs in the context of a sexual relationship for most adolescents and emerging adults. Oral sex is an important aspect of the sex lives of LGBTQ adolescents.

■ VIRGINITY AND SEXUAL ABSTINENCE

A high proportion of adolescents have not engaged in sexual intercourse when they enter high school, a percentage that decreases each year they are in school. There are many reasons why adolescents are abstinent, including not being ready for sexual intercourse, fear of the possible negative consequences of sex, holding beliefs about the importance of remaining abstinent, not having the right partner, and a lack of opportunity.

Making the transition from virginity to nonvirginity is an important psychological process for most adolescents. There are many similarities and some differences in the reasons why males and females are virgins. In general, virginity is more of a choice for females, and a reluctant outcome for many males. The meaning of losing one's virginity is captured by three themes, including viewing virginity as a gift, a stigma, and a transitional process. LGBTQ adolescents focus less on virginity and more on the first time they have a particular sexual experience.

■ SEXUAL INTERCOURSE

About 30% of 9th graders and 64% of 12th graders in the United States have had sexual intercourse. Many social, psychological, and biological factors are responsible for age differences in sexual intercourse. Slightly fewer adolescents today have had intercourse than in the 1990s.

■ GENDER AND ADOLESCENT SEXUALITY

Gender differences in sexual behavior and attitudes are narrowing, but they continue to exist in the United States and around the world. These differences likely are the result of the interaction of biological and cultural factors. Many writers, especially feminists, argue that female sexual desire is stifled by cultural constraints that suppress female sexuality. Girls are taught to inhibit and control their sexuality, while popular culture sends the message to girls that they should look attractive and be sexy. Girls are taught to make themselves objects of desire. This objectification of the self leads females to be more concerned about the sexual pleasure of their partner than their own sexual desire.

SUGGESTIONS FOR FURTHER READING ████████

Carpenter, L. M. (2005). *Virginity lost: An intimate portrait of first sexual experiences.* New York: NYU Press.

Haydon, A. A., Herring, A. H., Prinstein, M. J., & Halpern, C. T. (2012). Beyond age at first sex: Patterns of emerging sexual behavior in adolescence and young adulthood. *Journal of Adolescent Health, 50,* 456–463.

Kann, L., McManus, T., Harris, W. A., Shanklin, S. L., Flint, K. H., Hawkins, J., et al. (2016, June 10). Youth risk behavior surveillance—United States, 2015. *Morbidity and Mortality Weekly Report, 65*(6). Retrieved December 7, 2017, from *www.cdc.gov/healthyyouth/data/yrbs/pdf/2015/ss6506_updated.pdf.*

Kellogg, N. D. (2009). Clinical report—the evaluation of sexual behaviors in children. *Pediatrics, 124,* 992–998.

Robbins, C. L., Schick, V., Reece, M., Herbenick, D., Sanders, S. A., Dodge, B., et al. (2011). Prevalence, frequency, and associations of masturbation with partnered sexual behaviors among US adolescents. *Archives of Pediatric and Adolescent Medicine, 165,* 1087–1093.

Tolman, D. L. (2005). *Dilemmas of desire: Teenage girls talk about sexuality.* Cambridge, MA: Harvard University Press.

CHAPTER 2

The Biology of Adolescent Sexuality

The etymology of the word *puberty* derives from the Latin *pubertas,* which means the "age of maturity" or, more colorfully, "to grow hairy." Of all the changes that occur around the time of puberty, it is odd that the ancient Romans focused on the growth of body hair, although the appearance of pubic hair is an early sign of the onset of puberty.

Puberty is much more than the appearance of body hair. It is not a single event, but a complex series of biological changes that occur over a period of 5–6 years in humans. The biological changes that occur during puberty alter the physiology, form, and function of the body more dramatically than during any other period of life except for the 9 months between conception and birth. During puberty, profound internal and external changes occur to the human body that transform biologically immature children into biologically mature adults capable of reproduction.

Puberty thrusts children into biological maturity through the development of *primary sexual characteristics* and *secondary sexual characteristics.* Primary sexual characteristics are those biological features of the body related to reproduction, such as the ovaries and the uterus in females and the testes in males. Secondary sexual characteristics are those biological characteristics that distinguish males from females, but are not related to reproduction, such as large breasts in human females and facial hair in males.

The main question in this chapter is Do the biological changes that occur during puberty only affect physiology and appearance, or do these changes have an impact on the sexual behavior of adolescents? This is a profound question that is examined in four areas including the association between gonadal hormones and adolescent sexuality, early and late physical maturation, brain development, and genetic influences on sexuality. Before studying these issues, however, it is useful to examine the specific biological changes that occur during puberty and map out the physiological events responsible for those changes.

■ PUBERTY

What Determines the Onset of Puberty?

Scientists do not completely understand the mechanism that initiates puberty, but there is mounting evidence that genetic, metabolic, and even social events all play important roles. Most of the variation among animals, including humans, in the onset of puberty is due to genetic differences (Abreu et al., 2013). Age of puberty is not determined by genetic factors alone, but the timing and tempo of the pubertal clock is largely set when sperm meets egg. Some clocks tick faster than others, with some adolescents maturing before most of their peers, while others remain stuck in a prepubertal limbo, neither child nor adolescent, for a longer period of time.

The onset of puberty is not simply the result of a genetic trigger, immune from environmental influences. The beginning of puberty is an interaction between genetic and environmental factors, with the most important environmental influence being amount of body fat. The connection between body fat and puberty has been demonstrated for *menarche,* which is the first menstruation. Typically, when the body fat on a young U.S. female reaches about 17% of her total body weight menarche occurs, while regular menstrual periods are correlated with a body fat index of at least 22% (Kaplowitz, 2008). The association between body fat and menarche may have evolved as a natural form of birth control, reducing the likelihood of a pregnancy to females with inadequate fat stores, a condition that would endanger both the life of the mother and the life of the developing fetus.

What Are Hormones?

Hormones are chemical substances produced by endocrine glands that control and regulate the activity of particular cells and organs. One group of hormones that have potent effects on our physiology, appearance, and perhaps even our behavior are sex steroids produced by the gonads, called *gonadal hormones.* This group includes the "male" hormones, called *androgens,* such as testosterone (T), produced by the testes, and the "female" hormones, classified as *estrogens,* such as estradiol, produced by the ovaries. Male and female hormones are present in both genders, but in vastly different amounts. For example, adult men produce 6–8 milligrams of T each day, compared with 0.5 milligrams produced by adult women.

Unlike other hormones, which act on specific organs, sex steroids lead to many cellular changes. A single hormone, such as T, released into the bloodstream of boys during puberty, will produce cellular changes leading to the production of sperm, an increase in muscle mass, lengthening of a boy's penis, and facial hair growth. Estradiol jump-starts a girl's sex organs and regulates the functioning of the menstrual cycle. It also leads to the growth of pubic hair and to breast development.

What Physical Changes Occur during Puberty?

Although small amounts of T and estradiol circulate in the blood of prepubescent boys and girls, the amount of T in boys and estradiol in girls increases dramatically during puberty. The increase in sex-specific gonadal steroids and the production of new growth hormone during puberty significantly alter the appearance and physiques of young males and females. Variation exists in the ages when physical changes occur, but the sequence of changes is universal. The sexual maturation of females typically starts 1½–2 years before males with the emergence of breast buds. Pubic hair begins to grow at about the same time, followed by the growth spurt, menarche, and regular menstrual cycles. The first stage of puberty in boys is testicular growth, accompanied by the appearance of pubic hair. Next, a boy's penis begins to grow, followed by an adolescent growth spurt, with a deepening of the voice after growth begins. Notice that menarche occurs late in pubertal development among females, after the

The anticipation of menarche and its experience can produce anxiety in some young girls, which dissipates with time as the maturing girl becomes more comfortable with her monthly menstrual period, as the following story reveals.

IN THEIR OWN WORDS

When my breasts started growing, I was very nervous and anxious of when it was going to start my period. I would wonder when it would happen, if it was going to be during school, if I would be embarrassed if I bled through my pants, and I was worried how much blood I was going to have. The few days before the last day of school, I was eating a lot. I just didn't feel like I was full. My mother said I was very moody and wondered if I had already started my period. I had already bought pads and tampons so I was prepared when it did happen. While I was at school, everything was going normal. It was a typical last day of school. We had yearbook signing, saying good-bye to teachers and friends for the summer, and doing activities such as kickball with everyone in my graduating class. At the end of the day,

before getting on the buses to go home, I went to the bathroom, and discovered that I was on my period. I had blood in my urine and I knew this had to be my period. I did not have pads or tampons with me so I was unsure of what to do. So I grab a bit of toilet paper and put it into my underwear. When I went home I rushed straight into my bathroom and grabbed a pad. My mom was super confused and so she went up to my room to where I was. I told my mom what had happened. She said, "Congrats, you have started your period." I laughed and smiled. I was very uncomfortable about everything so when my mom joked about the situation, it made me feel a lot better. During the summer, each month I would have my monthly "friend." Each month it got a little easier for me to know what to expect.

growth spurt, but testicular growth, which is correlated with the production of sperm in males, occurs early in puberty, before the growth spurt. From an evolutionary perspective, it is critical that a female begins to grow and accumulate fat deposits before she becomes pregnant, increasing the probability that she and her fetus will survive pregnancy. Putting on height and weight before reproductive capability is unnecessary for the survival of males or their offspring, so sperm production occurs early in pubertal development, increasing the likelihood that males will produce offspring.

■ GONADAL HORMONES AND ADOLESCENT SEXUALITY

The fact that sex steroids transform the physiology and form of the human body during puberty is noncontroversial, but there is disagreement about whether gonadal hormones influence the thoughts, emotions, and behaviors of adolescents. The idea that adolescents are in the throes of hormonal turmoil is a long-held, popular belief and a convenient explanation for the sometimes odd behavior and inscrutable emotions of teenagers (Hollenstein & Lougheed, 2013). In the words of one group of researchers, however, the answer to the question "Are adolescents the victims of raging hormones?" is a resounding "No!" (Buchanan, Eccles, & Becker, 1992). The evidence for the effect of hormones on adolescent mood and behavior is not as strong as many believe, and where such a relationship does exist, the effect of hormones on behavior is complex (Nelson, 2011). The question examined in this section is Do hormones influence adolescent sexuality?

Why Does Sexual Behavior Begin in Adolescence?

Research on childhood sex play, which was discussed in Chapter 1, indicates that sex play is common in childhood, but sexual intercourse and behavior oriented toward the goal of achieving sexual intercourse is rare in prepubescent children all over the world (de Graaf & Rademakers, 2006; Lopez Sanchez, Del Campo, & Guijo, 2002; Sandfort & Cohen-Kettenis, 2000). Beginning in early adolescence, corresponding with the onset of puberty, true sexual behaviors appear.

Social scientists have developed two competing but not mutually exclusive theories to explain the appearance of sexual behavior in early adolescence. According to the biological explanation, prepubertal children have low sexual desire because of low gonadal hormones, which increase during puberty, creating the motivation for adult sexual behavior. The social model proposes that the development of sexual motivation during early adolescence is the result of social processes that inhibit the expression of sexuality during childhood, but allow and even encourage, sexual expression during adolescence. Based on this model, gonadal hormones are relegated to the role of producing primary and secondary sexual characteristics, which are signals to adolescents and to others that it is a developmentally appropriate time to express one's sexuality. Based on the social model, the expression of sexual behaviors is culturally determined; puberty is a sign of sexual readiness, but not a cause of sexual behavior. An integration of these two theories is possible, and adolescent sexual behavior may be the result of an interaction between biological and social factors; biology stimulates sexual development, which arouses sexual desire, but whether and with whom an adolescent acts on that drive is highly socially determined (Suleiman, Galván, Harden, & Dahl, 2017).

What Is the Relationship between Gonadal Hormones and Male Adolescent Sexuality?

An important series of studies on the relationship between sex steroids and adolescent sexual behavior was conducted in the mid-1980s and 1990s by Richard Udry and Carolyn Halpern and their colleagues at the University of North Carolina. An early study of ninth- and tenth-grade boys revealed a strong association between hormones and sexuality (Udry, Billy, Morris, Groff, & Raj, 1985). Specifically, T was highly related to reports of sexual intercourse, masturbation, general sexual experience, and sexual arousal. For example, only 16% of boys in the lowest quartile of circulating T had sexual intercourse, compared with almost 70% of boys in the highest quartile.

Further research on the possible connection between T and sexuality among boys reveals that the relationship between T and male sexual behavior is neither direct nor simple. In one investigation, T was positively related to the occurrence of sexual intercourse (Halpern et al., 1998), while in another study, T was unrelated to sexual ideation, or to the transition to nonvirginity (Halpern, Udry, Campbell, & Suchindran, 1993). Differences in study methodologies may account for these inconsistent findings, which require further research and theorizing to explicate. T appears to play some role in the initiation and maintenance of male adolescent sexuality, but that role is not straightforward or fully understood.

Additional research examined the joint effects of T and the social environment, specifically religious participation, on sexual ideation, motivation, attitudes, and activity among adolescent boys (Halpern, Udry, Campbell, Suchindran, & Mason, 1994). The authors hypothesized that T and religiosity act in opposite directions. The findings support the hypothesis. High-T boys who never or rarely attended religious services have the highest levels of sexual ideation, motivation, and activity. Conversely, boys with low T who frequently attend religious services have the lowest level of sexuality. The results suggest that sexual behavior is the result of an interaction between T and religiosity with T stimulating sexual behavior, but religious involvement constraining it (Regnerus, 2007).

In the following story, a young man recounts his experience with his sex drive during adolescence and attributes his frequent desire to have sex to biology, which may or may not be true. Whatever the reason, the young man perceives himself to be controlled by his sex drive rather than to be in control of it, a situation that leads to frustration and to the end of a relationship.

IN THEIR OWN WORDS

When I was a teenager, I had a relationship that lasted around a year and a half or so. This most recent and longest relationship was great, and I truly believed that I loved her, as opposed to how unsure I had felt in previous relationships. We did almost everything together, and were well accustomed to each other's company and support.

Despite this, however, there was a major problem in the relationship—I had a desire to have sex more often than she did. This made me unhappy some days, because I had a strong desire to have intercourse, and seeing as how we were dating, I was focusing all of my sexual desires on her. This made her feel pressured, and subsequently less likely to want to have sex on some days, in addition to the days that she felt no desire at all.

An important part of this story is that I felt as if my sex drive was a part of me that I could not control. Biology often dictates how often people want to have sex, and for me that setting was much higher than my partner's. Despite my best efforts to restrain myself, I was unable to keep my sex drive from becoming something that hurt the relationship that I was in. At the same time that I failed to control it, this may be a sign that the relationship was not set up to succeed. If partners do not have similar sex drives, this can lead to major problems, as it was demonstrated in my example.

Further work by Udry (1990) examined the relationship between T and attachment to church, home, and school and adolescent problem behaviors, including early sexual activity, getting drunk, smoking cigarettes, and other norm-violating behaviors. The results reveal that problem behaviors are highest among boys who are high in T and low in attachment to church, home, and school, which are social institutions that inhibit the expression of adolescent problem behaviors. Among all the variables, T is the best predictor of problem behaviors, including early sexual activity, especially when high T occurs in conjunction with low attachment to social institutions.

Other research reveals that the relationship between T and adolescent problem behaviors, including risky sexual behavior, is stronger during early adolescence, but decreases as boys get older and other social factors, such as peer influence, become more salient (Drigotas & Udry, 1993). The authors suggest that for early adolescents, high T by itself is a risk factor for sexual activity. High T might also be a risk factor for the formation of friendships with other high-T adolescents who take part in many unconventional behaviors, such as early sexual activity, alcohol and drug use, and delinquency. One can imagine high-T young males seeking one another out and forming peer groups that model and reinforce problem behaviors, creating a group culture that supports risky sexual activity.

What Is the Relationship between Gonadal Hormones and Female Adolescent Sexuality?

The limited amount of research on the relationship between hormones and adolescent sexuality in girls reveals findings that are inconsistent and difficult to interpret. In one study, the occurrence of intercourse was unrelated to gonadal hormones (Udry, Talbert, & Morris, 1986), while in another study, T was positively associated with sexual intercourse (Halpern et al., 1997).

It may be that androgens prime girls for sexual behavior, but whether a girl acts on her feelings is highly dependent on psychological and social factors (Fortenberry & Hensel, 2011; Halpern, 2006). Gonadal hormones may set the stage for sexual activity, but sexual behavior is more deeply tied to a girl's psychosocial characteristics, such as the relationship she has with her partner, than to the influence of gonadal hormones (Collins, Welsh, & Furman, 2009).

In the following story, a young woman describes her idea that she may have high T, accounting for some of her physical qualities. She also writes about having a strong sexual drive, which she has not acted on, and indicates that it, too, might be the result of high T, a possibility that is by no means a certainty.

IN THEIR OWN WORDS

As I remember back to my early childhood days I can't help but to think how different I felt from my female classmates. Around the time I went to middle school I can remember my female peers developing breasts, acquiring more body fat, and starting to look like women. I was not late on hitting puberty, around age 13 I finally got my period but none of these "womanly" changes were hitting me as hard as my friends. I was still scrawny with no hips and no breasts but my body hair did develop and I was having what I thought were traditional adolescent heterosexual thoughts.

. . . upon reaching the section of the class describing females who have been exposed to more testosterone, I could strongly relate to the scenarios presented on the screen. I texted my mom in a joking way saying, "We are learning about females with excessive testosterone in class and I swear it is describing me to a T!" She texted back saying, "No way, call me when you're out of class."

I called my mom to suggest all the women in our family have excessive testosterone because we are all so similar in our personalities. The women on my mom's side of the family are very level headed, non-emotional people who have all made strong independent lifestyle choices. As we chat back and forth about how we never have felt like other women, my mom reveals to me her doctor suggested getting a hormone test because of her thinning hair. Sure enough, my mother got tested and carries more testosterone than usual, therefore, her thinning hair and development of some facial hair in her early 40s.

To this day I live a heterosexual lifestyle still with strong sexual urges, which I don't act on but think about and make decisions based on like we learned in class and am thankful for my personality style. I feel that, if this is all true, having a higher level of testosterone has given me an advantage in life because I do not make emotion-based decisions . . . I'm not sure if my boyish stature is due to this, but for some reason it all falls into place somewhere that makes sense in my head. Now only if I could avoid the thinning hair and beard when I hit 40, that would be ideal!

Another reason why T might not have a strong association with sexual behavior in girls is that the absolute level of T in a girl's blood is low. Further work is needed to untangle the complex relationship between gonadal hormones, including T and estradiol, and sexuality among girls to gain a better understanding of how gonadal hormones influence female sexuality.

■ PHYSICAL MATURATION AND ADOLESCENT SEXUALITY

How Do Hormones Affect Adolescent Sexuality?

One pathway by which hormones might affect adolescent sexuality is by directly activating brain mechanisms that control sexual expression. Scientists call this pathway from hormones to brain to behavior a *direct effects model*. Another route by which hormones might have an impact on adolescent sexuality is more indirect, acting not on the brain but on physical appearance. From this perspective, hormones matter because they affect one's appearance through the timing of physical maturation. This perspective is called the *indirect effects model*. During early adolescence, early-maturing boys begin to look older and more masculine than late-maturing boys, and girls who are early maturers look older and more feminine than late-maturing girls. According to the indirect effects model, these differences in appearance have an impact on the expectations adolescents have for their own behavior and on the ways they are treated by others. It is these expectations and social interactions that are different for early- and late-maturing adolescents that affect sexual behavior. This indirect effects model has guided much of the research on the relationship between physical maturation and adolescent sexuality.

Do Masculine-Looking Boys and Feminine-Looking Girls Have More Sex?

The indirect effects model is built on the idea that appearance matters. A prediction from the indirect effects model is that adolescents who are the same age but who look older will be more sexually active than adolescents who look younger. Several sex-specific changes in physical appearance during puberty make early-maturing adolescents more attractive to the opposite sex. Increases in male attractiveness are related to increases in height, weight, and muscularity; having more prominent jaws and cheekbones; the emergence of body and facial hair; and having broader shoulders (Ellis, Schlomer, Tilley, & Butler, 2012). In one study of boys, the frequency of dating was positively related to a perceived increase in muscle mass and a decrease in voice pitch (Bulcroft, 1991). Boys who were beginning to resemble young men were more socially popular and attractive to girls than boys with a less manly appearance.

In another study of teen boys, researchers examined sexuality and its relationship to physical appearance, including pubertal development, facial dominance, and attractiveness (Mazur, Halpern, & Udry, 1994). All three aspects of physical appearance were related to sexual behavior, but having a dominant-looking face was the best predictor of sexual activity. It is not possible to determine whether dominant-looking boys have more sexual success because of what girls do or because of what boys do. Perhaps it is some combination of both. Girls may be especially attracted to dominant-looking boys because girls are attracted to boys who look like they would be good providers and protectors. Girls may also enjoy the reflected status they receive from going out with high-status, dominant boys. Alternatively, a boy with a dominant look may be more likely to approach a girl for a date or to assert his desire for sex in comparison to a boy who looks more timid. In general, advanced pubertal development in boys is associated with a high level of T and a dominant-looking face, which are related to more sexual activity.

For boys, bigger is better, in terms of being tall and muscular and having a prominent jaw, all of which are related to success in the dating world and to more sexual activity, but the relationship among physical development, dating, and sexuality is more complex for girls. Changes in physical appearance that make females more sexually attractive and desirable to young men include larger breasts, fuller lips, widening of the hips, and slender bodies (Ellis et al., 2012; Singh & Young, 1995). Further, slim girls are more likely to date, date at an early age, and engage in noncoital and coital activity than heavier girls (Halpern et al., 1999). Among girls, dating and sexual behavior in casual and romantic relationships are more strongly related to physical changes that can be seen by others, such as breast development, height, and weight than to the unobservable changes of puberty such as menarche (Moore, Harden, & Mendle, 2014). Thus, sexual activity among young females is not as connected to the direct effects of gonadal hormones as it is to the appearance of observable physical characteristics that signal the development of sexual maturity.

What Is Pubertal Timing?

Variation in the timing of physical maturation provides a natural experiment that allows researchers to study the indirect effects of puberty on adolescent sexuality. During early adolescence, roughly between about ages 10 and 14 years, great differences exist among adolescents in height and weight, and in the appearance of secondary sexual characteristics. Some early-maturing girls start to grow, develop their breasts, and accumulate fat around their hips before most of their peers, giving them a mature, feminine appearance in comparison to late-maturing girls, who retain their childhood height and shape for another 2–3 years. Similarly, some early-maturing boys will shoot up in height and add upper-body muscle mass years before some of their late-maturing peers, giving them the early appearance of manliness. This natural variation in the timing of physical maturation allows researchers to study the indirect effects of puberty on sexuality by comparing the sexual behavior of early maturers with late maturers. What differences are found are presumed to be the outcome of timing differences in physical maturity.

Why Might Pubertal Timing Affect Adolescent Sexuality?

Two theoretical perspectives have been offered to explain the effects of pubertal timing on adolescent psychological development in general, and on sexuality in particular (Susman & Rogol, 2004). The first is referred to as the *maturational deviance hypothesis,* which is the idea that adolescents who are off time, either maturing earlier or later than their peers, experience more psychosocial stress than adolescents who are on time (Caspi & Moffitt, 1991). Being off time is stressful for adolescents because early- and late-maturing adolescents perceive themselves, and are perceived by others, to be different from their peers. The difficulty late maturers experience is feeling left behind and being uncertain about when they will catch up with their peers. Early maturers have it hard because they do not have a same-age peer group to look to for guidance about how to behave. In addition, because early maturers look older, they may become members of older-age peer groups where they find it difficult to resist the older-age temptations of sex, drugs, and alcohol.

In the following story, an early-maturing boy describes another reason early maturers might become sexually active at an early age, which is that girls are attracted to them.

IN THEIR OWN WORDS

I reluctantly took one drink [of alcohol], and that's where the night changed completely. Not because I became intoxicated, but because the whole mood of the experience changed. It was my first time having more than a few small sips of beer and I was unaware of how it would affect me so I was nervous. We didn't get drunk but the aspects of partying and drinking and then hooking up seemed so in line with each other at the time. I ended up spending quite a bit of time with her that night and then we went upstairs as the party died down. We started kissing and one thing led to another in her bedroom. She asked if I wanted to go a little further than making out and I said, "Sure, why not." Eventually, she got undressed and so did I. She gave me oral sex and I "returned the favor." Surprisingly, neither of us was really bad at anything we tried even though we hadn't done anything even close to that before. It was a fun night and I went home wondering what it was that made her want to do those things with me even though I was younger than her.

Over time I came to realize that she was attracted to me because I was an early maturer. I was taller than my peers and I had always been athletic and lean, so she thought I looked a lot older than "my age." She liked that I was able to get along with older guys and girls regardless of the fact that I was much younger. Also, she thought that football players were attractive and that was one of the sports I played. Despite the fact that I hadn't expressed much sexual interest in her, she made moves on me because she expected me to know what to do (because she thought I looked older and was more popular with girls), and I kind of just went along with it. At the time, we didn't want to seem awkward but we later discussed the first time we hooked up and we both admitted we had absolutely no clue what we were doing; it just happened to end up being fun.

The maturational deviance theory is widely accepted as one explanation for the link between early maturation and problem behaviors, such as early sexuality. According to the maturational deviance theory, early-maturing adolescents are more likely to have older friends who pressure the younger, mature-looking adolescents to participate in age-inappropriate deviant activities (Felson & Haynie, 2002). Peers exert a powerful influence on young adolescents, an influence that may be especially strong on young, inexperienced adolescents who look older and who very much want to be accepted by their older friends.

The second theoretical perspective that connects physical development with adolescent problem behavior is the *stage termination hypothesis* (Peskin, 1973), also referred to as the *developmental readiness hypothesis* (Negriff & Susman, 2011), which focuses specifically on why early maturation might be an especially dangerous time for adolescents. The idea is that early-maturing adolescents spend less time in the relatively safe and secure world of childhood, and are thrust into the challenging world of adolescence before they are ready. Early maturers may look older than they are, even though cognitively, psychologically, and socially they are still children, and this discrepancy places early maturers at special risk to engage in risky adolescent behaviors and become sexually active before they have developed a mature understanding of the risks

---

In the following story, a girl describes her desire to have her breasts develop, and the satisfaction she had and the attention she received from boys when they did. Also, note the connection she makes between her breast development and her decision to have sex.

IN THEIR OWN WORDS

Middle school was terrible because I was unpopular with boys and physically awkward. I prayed every night that I would get boobs. For some reason, I thought that by possessing a large pair of breasts, all of my problems would be fixed.

My prayers were finally answered when I entered high school and walked down the hallway with an enviable set of boobs. I also made the cheerleading squad, which came with some popularity. However, as happy as I was about having boobs and being on the cheer squad, they came with a curse. Boys were finally interested in . . . my boobs. Great. Since I was only 14, I was not ready for the sexual attention I received from my male peers and even from male adults. My mother, noticing my physical changes, cornered me in the car every so often to ask me some awkward sexual question that never failed to make me uncomfortable. Luckily at

this point I was not sexually active and could safely report that back to my mom. My body was a constant focal point for me because I had to look good in my cheerleading uniform. I was always worried about how people were looking at my body and what they were thinking. I never felt good enough.

After months of deliberation, I finally mustered enough confidence to have sex with my first boyfriend at age 17. It was the exact opposite of magical. The relationship ended up blowing up and causing a lot of pain. However, I was glad that I had waited until then to have sex and only wished I had lost my virginity to a better guy. I didn't have sex for the remainder of high school. As a college student I have become more sexually open and less conservative. At age 20, I think I am finally done with puberty. Although I still think my boobs are growing. Seriously, be careful what you wish for.

and possible consequences of those behaviors (Mendle & Ferrero, 2012; Mendle, Turkheimer, & Emery, 2007).

What Is the Relationship between Pubertal Timing and Adolescent Sexuality?

A positive relationship exists between early maturation and a variety of romantic and sexual behaviors during adolescence, and this connection is especially strong during early adolescence (Baams, Dubas, Overbeek, & van Aken, 2015). Early-maturing adolescents in contrast to late maturers have an earlier age of kissing, dating, sexual touching, and sexual intercourse, and a higher rate of teenage pregnancy (e.g., Deardorff, Gonzales, Christopher, Roosa, & Millsap, 2005; Koo, Rose, Bhaskar, & Walker, 2012; Marceau, Ram, Houts, Grimm, & Susman, 2011; Michaud, Suris, & Deppen, 2006), findings not only true for U.S. adolescents but also for French-speaking Canadian adolescent females (Boislard, Dussault, Brendgen, & Vitaro, 2013) and Swedish female adolescents (Stattin, Kerr, & Skoog, 2011). Typically, the reverse is also true—fewer late-maturing adolescents of both genders engage in sexual intercourse—and if they do become sexually active, they usually start at a later age than early-maturing adolescents.

One explanation for the relationship between pubertal timing and sexuality is that peer associations matter, especially when adolescents hang out with older peers. In one study of girls in Finland, those girls who had older friends, especially older male friends, were more likely to be sexually active than girls who did not have older male friends (Savolainen et al., 2015). Both biological and social factors may play a role in this association. Boys are attracted to early-maturing girls with larger breasts and other signs of biological maturity that signify sexual development (Waylen & Wolke, 2004), while girls find older males more appealing (Marin, Kirby, Hudes, Coyle, & Gómez, 2006). In addition, older males have more freedom from parents, which exposes early-maturing girls who date older boys to situations that can lead to a sexual encounter. These findings are in accord with the maturational deviance theory and emphasize the important role older peers play in the expression of sexual behavior among early-maturing adolescents, especially early-maturing girls.

Does Timing of Puberty Matter for Emerging Adult Sexual Behavior?

Among emerging adults, timing of puberty is not related to sexuality, including strength of sex drive, virginity status, lifetime number of sexual partners, or frequency of intercourse for either males or females (Copeland et al., 2010; Lien, Haavet, & Dalgard, 2010; Ostovich & Sabini, 2005). Pubertal timing may matter during adolescence, but it diminishes in importance during emerging adulthood, when physical differences between early and late maturers disappear, and other more powerful social and psychological forces emerge as contributors to individual differences in adult sexual behavior (Lansford et al., 2010).

A FOCUS ON RESEARCH

One measurement problem that plagues researchers who study the relationship between puberty and adolescent behavior, including sexuality, is obtaining a reliable and valid assessment of puberty (Dorn & Biro, 2011). Puberty is not an event, but a series of complex biochemical and physical changes that occur over a period of several years in humans. Based on their research interests, researchers typically attempt to measure level of gonadal hormones, or amount of physical growth and development.

A typical study of the association between gonadal hormones and sexuality involves the comparison of adolescents high in the hormone—for example, T—with adolescents low in T, a comparison that requires the ability to accurately assess T levels. Level of T is determined by measuring the amount of T present in saliva, or more directly by assessing circulating T in a blood sample. Both approaches have their advantages and disadvantages, but the underlying problem is that gonadal hormones in the blood, including T, vary from day to day and even from hour to hour. A sensitive assessment of T requires multiple measurements over several days, a costly and cumbersome procedure that is rarely used in social science research. More typically, one sample of fluid is assayed and the result is treated as the T level in an adolescent. Measuring T in a single sample of spit or blood is at best an approximation of the average level of T for an adolescent. This imprecision may be partly responsible for the difficulty of replicating results from one study with findings from another study.

Another approach to the study of the puberty–behavior connection is to assess external, observable, physical changes as an index of underlying pubertal development. Researchers studying the indirect model of pubertal effects measure physical changes, such as the following: asking girls to indicate how old they were when they had their first menstrual period, asking teens to report on their age when pubic hair first appeared, and asking teens to indicate when their growth spurt began. These measures are easy to obtain, but they are based on memory and awareness of change and are far from perfect assessments of actual change. Another approach to assessing the stage of puberty has been to use pictures or line drawings of breast development and pubic hair growth for girls, and penis growth and pubic hair appearance for boys. Adolescents are asked to pick one of five pictures or drawings that best matches their own development for each characteristic that represents different stages of pubertal growth. One problem with this approach is that it is difficult to obtain parent and teacher approval to show adolescents explicit pictures or drawings of genital and breast development. Also, there is some question about the ability of young adolescents to choose pictures that accurately reflect their true biological development.

All these measures of pubertal development have some benefits, but they are not without their problems, especially in their agreement with actual change and with one another. These problems do not invalidate findings from research on puberty and sexuality, but the problems may partly explain some of the inconsistency in research findings.

■ FAMILY RELATIONS, PUBERTAL TIMING, AND ADOLESCENT SEXUALITY

In 1991, Belsky, Steinberg, and Draper published a landmark theory in which they used an evolutionary framework to link childhood family stress with accelerated physical maturation, and early, risky sexual behavior. Two novel, nonintuitive predictions emerged from this theory, both of which have received empirical support. First, a harsh, dangerous family environment accelerates physical development in preparation for early home leaving as an adaptive response to a potentially life-threatening situation. Second, accelerated physical maturation that emerges from early family conflict leads to risky sexual activity.

Is Early Family Stress Related to Pubertal Timing and Sexual Risk-Taking?

Several studies of girls have shown a remarkable association between early family stress and pubertal maturation, confirming the prediction that the early social environment of the family can have an influence many years later on physical development. For example, in one study, poor father–daughter relations in childhood predicted early age of menarche (Tither & Ellis, 2008), and in a study of mothers and daughters, maternal harshness directed at preschool-age daughters was associated with earlier age of menarche among girls (Belsky et al., 2007). In another study, mothers who harshly controlled their young daughters when they were ages 4–5 years—for example, by spanking them and expecting unquestioning obedience—had daughters who experienced early menarche, which was related to sexual risk-taking at age 15 (Belsky, Steinberg, Houts, & Halpern-Felsher, 2010). In addition, girls who are sexually abused in childhood reach physical maturity 8–12 months earlier than nonabused girls (Noll et al., 2017).

Early family stress is more highly related to earlier maturation and sexual risk-taking in females than in males (James, Ellis, Schlomer, & Garber, 2012). Young females may be more sensitive to stressful family living conditions, while males are less susceptible because they have a stronger peer orientation than do females. Consequently, females should be more sensitive to harsh family living conditions than males, whose sexual behavior is less constrained by family stress (Ellis, 2013).

Research on African American male adolescents found that community stress is a more important predictor of early puberty and risky sex than family stress (Kogan, Cho, et al., 2015). Boys who grow up in disordered and dangerous neighborhoods grow up fast and go through puberty at an earlier age and are more likely to engage in risky sexual behavior than boys who grow up in stable, low-stress neighborhoods. This study shows the powerful influence the nonfamily environment can have on boys, affecting not only their behavior but also their physical development.

The following student describes the discomfort she experienced being an early maturer, and attributes her early maturation to stress in the home. She writes that family stress made her want to leave home as soon as possible.

IN THEIR OWN WORDS

During my adolescence, I was considered an "early bird," in fact, it was too embarrassing for me because I was the youngest girl in my grade throughout my education. Where I lived, all of my peers grew up with me from kindergarten to graduation. We all saw each other throughout our adolescent changes. For me, it was the most embarrassing time of my life, because I was the first one to develop before any other girl and definitely every other boy too. My world changed as soon as I went through breast development.

First day of fifth grade—usually first day of school was exciting, not nerve-racking—I got to see my friends and talk about what we did over the summer and also have recess. However, that day was not exciting at all. I was nervous about what to wear, usually my mom picked out my clothes, but I had to make sure I was wearing something that could make my breasts disappear. Nothing was working. So, I put on a shirt that my mom had picked out for me, did my hair, and put on makeup (mother's idea), but the bra was so uncomfortable.

I walked in my classroom, late, with my Lisa Frank trapper-keeper and I was the last student to arrive. Of course, I remembered everyone, hopefully they still remembered me. So, I walked in, and all of the girls dropped their jaws, but all of the boys cheered. I noticed that they were not cheering because I had arrived, they cheered because my new pair of boobs tagged along with me. I was mortified. Speedily, I put my trapper-keeper up to my chest and that's where that object stayed for the next school year.

In my analysis, I developed earlier than most, because I had more body fat than most girls and boys. My theory was that that year was the year my parents were starting to have marriage issues. They would argue and never get along. As the oldest child of three, I found that very stressful. All the stress was burrowing down on me, so I developed faster to grow up faster and to leave the "nest" earlier to get away from the burden of my family's crisis.

Why Is Early Family Stress Related to Early Maturation and Early Sexual Debut in Females?

One explanation for the impact of early family conflict on physical maturation and sexual risk-taking in females is through weight gain. One response to early family stress might be an increase in food intake, with a corresponding increase in body fat that would be related to early maturation and open the door to involvement with older sexually active peers. This involvement could increase the odds that the early-maturing girls will, themselves, become sexually active (Dishion, Ha, & Véronneau, 2012).

A second possibility is that girls with poor relations with parents hope to find an emotional substitute in the romantic world for the closeness they do not receive at home. When these same girls are early maturers, they are likely to become sexually active at an early age as they search for a meaningful emotional bond with a boy to make up for the lack of love and attention they experience from their parents (Scharf & Mayseless, 2008).

A third possibility is that genetic factors account for the pattern of early family stress, accelerated puberty, and early sexual debut (Comings, Muhleman, Johnson, & MacMurray, 2002; Rowe, 2002). Consider the possibility that one or both parents might possess genes related to irritability and impulsivity. Parents may pass their genetic makeup on to their children, who are also irritable and impulsive, increasing the frequency and intensity of parent–child conflict. Further, some of these same parents may carry genes for early maturation that they pass on to their children. Girls who receive this constellation of genes that includes impulsivity and early maturation are at risk for early sexual behavior, especially when they live in a stressful, high-conflict family environment (Carlson, Mendle, & Harden, 2014).

■ SEX AND THE ADOLESCENT BRAIN

What Changes Take Place in the Brain during Adolescence?

Using brain mapping technologies, such as functional magnetic resonance imaging (fMRI), scientists have discovered that the teen brain is not just a smaller version of an adult brain but has its own unique structure and functioning. Two major differences between the teen brain and the adult brain are in the development and functioning of the prefrontal cortex, and with the early development of the limbic system. The prefrontal cortex is the rational part of the brain associated with judgment and reasoning, which is not fully developed during adolescence but continues to mature until the mid- to late 20s. In contrast, the limbic system, the seat of our emotions, is more fully formed and develops more quickly during adolescence. As a consequence of this imbalance during adolescence, emotions are strong and rewards are potent, but the ability to control one's emotions and to delay rewards is relatively weak (Casey, Jones, & Hare, 2008; Dreyfuss et al., 2014; Steinberg, 2008). The different timetables of these two developments put adolescents at a heightened risk for acting without thinking (DeWitt, Aslan, & Filbey, 2014), or at least for not thinking clearly, leading to reckless behavior in many areas, including engaging in risky sexual behavior (Conradt et al., 2014; Khurana, Romer, Betancourt, Brodsky, Giannetta, et al., 2015).

Is There a Relationship between Teen Brain Development and Risky Sex?

There is increasing evidence that neurological development and brain activity are associated with risky sexual behavior during the teen years (Feldstein Ewing, Ryman, Gillman, Weiland, Thayer, et al., 2016). During adolescence, emotional centers in the brain are highly sensitive to social rewards at the same time the seat of rational thought in the prefrontal cortex is not fully mature (Eckstrand et al., 2017; Urošević, Collins, Muetzel, Lim, & Luciana, 2012). Some have proposed that this unevenness contributes to a focus on immediate rewards and a neglect of possible long-term negative consequences (Casey, Getz, & Galvan, 2008).

In one study, researchers investigated the joint effects of reward-seeking and cognitive control on early adolescent sexual behavior (Wasserman, Crockett, & Hoffman, 2017). Reward-seeking is a measure of how strongly adolescents pursue rewards, while cognitive control is a measure of teens' ability to control their behavior. The results reveal that both high reward-seeking and low cognitive control predict early adolescent sexual behavior. The findings support the idea that teens who engage in risky sexual behavior are highly influenced by the possibility of sexual rewards and have difficulty controlling their behavior.

Another example of the power of emotional arousal to override rational thought is shown in a study of the relationship between sexual arousal and contraceptive use. Before adolescents become sexually aroused they are more likely to engage in rational planning of their sexual activity, such as having and using a condom, but after they are aroused they are more likely to throw caution to the wind and have sex, even if some form of contraception is not available (Goldenberg, Telzer, Lieberman, Fuligni, & Galván, 2013). Even adults find it difficult to control their emotions after they are aroused, but adolescents find it especially difficult to act rationally when they are in an aroused state (Casey, 2015; Dir, Coskunpinar, & Cyders, 2014).

In one important study of adolescent girls, data on brain activity from fMRI scans were coupled with reports of sexual decision making. The researchers found that the prefrontal cortex was more active among girls who made thoughtful decisions about having sex, while neural activity was greater in the ventral striatum—which functions as part of the reward center of the brain—among girls who acted more impulsively (Hensel, Hummer, Acrurio, James, & Fortenberry, 2015). The findings support a dual systems model of brain development in which emotional reward centers in the limbic system mature earlier than cognitive control centers in the prefrontal cortex.

■ THE GENETICS OF ADOLESCENT SEXUALITY

Biology affects adolescent sexuality in a multitude of ways, but one important route that is often ignored in research and discussions about the causes of teen sexuality is through the operation of genes. Findings from recent research suggest that a relationship exists between genes and age of first intercourse, sexual desire, and interest in sexual variety (Halley, Boretsky, Puts, & Shriver, 2016). How important are genetic influences on the sexual behavior of adolescents?

How Do Researchers Determine the Impact of Genes on Behavior?

How do researchers estimate the strength of genetic influences on behavior? The formula for determining the impact of genes on behavior involves comparing monozygotic (identical) twins with dizygotic (fraternal) twins. If a characteristic, such as sexual behavior, is highly influenced by genetic factors, then the sexual behavior of identical twins should be highly similar and more alike than the sexual behavior of fraternal twins. On the basis of this type of comparison it is possible to calculate a number that is an estimate of the degree of influence of genetic factors on the behavior in question. That number is referred to as *heritability,* which can range from 0%, meaning that genes have no influence on the behavior, to 100%, meaning that the behavior is completely determined by genetic factors. Heritability is low for the type of movies one enjoys, for example, but scientists have shown that heritability is high for the etiology of many psychological problems, such as schizophrenia, autism, and alcoholism. Where does adolescent sexuality fall on this continuum?

Do Genes Affect Adolescent Sexuality?

K. Paige Harden at the University of Texas at Austin conducted a thorough and masterful review of behavior genetic studies of adolescent sexuality and concluded that the heritability of sexuality was "significant and nontrivial" (Harden, 2014a, p. 437). The median heritability for age of first intercourse was 34%, while the heritability of other aspects of sexuality, such as lifetime number of sex partners, teenage pregnancy, and risky sexual attitudes, was about 46%. These results indicate that a modest relationship exists between genetic factors and adolescent sexuality, which is also influenced by the psychosocial environment.

When It Comes to Sex, Why Are Adolescents Like Their Parents?

Family resemblance in sexual behavior is one area in which genes matter, but is rarely included in explanations for family similarity in sexual behavior. Sex runs in families. There is similarity in the sexual behavior of parents and their adolescent children, and between adolescent siblings. For example, the daughter of a mother who gave birth to a child when the mother was a teenager is two to three times more likely to become a teenage mother herself, even if the daughter is not the child born to the mother during her teen years (Meade, Kershaw, & Ickovics, 2008). Similarly, a high percentage of sons with fathers who were teenage fathers become teen fathers themselves (Sipsma, Biello, Cole-Lewis, & Kershaw, 2010). This intergenerational transmission of sexuality is typically attributed to modeling or ineffective parenting, without regard to the obvious genetic relationship between parent and adolescent. One possible genetic route between parent and adolescent is through the inheritance of traits such as sensation-seeking and impulsive behavior, which have a high genetic loading and are implicated in risky sex and inconsistent contraceptive use (Donohew, Zimmerman, Cupp, Novak, Colon, et al., 2000). One can easily imagine the trouble adolescents might get into if they are impulsive risk takers being raised by overwhelmed single mothers who also are impulsive risk takers.

In addition to parent–child similarity in sexual behavior, siblings also have like-minded sexual attitudes and similar sexual histories (East, 1998; Haurin & Mott, 1990). As was true for parent–adolescent resemblance in sexual behavior, explanations for sibling similarity usually focus on modeling and social influence, while ignoring the strong genetic connection between siblings. McHale, Bissell, and Kim (2009) showed that the more genetically similar siblings are— going from genetically alike monozygotic twins to dizygotic twins to full siblings, half siblings, and genetically unrelated adopted siblings—the more alike they are in their attitudes about risky sex, and their participation in risky sexual behavior. Genes are not the whole story, however. Siblings who are emotionally close to each other and who live in an emotionally warm family environment are more alike sexually than siblings who are not close to each other and who live in an emotionally distant family environment. The pattern of results suggests that genes do not automatically lead to a particular outcome, irrespective of social influences, but that the strength of genetic influences is moderated by the environment.

How Important Are Genes to Males and Females?

Heritability of the sexual behavior of males is higher than the heritability of the sexual activity of females (Harden, 2014a). As Harden points out, this difference may occur because female sexuality is more strongly regulated by nongenetic factors, such as parent socialization and peer pressure, increasing the importance of the social environment for females and decreasing the significance of genetics. Males live in a more laissez-faire social world when it comes to their sexual behavior, which means that the environment has less of an effect on male sexuality, than on female sexuality, while genes play a more prominent role in differences in sexuality among males than among females.

How Could Genes Affect Adolescent Sexuality?

There are good reasons to expect that genes play some role in the expression of adolescent sexuality. As was discussed in a previous section, T is related to sexual behavior, at least for boys. Adolescents differ in how much circulating T is present in their blood, a difference that is at least partly the result of genetic factors (Harris, Vernon, & Boomsma, 1998). A group of researchers at the University of Amsterdam showed that in a sample of boys and girls in the Netherlands, T levels are related to both genetic and nongenetic influences, one of the most important environmental influences being sexual behavior itself (Hoekstra, Bartels, & Boomsma, 2006). In other words, the relationship between T and sexuality is reciprocal. T has an impact on sexual behavior, but sexual activity also has an impact on level of T. So the impact of genes on sexual behavior is through their effect on T, which affects sexuality and which itself has an impact on T.

Further, genes play an important role in pubertal timing and family relations, both of which are tied to early sexual behavior. Research has demonstrated that variation in pubertal maturation in boys and girls is at least partly influenced by genetic factors, and early pubertal timing is related to early sexual activity (Ge, Natsuaki, Neiderhiser, & Reiss, 2007; Silventoinen, Haukka, Dunkel, Tynelius, & Rasmussen, 2008). In addition, genes affect parent and adolescent characteristics, such as impulse control and sensation-seeking, which have an impact on the social environment of a family. When the family environment is stressful and high in conflict, adolescents mature earlier, which makes it more likely that they will engage in early sexual activity.

Taken as a whole, results of studies of the influence of genes on adolescent sexuality point to the conclusion that genes exert some influence on adolescent sexual behavior, especially for males, but considerably more research is needed to elucidate the mechanism by which genes affect sexuality.

SUMMARY

■ PUBERTY

The physical changes that occur during puberty alter the form and function of the growing adolescent's body, transforming biologically immature children into biologically mature adults capable of reproduction. What triggers the onset of puberty is not entirely understood, but it is the result of a combination of genetic and environmental factors acting in conjunction with each other. Menarche typically occurs among U.S. females when body fat reaches about 17% of total body weight. An increase in the production of sex steroids occurs during puberty, two of the most important classes of steroids being androgens, such as T in males and estrogens in females. During puberty, many changes occur in the development and appearance of primary and secondary sexual characteristics, changes that differentiate the functioning and appearance of the bodies of males and females.

■ GONADAL HORMONES AND ADOLESCENT SEXUALITY

The literature on the relationship between gonadal sex hormones and adolescent sexuality is neither extensive nor simple to summarize. Further, many of the key studies are 20–30 years old, done before the development of modern, more sensitive hormone assay techniques and more sophisticated types of data analyses. Even with these limitations, however, it is still possible to arrive at a few tentative conclusions. The relationship between gonadal hormones and adolescent sexuality is subtle and complicated, and no simple, linear relationship exists between hormones and adolescent sexual thoughts, emotions, and behaviors. Hormones interact with social-psychological factors, which exert a powerful effect on every aspect of adolescent sexuality. The sexual behavior of both genders is influenced by the interaction of hormones and environment, but hormones exert a somewhat stronger effect on males than on females, while the environment is to some degree more important for females than for males. Udry et al. (1985) suggests that androgens may matter for males more than for females because young adolescent males have 10–20 times more T circulating in their blood than do females. In addition, female sexuality is more highly regulated and socially controlled than male sexuality, thus the social environment has a stronger effect on females. These conclusions are the beginning but not the end of an ongoing effort to understand the complex relationship between pubertal hormones and adolescent sexual behavior.

■ PHYSICAL MATURATION AND ADOLESCENT SEXUALITY

The relationship between early pubertal timing and risky sexual behavior is usually explained as the result of accelerated physical growth among adolescents who are still psychologically and socially young, coupled with an association with older peers who have older norms about sexual behavior and who may be engaged in a variety of risky behaviors, including early sex. This explanation has three components. First, early-maturing adolescents perceive themselves and are perceived by others to be older and more mature than their age-mates. Second, early maturers often become members of peer groups comprising older teens. Third, because early maturers have many older friends, they have more opportunities to engage in behavior that is typical of older adolescents, including risky behavior such as early sex.

■ FAMILY RELATIONS, PUBERTAL TIMING, AND ADOLESCENT SEXUALITY

For girls, early family conflict predicts early pubertal timing, which is associated with risky sexual behavior. Several explanations have been offered for the relationship between family stress, early maturation, and risky sexual behavior, including weight gain; associating with older peers; a search for a close, supportive relationship that is absent at home; and genetic influences.

■ SEX AND THE ADOLESCENT BRAIN

Profound changes occur in the brain during adolescence, two of the most important being the rapid development of the limbic system and the slower development of the prefrontal cortex. In combination, these two sets of changes mean that during adolescence emotions are strong, while the capacity of the adolescent to exert control over those emotions is not fully formed. These developments put adolescents at a heightened risk for acting without thinking clearly, leading to reckless behavior, including engaging in risky sexual behavior.

Although research on the relationship between brain development and adolescent sexuality is in its infancy, there is suggestive evidence that the still-developing teen brain is implicated in the willingness of some adolescents to engage in sexual risk-taking.

■ THE GENETICS OF ADOLESCENT SEXUALITY

The interplay of genetics and the social-psychological environment on adolescent sexuality is complex, and no simple relationship exists between genes and adolescent sexuality. Two conclusions are strongly supported by the evidence currently available: first, genes have a direct effect on adolescent sexuality, operating through gonadal hormones and neurotransmitters; and second, genes play a role in the social-psychological factors related to sexuality, such as impulsivity and family and peer relations, factors often incorrectly thought of as existing apart from genetic-biological factors. The inclusion of genetic factors in a biosocial explanation of adolescent sexuality does not diminish or simplify our general understanding of the sex lives of adolescents, but adds to and enriches our appreciation of this important and multifaceted issue.

SUGGESTIONS FOR FURTHER READING

Belsky, J., Steinberg, L., Houts, R. M., & Halpern-Felsher, B. L. (2010). The development of reproductive strategy in females: Early maternal harshness → earlier menarche → increased sexual risk taking. *Developmental Psychology, 46,* 120–128.

Deardorff, J., Gonzales, N. A., Christopher, S., Roosa, M. W., & Millsap, R. E. (2005). Early puberty and adolescent pregnancy: The influence of alcohol use. *Pediatrics, 116,* 1451–1456.

Halpern, C. T. (2006). Integrating hormones and other biological factors into a developmental systems model of adolescent female sexuality. In L. M. Diamond (Ed.), *Rethinking positive adolescent female sexual development* (pp. 9–22). San Francisco: Jossey-Bass.

Halpern, C. T., Udry, J. R., & Suchindran, C. (1998). Monthly measures of salivary testosterone predict sexual activity in adolescent males. *Archives of Sexual Behavior, 27,* 445–465.

Harden, K. P. (2014). Genetic influences on adolescent sexual behavior: Why genes matter for environmentally oriented researchers. *Psychological Bulletin, 140,* 434–465.

Hensel, D. J., Hummer, T. A., Acrurio, L. R., James, T. W., & Fortenberry, D. (2015). Feasibility of functional neuroimaging to understand adolescent women's sexual decision making. *Journal of Adolescent Health, 56,* 389–395.

CHAPTER 3

Parents and Adolescent Sexuality

Several years ago, the Public Broadcasting System released a disturbing 90-minute documentary entitled *The Lost Children of Rockdale County* that chronicled the reckless sexual behavior of a group of well-to-do teenagers living in a suburb of Atlanta, Georgia (Frontline WGBH, 1999). For a number of years, the teens had been engaged in unrestrained sexual behavior that included multiple sex partners and group sex, the unfortunate outcome of which was an outbreak of syphilis, a disease rarely found among white, affluent teens. The program explores the influence of alcohol, boredom, and peer pressure on adolescent sexuality, but the point that comes across most strongly is the distressing impact that absent parents and a lack of parental supervision had on these adolescents. All too often, these professional, overscheduled parents left their teens to care for themselves, believing that they had done all they could do to raise their children well. A common attitude among many of the parents was that they no longer could influence their adolescents, who were beyond parental control and on their own. As one father of a young daughter heavily caught up in a world of alcohol-fueled group sex glumly remarked:

> "But what can you do about it? You know, you can't lock a kid in a closet, 13, 14, 15 years old. No, they don't want their parents to go with them and their friends, and you've got to understand that. You've just got to hope that you've instilled the kind of values in them or that you've taught them the kind of values, what is important, and when they get that old, they will respect that." (Frontline WGBH, 1999)

The extreme behavior of these teens is rare, although the belief that adolescents are beyond the control of parents is common. Many parents mistakenly believe

> *In the following story, a daughter is certain her mother had an impact on her sexuality, not only during adolescence but even into emerging adulthood.*

IN THEIR OWN WORDS

My mother . . . has made it extremely clear to me that sex before marriage is absolutely taboo in her eyes. Her sex talk comprised several bible verses stating the evils of nontraditional sex, as well as the medical breakdown of many sexually transmitted diseases. I remember being appropriately horrified and unwilling to partake of premarital sex as a child. However, as I grew older, garnered rosy descriptions of sex from more experienced friends, and grew more distant from my mother, her opinions started to matter less to me. By the time I was 16, I had completely different views about premarital sex, as well as quite a few other things, than my mother.

Despite my different views, I know that her opinion indeed impacted my life because of how I approached sex and still approach it today. First, I made sure I hid all evidence of sexual activity from my mother, as I was terrified of what her reaction would be. Second, I was and am always very careful to be protected from sexually transmitted diseases as well as pregnancy, mostly because I am still terrified of what her reaction would be. Third, although I do not believe waiting to have sex until marriage is important, I am of the opinion that one should wait to have sex until they are in love. I believe that my opinions would have been somewhat different, and probably more liberal, if my mother's influence had not been so powerful to me in my childhood.

they can have little effect on their children when they become adolescents and are swallowed up by the exciting world of peers and social media (Albert, 2012). Is it true that parents disappear into the background of the increasingly peer- and media-centered lives of adolescents? Do parents have an impact on the sexuality of adolescents? This chapter explores these questions and examines the relationship between adolescent sexual behavior and family structure, fathers, divorce, and parenting.

■ FAMILY STRUCTURE

Is Family Structure Related to Adolescent Sexuality?

Living in a two-parent family protects adolescents against risky sexual behavior, not only among teens in the United States but also among those in the developed and developing world (Jovic et al., 2014; Pilgrim et al., 2014). Teens in two-parent families are less likely to engage in risky sexual behavior than teens in other family configurations (Bámaca-Colbert, Greene, Killoren, & Noah, 2014; Halpern & Haydon, 2012). There are no differences in the sexuality of adolescents living in mother-only families or in father-only families, suggesting that the gender of the parent has less of an influence on teen sexual behavior than having two parents (Dufur, Hoffmann, & Erickson, 2018).

Sexual Debut

Family structure is related to the age when adolescents first become sexually active. Age of sexual debut among adolescents living in different family types occurs in the following order from youngest to oldest: living with neither parent, living with a single biological parent, living in a family with a stepparent, and living with two biological parents (Sturgeon, 2008). Further, living in a two-parent family rather than another type of family matters more for younger adolescents, especially for those under the age of 15 years, but as adolescents get older, family structure is less strongly related to age of sexual debut (Donahue et al., 2010).

Number of Sexual Partners

Family structure is also related to the number of sexual partners an adolescent has. In general, adolescents from two-parent families have fewer sexual partners than adolescents in other family types (Cleveland & Gilson, 2004; Ku et al., 1998). The main reason for this difference is that a higher proportion of adolescents in two-parent families have never had sexual intercourse, so they have zero number of sexual partners. When the association between family structure and number of sexual partners is examined among sexually active adolescents only, there is little difference in number of sexual partners between adolescents in two-parent families in comparison to adolescents in other types of families. In other words, family structure has little effect on number of sexual partners, once adolescents begin to have sex.

Contraceptive Use

Sexually active adolescents from two-parent families are more likely to use some form of contraception than adolescents from other family types (Manning, Longmore, & Giordano, 2000). This difference is due to the fact that adolescents in two-parent families start to have sex at a later age than adolescents in other family types. Older adolescents are more likely to consistently use contraception than younger adolescents, so the effect of family type on contraceptive use is mainly explained by the fact that sexually active adolescents from two-parent families are older than sexually active adolescents from other family types (Martinez, Copen, & Abma, 2011).

Sexually Transmitted Infections

The prevalence of STIs is lower among adolescents in two-parent families than in other family types. That difference is accounted for by the fact that in two-parent families, fewer adolescents are sexually active, and those who are tend to be older and more likely to use condoms consistently than adolescents in other family types (Upchurch, Mason, Kusonuki, & Kriechbaum, 2004).

Pregnancy

Adolescent females who have the lowest probability of becoming pregnant or giving birth to a child during their teen years are females who have lived all their lives with two biological parents (Amato & Kane, 2011). Living in a two-parent family also protects adolescent males, who are less likely to father a child in comparison to males from other types of family structures (Ku, Sonenstein, & Pleck, 1993). As was true for number of sexual partners and STI rates, comparing pregnancy and birth rates across family types is confounded by the fact that fewer adolescents in two-parent families are sexually active in comparison to adolescents in other family types. When only sexually active teens are examined, the effect of family structure on teen pregnancy and birth rates diminishes, but does not disappear (Brückner, Martin, & Bearman, 2004).

In general, adolescents in two-parent families have fewer sexual partners, more consistent contraceptive use, and lower rates of STIs, pregnancies, and births than teens in other family types. These differences are largely accounted for by the fact that adolescents in two-parent families begin to have sex at a later age than adolescents in other family types and so are more cautious and responsible than sexually active younger adolescents. Once adolescents begin to have sex, the association between family structure and adolescent sexual behavior decreases but does not disappear (Garneau, Olmstead, Pasley, & Fincham, 2013; Stark et al., 2016).

Is Family Income Related to Teen Sexual Behavior?

One critical difference between one- and two-parent families is that the income level of single-parent families is generally lower than it is in two-parent families. In 2016, the median household income for three family types with children in the United States was $86,811 for married couple families, $51,568 for male-headed families, and $36,658 for female-headed families (U.S. Census Bureau, 2017). Adolescents not living with both parents have fewer economic resources, which is viewed by economists as largely responsible for the risky adolescent sexual behavior associated with living in a family without a father (Crowder & Teachman, 2004). Growing up with only one parent deprives adolescents of important economic resources, which increases the risk of early sexual debut, pregnancy, and childbearing (Thomson & McLanahan, 2012). Adolescents who grow up in two-parent families are more likely to live in more affluent neighborhoods, attend good schools, do better in school, and have friends who are less likely to be involved in deviant activities, all of which support the development of long-term goals and high educational attainment that in turn decrease the likelihood of early sex, inconsistent contraceptive use, adolescent pregnancy, and early childbearing (Upchurch, Aneshensel, Sucoff, & Levy-Storms, 1999).

Family finances matter but they do not account for all of the differences between one- and two-parent families in the sexual behavior of adolescents

(Ziol-Guest & Dunifon, 2014). Even after statistically controlling for differences in household economic resources, adolescents living in one-parent families are more likely to engage in risky sex than adolescents in two-parent families, although the relationship between family structure and adolescent sexuality is weaker (McLanahan & Sandefur, 1994). There are psychological and social costs that go beyond economics to growing up in a one-parent family that are related to the sexual behavior of adolescents.

Is the Dating Behavior of Single Mothers Related to Adolescent Sexuality?

There are many ways in which single parenthood may influence the sexual behavior of adolescents, such as an increase in parent–adolescent conflict or a decrease in parent monitoring. The dating behavior of the parent is another influence on risky adolescent sexual behavior, one that many parents, especially custodial mothers, are particularly worried about. Sons and daughters who live with their mothers are more likely to be sexually active if the mothers date, especially if they date frequently (Zito & De Coster, 2016). Further, mothers who date have more permissive attitudes about teen sexuality than mothers who do not date, which increases the probability that the teens will be sexually active. The majority of adolescents in single-parent families live with a

The following story reveals the tension between a divorced mother and her daughter about sex, and the change that occurred after the daughter heard her mother having sex.

IN THEIR OWN WORDS

My parents are divorced, thus I have had two very different experiences with "the talk." Throughout my adolescence, my mom was exactly the parent I do not want to be. She was very secretive when it came to sex. She seemed as if she did not want my sister and I to know that sex even existed. We had many questions, but every one of them was answered with "Why do you want to know? Are you having sex?!?!" She also thought that my sister and I "wouldn't do something like that." This was not helpful to our learning process. If anything, it made us more curious about sex, what it felt like and what was so special. I feel that her choice in approaching the sex talk is what made my sister and I lose our virginities at a rather young age. I lost mine at 15 and she lost hers at 14. Now

that I am 18, my mom is much more open about sex. Unfortunately, this comes at a pretty late time. She is more open now because she has started dating again, 10 years after her divorce. She was forced to be more open about sex because my boyfriend and I overheard her having sex one night, thus her notion of premarital sex is a sin was thrown out the window. Now, she has almost reverted into a teenager and is completely accepting of my sexual activity. She has even asked me personal questions about my sex life. This hasn't really affected my responsibility in my sex life, but my sister has been negatively affected. She is fairly promiscuous and I feel that my mom's inability to talk to us about sex played a role in that.

custodial mother who is often in her late 30s or early 40s. Most of these mothers are interested in forming romantic relationships with men, relationships that sometimes become sexual (Gray, Garcia, Crosier, & Fisher, 2015). Adolescents know that their mothers date and, at some level, even may be aware that their mothers are sexually active, all of which occurs during the time adolescents are beginning to date, forming romantic relationships, and developing their own sexual attitudes. It is difficult for most mothers to keep their romantic lives separate from the romantic lives of their adolescents, which is not to suggest that mothers with adolescents should be stay-at-home recluses, but mothers need to know that what they do affects their adolescents, so it is important for mothers to act responsibly and to have open and honest talks about dating and sex with their teens.

How single parents handle their romantic lives sends a powerful message to their adolescents about what is appropriate dating and sexual behavior. As one young woman once said to me, "Most of what I know about flirting, I learned from my mother," a statement that says something about the mother, the daughter, and the mother–daughter relationship. Single parents who are sexually active may send a message to their adolescents that teen sex is acceptable, and the more sexually active the parent is, the stronger that message.

■ FATHERS

Do children, including adolescents, need a father? Biologically, of course, they do, and most are greatly helped economically if they grow up in a household with a mother and an employed father. But is a father more than a chromosome and a paycheck? Does he uniquely contribute to the cognitive, psychological, and social development of his children, especially his adolescent-age children? The obvious answers to these seemingly simple questions are neither obvious nor simple, as will be seen in this section.

There is no uncertainty about the importance of fathers in the mind of President Barack Obama, who in 2008 gave a Father's Day speech in which he urged fathers, especially African American fathers, to be more engaged in raising their children. To quote President Obama:

> "Of all the rocks upon which we build our lives, we are reminded today that family is the most important. And we are called to recognize and honor how critical every father is to that foundation. They are teachers and coaches. They are mentors and role models. They are examples of success and the men who constantly push us toward it."

In contrast to the idea that fathers matter, several social scientists argue that the association between fatherlessness and poor child outcomes is not due to the absence of fathers, but to the absence of a second parent and to the loss of economic resources (Biblarz & Stacey, 2010; Silverstein & Auerbach, 1999). These social scientists provocatively conclude that fathers are not essential to healthy child development.

What Impact Do Nonresident Fathers Have on the Sexual Behavior of Their Adolescents?

Fathers are associated with a delay in the age at which their adolescents become sexually active. For example, in one investigation of the sexual behavior of adolescents, approximately 14% of youth in father-present families had sexual intercourse before the age of 15 years in comparison to about 32% of adolescents with nonresident fathers (Abma & Sonenstein, 2001). Fathers matter when it comes to the sexual behavior of their adolescents, primarily by slowing down the sexual debut of their adolescents.

The risk of early sexual debut is highest among adolescents with an unstable background that includes fathers or father figures repeatedly moving in and out of the home (Hogan, Sun, & Cornwell, 2000). Further, the earlier in their lives adolescents experience the loss of a father, the earlier they engage in sexual intercourse for the first time, and the more likely girls are to become pregnant during adolescence (Ellis et al., 2012; Quinlan, 2003).

Is Teen Sexuality Related to Father Genes?

One avenue by which nonresident fathers might affect risky adolescent sexuality is genetic. Teens may inherit dysfunctional personality traits from their absent fathers (Moffitt, 2005; Raeburn, 2014). Specifically, men who have externalizing behavior traits—such as negative emotionality, acting-out behaviors, and impulsivity—are at risk for divorce, desertion, and becoming nonresident fathers (Mendle et al., 2009). Adolescents with this type of father

---

Some fathers may be awkward in the way they approach the subject of sex, but the daughter in the following story appreciated the effort her father made, and it made a difference to her.

IN THEIR OWN WORDS

My mom was the one who had the biggest influence on me when it came to sexuality. She was the one who talked about it frequently and I don't remember my dad saying much of anything . . . until my 16th birthday. On my 16th birthday, my dad took me out to a nice dinner. . . . Halfway through dinner he gave me two presents. One was a pink sapphire and diamond ring and the other was a small cactus. He explained the meaning of the cactus as "You have to take care of a cactus like you have to take care of your virginity." I don't remember the whole conversation or the exact words after that. And while it may sound cheesy, I really respected him for doing that for me. I always heard him in the back of my head if I was getting a little carried away and would immediately stop what I was doing and really think about it.

are likely to possess these traits themselves, traits associated with sexual risk-taking (Timmermans, van Lier, & Koot, 2008). One route by which adolescents may acquire these dysfunctional traits is genetic (Rhee & Waldman, 2002). In fact, an androgen receptor gene has been identified that is associated with impulsivity, a high number of sexual partners, and family abandonment in males, confirming the idea that these traits have some genetic basis (Comings et al., 2002).

Do Nonresident Fathers Have the Same Effect on the Sexual Behavior of Boys and Girls?

The association between nonresident fathering and adolescent sexuality is different for boys and girls. Girls are more likely to engage in sexual risk behavior than boys when a father is not present in their family (Ryan, 2015), an effect that is due to an earlier age of menarche among father-absent girls, leading to an earlier sexual debut (James et al., 2012). Nonresident fatherhood does not have an effect on the age when puberty begins for boys. Father absence has a greater effect on the reproductive development of girls than of boys, perhaps because girls are more sensitive to a disrupted family environment and to poor family relationship dynamics than boys, who are more oriented to peers for support and companionship.

How Do Nonresident Fathers Affect Their Daughters?

The role of nonresident fatherhood in the sexual and reproductive behavior of daughters has been of considerable interest to evolutionary psychologists, who have proposed that early childhood experiences with a father shape future sexual behavior and reproductive strategies for females (Belsky et al., 1991). According to Belsky et al., the presence or absence of a father during childhood leads to the development of two very different strategies for reproduction among females. Girls from father-present families develop a *parenting reproductive strategy* that starts with a delayed onset of puberty, a late age of sexual debut, having stable long-term relationships, and not having children in adolescence, all of which leads to having a fewer number of children and more investment of time and energy in each child (Ellis et al., 2003). Conversely, girls in father-absent families develop a *mating reproductive strategy* that starts with early physical maturation, early onset of sexual activity, and many short-term sexual partners (Quinlan, 2003). Girls with these characteristics are more likely to engage in risky sex and therefore, are more likely to become pregnant when they are teens (James et al., 2012).

How Do Fathers Affect Teen Sexuality?

A family without a father is structurally different from one with a father, but a father's impact on his adolescents, especially on their sexual behavior, extends beyond his mere presence or absence. In order to better understand the effects of fathers on adolescent sexuality, it is important to go beyond merely looking at whether fathers are present or absent and look at what fathers do—the impact of their parenting—on adolescent sexuality.

Father–Adolescent Closeness

The aspect of the father–adolescent relationship that has the greatest impact on adolescent sexuality is the quality of the relationship fathers have with their adolescents. Fathers who have good relations with their teens, which includes closeness, warmth, and connectedness, are more likely to have adolescents, especially daughters, who are not sexually active, who wait until they are older before they become sexually active, and who have a fewer number of sexual partners (Regnerus & Luchies, 2006; Rink, Tricker, & Harvey, 2007).

Father–adolescent closeness can be a deterrent to early adolescent sexual activity, but early adolescent sexuality also may reduce father–adolescent closeness (Ream & Savin-Williams, 2005). Thus, adolescent sexuality may drive a wedge between fathers and adolescents, perhaps because sexually active adolescents pull away from their fathers, or because the fathers react negatively to the sexual behavior of their adolescents.

Adolescents who spend time with their fathers are less likely to be sexually active than adolescents who spend little time with their fathers (Coley, Votruba-Drzal, & Schindler, 2009; Ream & Savin-Williams, 2005). Spending time together may be one manifestation of a close relationship and a building block for further closeness.

The following story by a daughter reveals how awkward it can be for an adolescent to talk to her father about sex, but also how important it is for the adolescent to feel understood and cared for by her father.

IN THEIR OWN WORDS

During high school I started to become closer with my dad. One night as he was dropping me off at my first boyfriend's house, he found the opportunity to talk to me about sex. He told me that it was OK to say no and not to feel pressured. He assured me that if anyone tried anything without my consent that he would have my brother take care of it. And he kind of just left it at that. Later in high school, my dad became better with his sex talks. He talked more to me about coming to him if anything went wrong or if I had any questions.

When I was younger my parents talked to me about sex together. My mom, shortly after, took control when it came to more stuff about dealing with puberty and my own body. As I got older, dad took over making sure I had no questions. This approach worked because it assured me that I had two people who cared and understood to go to for any questions or issues I had.

The following story illustrates the rift that developed between a father and his daughter after the daughter became pregnant.

IN THEIR OWN WORDS

When I was 15, about 9 months after I lost my virginity, I got pregnant. My father was hurt, angry, and demanded that I get an abortion. My mother was supportive in dealing with my emotions, but she never offered any opinions about how she felt at the time. After my abortion, my mother put me on the pill, but we did not discuss other birth control options or STI prevention. My father did not discuss the situation with me. He just told me, "This is what happens when you have sex before you're ready." He also told me that I was not allowed to have anymore boyfriends until I was 18.

Discipline and Monitoring

Paternal discipline and monitoring also influence adolescent sexuality. Fathers who are lenient disciplinarians and fathers who are very strict have adolescents who are likely to initiate sex at an early age in comparison to adolescents with fathers who exert a moderate degree of discipline over their adolescents (Jemmott & Jemmott, 1992; Kao & Carter, 2013). Fathers matter by setting and enforcing family rules and curfews, which have the effect of curtailing adolescent sexual behavior (Langley, 2016), but rules and curfews need to be appropriate or else adolescents may take advantage of their freedom or rebel against their restrictions. In addition, fathers who are poor monitors of their adolescents have teens who are more likely to engage in risky sexual behavior (Manlove, Wildsmith, Ikramullah, Terry-Humen, & Schelar, 2012; Ryan, 2015). Discipline and monitoring act in conjunction with each other, and adolescents with fathers who exert little control over their adolescents and who do not monitor them provide the opportunities for adolescents to engage in sex with little chance of getting caught and with few, if any, consequences if they are caught.

Paternal Attitudes about Adolescent Sexual Behavior

Fathers who have lenient attitudes about adolescent sexuality have teens who are more likely to be sexually active and have more sexual partners, while paternal disapproval of adolescent sexuality is associated with delayed sexual debut and fewer partners (Kao & Carter, 2013). Paternal attitudes matter, but what matters more are adolescents' perceptions of those attitudes, along with the quality of the relationship between adolescents and fathers. Adolescents who believe that their fathers disapprove of adolescent sexuality are less likely to be sexually active, especially if the father–adolescent relationship is close, since adolescents with these perceptions may not want to disappoint their fathers.

Communication about Sex

One final aspect of the father–adolescent relationship associated with a later age of sexual debut among adolescents is communication about sex. Fathers who talk to their teens about sex have adolescents who are less likely to be sexually active than adolescents with fathers who do not talk to them about sex. Typically, fathers emphasize the importance of waiting to have sex until the adolescents are older and more mature. In addition, fathers with daughters often caution their daughters about the questionable motives of young men (Brown, Rosnick, Webb-Bradley, & Kirner, 2014).

The age when fathers talk to their adolescents about sex is related to adolescent sexual behavior, but not in a straightforward way. Father–adolescent communication about sex is associated with *less* sexual activity among younger adolescents but, paradoxically, *more* sexual activity among older adolescents (Somers & Paulson, 2000). The finding that father–adolescent communication about sex is related to more sexual activity among older adolescents is peculiar. One explanation for this odd finding is that communication with young teens occurs before the teens become sexually active and focuses on delaying sexual debut, but communication with older adolescents often occurs after the adolescents have become sexually active and emphasizes the importance of practicing safe sex. The association between father–adolescent communication about sex and teen sexual behavior not only depends on whether communication occurs but also on what is said and when.

■ PARENTAL SEPARATION AND DIVORCE

A divorce does not take place at the single point in time when a judge grants a final divorce decree dissolving the marriage—rather, it is a series of unsettling events for parents and children that take place over a period of months and even years before and after the divorce. A divorce may bring relief through the end of an empty relationship, a loveless marriage, or an abusive relationship, but whether the divorce is a source of sadness or relief, it can be a long-term disruptive experience for all involved, especially the children. Long before the divorce occurs there may be a deterioration of family relations. Frequently, there is an increase in stress and conflict between spouses and between parents and children before, during, and after the divorce, all of which may contribute to adolescent problem behavior.

Why Is Parental Divorce Related to Teen Sexuality?

Parental separation and divorce are risk factors for early sexual intercourse, having many sexual partners, premarital pregnancy, and early childbearing among adolescents in every country in which this issue has been examined (Lansford, 2009; Orgilés, Carratalá, & Espada, 2015). The consistency of the association between divorce and adolescent risky sex is impressive and cries out for explanation, given high divorce rates in Western countries such as the United States, where between 30 and 50% of all children will experience a parental divorce (Vespa, Lewis, & Kreider, 2013).

Family Change

Family change is one factor that is related to adolescent sexual activity, with more change associated with an increase in risky sex (DeLeire & Kalil, 2002). Significant changes in the family during and after divorce disrupt the lives and tax the coping skills of even the most resilient adolescents who are faced with an uncertain future. Major disruptions in family economic conditions, parental employment, place of residence, schools, relations with fathers, and family composition often occur after a divorce. There is a decline in family income that leads to the disappearance or decrease of some family resources. Sometimes parents are forced to change jobs, or a stay-at-home parent may begin working. In addition, divorce often entails unwanted moves from home, school, and neighborhood to new, unfamiliar environments (Astone & McLanahan, 1994). There is the loss of neighbors, friends, and classmates and, most importantly, a significant loss of daily contact with one parent, usually the father. In addition to the stresses that are the result of the process of divorce, the formation of a postdivorce life may include cohabitation and remarriage, with the addition of a stepparent, and sometimes stepsiblings, further complicating life at home.

Family Transitions

Another factor related to the effect of divorce on adolescent sexual behavior is the number of *family transitions,* which are defined as the number of times a child experiences a parental separation, divorce, remarriage, or the entry or exit of a live-in romantic partner of the parent. Adolescents who experience multiple transitions in their family structure are more likely to begin to have sex at an earlier age and to have an unplanned pregnancy than adolescents raised in stable, two-parent families, or even stable, single-parent families (Fergusson, McLeod, & Horwood, 2014). Each transition requires a reorganization of family roles, relationships, and functioning, and may diminish the quality of parenting that adolescents receive. Adolescent risky sex is higher among teens who have experienced multiple family transitions, which suggests that family transitional events have a cumulative effect on adolescent sexual behavior (Belsky, Schlomer, & Ellis, 2012; Capaldi, Crosby, & Stoolmiller, 1996). Hetherington and Kelly (2003) propose that family transitions lead to a deterioration of the parent–adolescent attachment bond, especially between mothers and daughters, who may seek emotional support and intimacy from a boyfriend rather than from the mother, increasing the risk of early sexual debut, casual sex, and adolescent pregnancy. In addition, adolescents who experience several instances of different adult males moving in and out of a female-headed household may come to view romantic relations as temporary and short-lived, attitudes that may carry over into their own dating relationships, accelerating sexual involvement and leading to a high number of sexual partners.

Monitoring

Another factor related to risky sex among adolescents in divorced families is that the always demanding task of monitoring teens who can be rambunctious or secretive is made even more difficult for a custodial parent, usually the mother, during and after a divorce when surveillance decreases from four watchful eyes to two. A decrease in the ability of mothers to monitor their adolescents often occurs as families go through the upheaval of a divorce, and adolescents are given more freedom and independence (Wallerstein, Lewis, & Blakeslee, 2001).

The effect of a divorced mother moving in with her boyfriend has a greater impact on the sexual behavior of the daughter and on the relationship the daughter has with her mother than the mother's words about sex, as the following story illustrates.

IN THEIR OWN WORDS

My parents got divorced when I was in high school. I remember sitting at a table with my mother and adult, college-graduated sister (she is 8 years older than I am) at my mother's house. My sister was telling my mother that she was moving in with her boyfriend, whom my mother did not like at all. My mother looked at her with what can only be described as religious disapproval. She reminded my sister that the bible does not approve of her decisions and that she should not move in with him; they are not married, which my mother went on to imply they were not ready for. My sister's defense was that it was because my mother did not like him. My mother said "that's not true." The conversation ended with my mother unable to do anything more than disapprove and be disappointed since my sister was an adult. She moved in with him.

I went to boarding school but agreed to spend part of my break with my mother. It was only about a year after the discussion with my sister. Now, however, my mother was living with her boyfriend. There was almost immediate talk of marriage, but she was, nonetheless, living with him, unmarried. I remember my mother making a point of showing me her room in the house, which I was to be sleeping in. Furthermore, when I woke up around 10 a.m., my mother made a show about how she was just getting up from her make shit [sic] bed on the couch in the living room. I didn't buy it for a minute; that woman got up before 6 every day of my life and now she suddenly is sleeping past 10. On the couch. I was a virgin at the time and was planning to wait until marriage but nonetheless thought she was absolutely ridiculous. I thought that if she seriously was sleeping in a separate room that she was absurd and if she was putting on a show her efforts were wasted in the hilarity of the situation. Either way, I thought about the conversation with my sister and knew if nothing else she was hypocritical. I think she recognized that; it was nice to see her knocked off her high horse.

Could Marital Problems before a Divorce Affect Teen Sexuality after a Divorce?

Besides the real effects of divorce on adolescents, factors that may exist prior to the divorce can also have an influence on adolescents. Risky sexual activity may be a manifestation of problematic adolescent characteristics present before the divorce occurs, referred to as *predisruption problems*. Data from some longitudinal studies show that children with parents who would later divorce exhibited behavior problems during the time the parents were still married, long before the eventual divorce (Peris & Emery, 2004; Strohschein, 2012). At least two explanations are possible. The first is that these children were different from other children before the marital disruption, and they might have been on a pathway that would put them at risk for early sexual activity, having many sexual partners, and a premarital pregnancy even if the marriage had not dissolved. A second related explanation is that the gradual deterioration of the marital relationship negatively affects children long before the actual divorce. The escalation of adolescents' sexual development may be due to the gradual disintegration of the parent–child relationship that has its beginnings months or even years before the divorce.

Another predisruption problem related to risky sexual behavior during adolescence is conflict between parents during the marriage (Orgilés et al., 2015). Adolescents living in a two-parent family high in parental conflict are more likely to be involved in risky sexual behavior than adolescents living in a two-parent family low in family conflict (Fergusson et al., 2014). Conflict between parents may be especially difficult for teens to cope with because the adolescents rightly perceive it to be a threat to family stability and cohesion.

Are Custody Arrangements Related to Adolescent Sexuality?

One factor related to adolescent sexual behavior after a divorce is the postdivorce custody arrangements for the adolescents. Historically, mothers were awarded sole custody of children, an outcome still typical today, although approximately 30% of divorced parents in the United States share custody of their children, a percentage that has been increasing over the past several years (Cancian et al., 2014). Shared custody is thought to benefit children because it allows them regular contact with both parents, who continue to share the responsibilities for raising the children. In one study of Swedish adolescents, the age of sexual debut was lower in one-parent families than in shared-custody families and two-parent families, which were not different from each other (Carlsund, Eriksson, Löfstedt, & Sellström, 2012). The results support the idea that regular contact with both parents through a shared-custody arrangement can have a beneficial effect on adolescent sexual behavior as great as living in a two-parent family (Bergström et al., 2015).

Studying the effects of divorce on adolescent sexual risk-taking is not as simple as comparing adolescents from divorced families with adolescents from nondivorced families. Adolescents in families in which the parents will later divorce often exhibit predisruption troubles before the divorce that are more severe than the troubles adolescents in families not headed toward dissolution exhibit. In addition, poor-quality family relations are more common in families with spouses who will eventually divorce than in families with spouses who will not divorce. These predisruption problems can have an influence on the expression of postdivorce risky behavior by adolescents that can be as important as the divorce itself.

The best investigations of the relationship between divorce and adolescent problem behavior are prospective studies that assess adolescent problem behavior before and after a divorce in order to untangle the effects of predisruption adolescent characteristics from the actual impact of the divorce itself. Research indicates that the well-established relationship between divorce and adolescent problem behavior, including risky sexual behavior, is partly accounted for by predisruption characteristics of adolescents and by dysfunctional family dynamics that exist before the divorce occurs. Without

taking into account the behavior of adolescents and the family environment before the divorce it is possible to overestimate the impact of divorce on adolescent risky sexual behavior.

Researchers continue to search for those predisruption qualities within the adolescent and embedded in predivorce dysfunctional family dynamics that may contribute to postdivorce adolescent sexual risk-taking. For example, risky sexual behavior is more frequent among adolescents who are high in sensation-seeking and low in impulse control, characteristics that are more common among adolescents in families headed toward divorce than in youth in families that remain together. In addition, parental depression, marital dissatisfaction, and frequent and intense parent–adolescent conflict are more common in families in which the spouses will eventually divorce, and these dysfunctional family characteristics are related to adolescent risky sexual behavior, even in nondivorced families. Studies of the impact of divorce on adolescent problem behavior, including risky sexual activity, find that the effects of divorce on teens are lessened, but do not disappear, when adolescents do not have predisruption problems and when parents are able to maintain a healthy family environment before the divorce.

■ PARENTING AND ADOLESCENT SEXUALITY

A substantial minority of adolescents and parents believe that parents have an important influence on teens' decisions about sex. In one study of a nationally representative sample of U.S. adolescents and parents, 46% of adolescents and 41% of parents thought parents had more of an influence on teens' decisions about sex than friends, media, or any other group (Albert, 2012). Further analyses reveal the expected waning influence of parents as adolescents get older, with 57% of 12- to 14-year-old teens choosing their parents as the most influential group on their sexual lives, a figure that drops to 39% among teens ages 15–19 years.

Thinking something is true does not make it true, and researchers have gone beyond simply asking teens who they think has the most influence on their sexual decision making to examining the actual influence of parents on adolescent sexuality. Researchers have concentrated on four important aspects of parenting that might have an influence on the sexual behavior of adolescents: emotional support, control, monitoring, and parental attitudes about sex. *Emotional support* includes acceptance, warmth, connectedness, love, and closeness. It is often expressed through involvement, the amount of time parents and adolescents spend together, and the perceived quality of and satisfaction with the parent–adolescent relationship. *Control* refers to parents' attempts to direct and influence the behavior of their adolescents. Control encompasses the number of rules parents have for their adolescents, how strictly those rules are enforced, and the degree of autonomy adolescents have. *Monitoring* has been used synonymously with parental knowledge, which is traditionally defined as parental awareness of where their adolescents are, who they are with, and what they are doing when the parents are not present. *Parental attitudes about sex* refer to the parents' beliefs about how acceptable it is for their adolescent to be sexually active.

What Is the Relationship between Parent Emotional Support and Teen Sex?

The Impact of Emotional Support on Teen Sex

Higher levels of parental emotional support and warmth are associated with an increase in intentions to remain sexually abstinent (Cox, Shreffler, Merten, Gallus, & Dowdy, 2015) and a decrease in risky sexual behavior during adolescence (Markham et al., 2010). The relationship between high parental support and low risky sex during adolescence has been found not only among white, Asian American, and African American adolescents in the United States (Kao & Martyn, 2014; Kogan, Yu, Allen, Pocock, & Brody, 2015) but also among teens in other countries, such as the Netherlands (van de Bongardt, de Graaf, Reitz, & Deković, 2014) and Nairobi (Sidze, Elungata'a, Maina, & Mutua, 2015), showing the pervasive influence of parental emotional support on risky adolescent sexual activity.

Parental support sends a message to adolescents that they are loved and accepted, which makes it more likely that adolescents will internalize parental attitudes about sex that often emphasize the importance of waiting to have sex and engaging in safe sex if the adolescent does become sexually active (Longmore, Eng, Giordano, & Manning, 2009). Results from one study reveal that adolescents are less likely to become sexually active when they perceive their parents to have negative attitudes about teen sexual activity, but only when they feel emotionally connected to their parents (Kao & Martyn, 2014). As one 17-year-old girl stated:

"My parents do not want me to have sex right now . . . I thought that it was really good that my parents were attentive to who I was hanging out with or what I'm doing . . . this is different from some of my friends' parents." (Kao & Martyn, 2014, p. 11)

Another way in which a lack of emotional support is related to risky sexual behavior is through the formation of an insecure attachment bond to parents (Simons, Sutton, Simons, Gibbons, & Murry, 2016). An insecure attachment bond is characterized by weak emotional bonds to parents who are perceived to be unsupportive and emotionally unavailable. The authors of this study suggest that insecurely attached adolescents may engage in sex at an early age and have sex with many partners in a misguided attempt to compensate for a lack of emotional support at home.

Gender and Age Differences

The association between low parental support and adolescent risky sexual behavior varies by gender and age. Both boys and girls with a warm relationship with their parents are less likely to engage in risky sexual behavior than teens who have a cold relationship with their parents, but this effect is especially strong for girls (de Graaf, Vanwesenbeeck, Woertman, & Meeus, 2011; Kincaid, Jones, Sterrett, & McKee, 2012). Girls may be particularly sensitive to the type of relationship they have with their parents, especially their mothers, while boys are more affected by the amount of structure in their lives. In addition, the relationship between parental support and adolescent sexual behavior is stronger for younger than for older adolescents, reflecting the increasing orientation of adolescents toward their peers and away from their parents (Lammers, Ireland, Resnick, & Blum, 2000). Parental support still matters, even for 17- and 18-year-olds, but it matters less than it does for 12- and 13-year-olds.

What Is the Relationship between Parent Control and Teen Sex?

Research on the relationship between parental control and adolescent sexuality focuses on the dimension of strictness, which varies from lax to very firm. In some families, parents are lenient and give their adolescents a great deal of freedom, while in other families parents are very strict, limiting adolescent freedom and autonomy. Measures of parental strictness typically focus on adolescents' perceptions of how strict their parents are, or on the number of rules parents have for their adolescents.

The relationship between parental control and adolescent sexuality is not simple or straightforward, but some conclusions do emerge from this research. Very strict parents with many rules for their adolescents, including rules about dating and sexuality, tend to have adolescents with an elevated risk of engaging in sexual intercourse in comparison to adolescents with parents who are moderately strict (Coley, Medeiros, & Schindler, 2008; Mohammadyari, 2014). At the other end of the continuum, permissive parents also have adolescents who are more likely to engage in sexual intercourse than adolescents with parents who are moderately strict (Jemmott & Jemmott, 1992). Together these findings suggest that the relationship between parental control and adolescent sexuality is curvilinear; parents who are moderately controlling have adolescents with the lowest level of sexual activity (Miller, Benson, & Galbraith, 2001). Too much control or too much freedom are both detrimental to adolescent sexual development, and the critical task for parents is to find the appropriate level of control for their particular adolescent.

Besides being over- or undercontrolling, another way in which parental attempts to influence their adolescents may backfire is when parents use an insidious type of control called *psychological control,* which is the manipulative use of guilt by a parent to get an adolescent to comply with parental desires. For example, a parent might attempt to control the sexual activity of an adolescent by emphasizing the crushing sense of shame and failure adolescent sexual behavior might have on the parent. The use of psychological control often has the opposite effect from the effect the parent desires. The use of psychological control is associated with earlier adolescent sexual activity, not later (Oudekerk et al., 2014). One route by which psychological control might lead to an increase in risky sexual behavior is that the use of psychological control is associated with adolescent detachment from parents and attachment to peers, who are more likely to reinforce risky sexual behavior (Chan & Chan, 2011).

What Is the Relationship between Parent Monitoring and Teen Sex?

Definition of Monitoring

Imagine the following exchange between a mother and her 15-year-old son as he is about to go out the door of the house.

MOTHER: Where are you going?

SON: Out.

MOTHER: Who are you going out with?

SON: No one.

MOTHER: What are you going to do?

SON: Nothing.

This apocryphal conversation is an illustration of an ancient struggle between parents' need to know and adolescents' need for privacy. As difficult as these type of conversations can be for parents, they are the necessary first step of what is the foundation of good parenting during adolescence. As children move through adolescence, they spend more time away from the watchful eyes of parents, which makes it increasingly difficult for parents to keep track of their teens in order to head off and respond to adolescent risky behavior. Parents do not need to know where their adolescents are, who they are with, and what they are doing 24/7, but they do need to know that their adolescents are not some places, with some people, doing some things. How parents keep track of and acquire knowledge about their adolescents is called parental *monitoring,* which is defined as what parents know about their adolescents when the parents are not present, typically where the adolescents are, who they are with, and what they are doing.

The Impact of Monitoring on Adolescent Sexual Behavior

A higher level of monitoring is associated with lower adolescent sexual risk-taking (Guilamo-Ramos, Jaccard, & Dittus, 2010; Hadley, Houck, Barker, & Senocak, 2015). The relationship between high monitoring and low sexual risk-taking is robust and has been reported for adolescents of both genders and all races and ethnic groups in developed and developing countries (Karoly, Callahan, Schmiege, & Feldstein Ewing, 2016; Oliveira-Campos, Giatti, Malta, & Barreto, 2013; Roberts et al., 2012).

The effect of monitoring on adolescent sexuality is substantial. For example, in one large-scale study of a representative sample of U.S. adolescents, those teens with parents classified as low monitors on average began to have sex at age 14.7 years, in contrast to adolescents with parents classified as high monitors who initiated sex at 16.2 years, a difference of almost a year and a half (Huang, Murphy, & Hser, 2011).

Longitudinal research has shown that monitoring is not just correlated with low sexual risk behavior, but is predictive of it (Cabral et al., 2017; Ethier, Harper, Hoo, & Dittus, 2016). In one study, high monitoring during preadolescence was associated with a lower risk of sexual behavior during adolescence and a lower risk of problem behavior in general, including smoking cigarettes, drinking alcohol, using marijuana, and involvement in delinquency (Huang et al., 2011). The results show that early monitoring lays a foundation for later, more responsible sexual decision making and for avoiding a variety of risky behaviors (Longmore, Manning, & Giordano, 2001).

Effective Parent Monitoring

One way in which monitoring may reduce the probability of risky sex is that effective monitoring discourages teens from going to places where alcohol or drugs may be available, or where risky sex is a possibility. It is difficult to keep track of teens, especially those who can drive, but parents can continue to exert some control from a distance over their adolescents if they have a good relationship with the teens and if the parents are effective monitors.

Another explanation for the impact of parental monitoring on adolescent sexual behavior focuses on the involvement of adolescents with deviant peers who are sexual risk takers, drink alcohol, use drugs, and engage in antisocial activities. Having friends who engage in deviant activities is a risk factor for early sexual intercourse and multiple partners because adolescents generally choose their sexual partners from within their peer group (Capaldi, Stoolmiller, Clark, & Owen, 2002). Effective parental monitoring may deter adolescents from forming friendships with deviant peers, reducing the probability that they will engage in norm-breaking behavior, including early sex.

The following story shows how parental monitoring combined with supervision prevented what might have turned into a sexual encounter. Note how merely being scolded by her mother was enough to make this daughter feel guilty about what she did.

IN THEIR OWN WORDS

J. and I had been dating for about 3 months and we hung out at my house a lot. Since it was the beginning of our relationship, my parents felt more comfortable with us spending more time at our house rather than his. My dad used to work until 11 at night so it would be just my mom, J., and I at my house on Friday or Saturday nights. J. and I were getting more comfortable with each other so when we watched movies we could go to my room. This never bothered my mom because she knew that I was responsible and would not do anything inappropriate.

One of the Friday nights, J. and I were watching a movie in my room. We usually used to sit up and lean against my wall while we were on the bed, that way it would not be like we were laying in bed together, rather just sitting. Well, this night was different, we just decided to lay in my bed completely and get under the covers. I did not think much of it, I just felt that it was more comfortable.

During the movie, J. and I started kissing. It wasn't much, but as the seconds went on things heated up. I knew my mom was in her room and I would hear her door open if she came out so I didn't feel worried. Well, turns out that when you are more worried about hooking up with your boyfriend, you are not paying attention to whether your mom opens her door or not. All of a sudden I heard my mom at my door saying my name. I pushed J. away from me and I felt like I was going to die of embarrassment.

My mom called me into the kitchen. I thought about bringing J. with me so she couldn't yell at me but then I decided that would just make things worse than they already were. I walked into the kitchen and I felt her eyes glued to me. I acted as innocent as I could and asked her what was up. She asked me what I was thinking, how I could be so irresponsible. She told me that she wasn't going to allow us to behave that way under her roof. She said it was disrespectful to her, especially since she trusted us to behave. She said I should be embarrassed with myself and she never wanted to see that again. She also said J. and I weren't allowed to be in my room anymore and that we would have to start hanging out in the living room, aka in clear sight. While she was lecturing me, her face was red and her voice was stern. I didn't get grounded and J. didn't get yelled at, but her words were frightening enough. My mom is the type of person you don't want to push to her limits, so her warning was enough for me not to do it again.

Looking back at it, I just laugh. I got in trouble for such a little thing. . . . My mom, although she works a lot and I'm constantly home alone, raised me to be proper. She kept an eye on me even when she wasn't home. She also knows that her strongest weapon against me is yelling at me because I can't tolerate her being mad at me.

What Is the Relationship between Parent Attitudes about Sex and Teen Sex?

One final component of parenting related to low risky adolescent sexual behavior, especially early sexual debut, is parental disapproval of adolescent sexual activity. In particular, when parents communicate their disapprobation of adolescent sexual behavior to their teens and when adolescents perceive their parents to be disapproving, teens are less likely to be sexually active and more likely to wait until they are older before they become sexually active than teens with parents who approve of adolescent sexual activity (Zimmer-Gembeck & Helfand, 2008). The association between parental disapproval of teen sexual behavior and adolescent sexual activity is especially strong when adolescents have close relations with their parents.

Contrary to popular belief, children do not cast off parental bonds when they become teens and slavishly mimic the attitudes and behavior of their friends. Parental attitudes matter, especially for younger adolescents and for daughters who have good relations with their parents (McNeely et al., 2002). Young adolescents who believe that their parents would be proud of them if they remained sexually abstinent have more negative views about teen sexual activity and do not plan to have sex in comparison to adolescents who think their parents approve of adolescent sexual behavior (Sneed, Tan, & Meyer, 2015). Parents' attitudes about sexuality are a better predictor of the age of sexual debut for younger adolescents than the attitudes or behavior of friends (Maguen & Armistead, 2006). Among older teens, however, perceived peer attitudes about sex and the sexual behavior of friends are more strongly related to adolescent attitudes about sex and to their sexual behavior than perceived parent attitudes.

What parents say to their adolescents about sex makes a difference, especially when parents and adolescents have a close relationship. In one study of Latino mothers and adolescents, mothers who spoke to their adolescents about their hopes that the teens would abstain from sexual activity had adolescents

---

Sometimes parents do not even need to explicitly express their disapproval of sex before marriage for an adolescent to get the message that the parent thinks sex is wrong, as illustrated by the comments from the following daughter.

IN THEIR OWN WORDS

Growing up, my sexuality was affected most by my parents. They were the ones, who from the start, shaped my opinions, morals, and beliefs about sexuality.

The way I see it, the idea of sex before marriage was just a nonexistent thought for the majority of my younger adolescent years.

It seems to be one of those household rules that doesn't need to be discussed too much but that everyone knows. I have an older sister who also had an influence on me. I never wanted to disappoint her and knew that when it came to serious stuff like that, she would be very disappointed.

who waited longer to have sex than adolescents with mothers who did not discuss their personal values with their teens, and this effect was especially true when the mother–adolescent relationship was warm and close (Romo, Lefkowitz, Sigman, & Au, 2002). Many of the mothers who talked about the importance of remaining sexually abstinent tempered their abstinence message with the additional point that it is imperative to practice safe sex if the adolescent does become sexually active. These multifaceted messages about the importance of abstinence and the need for caution if the adolescent does have sex, reveal the sensitivity and realism of these mothers as they attempt to help their adolescents cope with the complexities of sexual activity.

SUMMARY

■ FAMILY STRUCTURE

Adolescents in two-parent families engage in less risky sexual behavior than teens in single-parent families. The main reason for this lower sexual risk is that adolescents in two-parent families begin to have sex at a later age and, therefore, act more responsibly than adolescents in single-parent families. Adolescents in single-parent families have fewer economic resources than adolescents in two-parent families, which contributes to their involvement with deviant peers and risky sexuality. One reason why adolescents in single-parent families are more likely to engage in risky sexual behavior than teens in two-parent families is that single-parent mothers often date and become sexually active themselves, modeling sexual behavior to their adolescents.

■ FATHERS

Nonresident fatherhood is associated with risky adolescent sexuality. The presence of a father in the family is associated with a delay in the age when adolescents become sexually active. One way fathers can negatively influence their adolescents is that adolescents may inherit dysfunctional personality traits from their fathers. Nonresident fatherhood has an especially powerful effect on girls, influencing their reproductive strategies. Several aspects of the father–adolescent relationship are strongly related to adolescent sexuality, and those include the quality of the relationship adolescents have with their fathers, along with paternal discipline, monitoring, and communication.

■ PARENTAL SEPARATION AND DIVORCE

Parental separation and divorce are related to adolescent risky sexuality. Three reasons for the effects of separation and divorce on teen sexuality include changes in the family situation, an increase in family transitions, and a decrease in a parent's ability to effectively monitor and control his or her adolescents during and after a divorce. One needs to be cautious about attributing adolescent risky sexual behavior to parental divorce, because predivorce disruption problems also contribute to risky sexual behavior. Joint custody lowers the risk of adolescent sexual activity over single-parent custody.

■ PARENTING AND ADOLESCENT SEXUALITY

Parents can influence the sexual behavior of their adolescents in several ways. First, parental emotional support matters, and its relationship to adolescent sexual behavior is linear—more support is associated with less adolescent sexual activity. Support is especially important for girls and younger adolescents. Second, the impact of control on sexual activity is complicated, and depends on the amount of control and on the type of control. Too much control or the use of psychological control is associated with high sexual activity, whereas a moderate degree of noncoercive control is related to less sexuality. Third, parental monitoring is related to less teen sexual behavior, especially to a delay in the age of first sexual intercourse. Effective monitoring discourages adolescents from becoming involved with peers who engage in risky behavior. Fourth, parents who disapprove of adolescent sexual activity have adolescents who are less likely to engage in sexual activity, especially when the parent–adolescent relationship is close. The importance of parental attitudes declines as adolescents get older, however.

SUGGESTIONS FOR FURTHER READING

Ellis, B. J., Bates, J. E., Dodge, K. A., Fergusson, D. M., Horwood, L. J., Pettit, G. S., et al. (2003). Does father absence place daughters at special risk for early sexual activity and teenage pregnancy? *Child Development, 74*, 801–821.

Guilamo-Ramos, V., Jaccard, J., & Dittus, P. (Eds.). (2010). *Parental monitoring of adolescents: Current perspectives for researchers and practitioners.* New York: Columbia University Press.

Kincaid, C., Jones, D. J., Sterrett, E., & McKee, L. (2012). A review of parenting and adolescent sexual behavior: The moderating role of gender. *Clinical Psychology Review, 32*, 177–188.

Sturgeon, S. W. (2008, November). *The relationship between family structure and adolescent sexual activity.* Washington, DC: The Heritage Foundation. Retrieved July 10, 2016, from *www.familyfacts.org.*

Zimmer-Gembeck, M. J., & Helfand, M. (2008). Ten years of longitudinal research on U.S. adolescent sexual behavior: Developmental correlates of sexual intercourse, and the importance of age, gender, and ethnic background. *Developmental Review, 28*, 153–224.

CHAPTER 4

Parent–Adolescent Communication about Sex

Not all parents agree on how children should be raised. For example, parents disagree about whether corporal punishment is an appropriate way to discipline children, on when adolescents should be allowed to date, and on how much autonomy adolescents should have. But there is one idea nearly all parents believe in, an idea that cuts across every demographic group, and it is this: Parents have a special obligation to talk to their children about sex (Wilson, Dalberth, Koo, & Gard, 2010). School-based sex education classes, health books, doctors, and the Internet may have much to offer children as they navigate through the murky waters of sexual development but, in the end, parents believe that they are primarily responsible for teaching their children about the facts of life and for instilling in them the values that will help their children make good decisions about their sexual behavior (Lagus, Bernat, Bearinger, Resnick, & Eisenberg, 2011).

■ PARENTS AND ADOLESCENTS TALKING ABOUT SEX

There are many reasons why parents are expected to play a pivotal role educating their children about sexuality. First, parents are primarily responsible for preparing their children for adulthood, and sex is an important component of responsible adult behavior. Second, sexuality is a highly charged moral issue and parents view themselves and are viewed by others as largely responsible for instilling appropriate standards of moral conduct in their children. Third, parents and others think that the information parents provide their teens about sex will facilitate responsible sexual decision making (Feldman & Rosenthal, 2000).

Consider the following story by a college student about the lesson her mother taught her about boys when she was an adolescent. The mother makes a general point about relations with boys, and her comments go beyond a narrow sex talk.

IN THEIR OWN WORDS

My mother sat down with me and decided to focus on the emotional side of sex instead of the physical act itself. She told me that the majority of boys will tell me all the things that I want to hear in order to get inside of my pants and not because he truly cared about me. She told me that most females put all their emotions in when they have sex with their significant other and become more emotionally attached to this individual. You have this eternal bond with this individual regardless if you stay with this person or not, you will always remember that experience with that person. I will always remember her saying that I should keep my virginity for that one special person (my husband) who will truly cherish me, my body, and all the emotions that are included in the act.

Do Parents and Teens Talk about Sex?

What parents believe they should do and what they actually do are two different issues. Results from studies of parent–teen communication about sex reveal that a sizable minority of parents do not fulfill their role as primary sex educators for their children (Lindberg, Maddow-Zimet, & Boonstra, 2016). For example, in 2011–2013 only 31% of males and 52% of females report that they have talked to their parents about birth control. Further, 49% of males and 58% of females indicate that they have discussed STIs with their parents. Between 30 and 40% of teens report that they have not talked to their parents about any aspect of sexuality. Little has changed since 2002, and the evidence indicates that the quantity and quality of parent–teen communication about sex has not improved over the past several years.

The percentage of U.S. parents who have talked to their children about sex is similar to the percentage of British parents who have discussed sex with their children (NHS Bristol, 2009), percentages that are considerably higher than the percentage of parents who have talked about sex with their children in more conservative countries, such as South Africa (Coetzee et al., 2014) and Singapore (Hu et al., 2012). In a conservative country such as Iran, only a small minority of parents have discussed sex with their children, mainly because the parents feel "incompetent" about sexual matters and also believe that their children are "sexually innocent" (Merghati-Khoei, Abolghasemi, & Smith, 2014). Although many American parents may not act on their beliefs that they should talk to their teens about sex, U.S. parents are as likely to talk about sex as European parents and more likely than parents in more traditional countries.

Parents and children often have different perceptions about whether communication about sex has occurred (Atienzo, Ortiz-Panozo, & Campero, 2015; Diiorio, Pluhar, & Belcher, 2003). For example, in one study of mothers and their teenage children, 73% of mothers strongly agreed with the statement, "I have talked with my teen about sex," but only 46% of teens strongly agreed with the equivalent statement, "My mother has talked to me about sex" (Jaccard, Dittus, & Gordon, 1998). One implication of this difference is that many parents may think they have discussed sex with their teens, although the teens either do not remember the conversation, or do not consider the discussion to be about sex.

Consider the following fictional conversation played for laughs between a father and his teenage son from the 1999 movie *American Pie,* a comedy about four high school boys determined to lose their virginity by prom night. Is this a sex talk? Would the father think it was? The son? What, if any, effect do you think this talk would have on the sexual behavior of the son?

> FATHER: I was just walking by your room and I was thinking it's been a long time since we had a little father–son chat. Oh, I brought some magazines. [Shows son the magazine *Perfect 10.*] If you want to, just flip to the center section. Well, this is the female form and they have focused on the breasts, which are used primarily to feed young infants, and also in foreplay.
>
> SON: Right.
>
> FATHER: This is *Hustler* [gives *Hustler* to son] and this is a much more exotic magazine. Now they have decided to focus more on the pubic region, the whole groin area.
>
> SON: Uh-huh.
>
> FATHER: Look at the expression on her face. You see that, you see what she's doing? She's looking right into your eyes saying, "Hey big boy, how are you doing?" You see?
>
> SON: Right.
>
> FATHER: *Shaved* is a magazine I'm not too familiar with, but again, if you flip to the center section, well, you see the detail that they go into in this picture here. It almost looks like a tropical plant of some kind, an underwater thing. Do you know what a clitoris is?
>
> SON: Oh my God! Dad, I know what a clitoris is.
>
> FATHER: Oh you do. Oh I forgot you've been there and back.
>
> SON: I learned about it in sex ed. I really don't need you to sit here and talk to me about a clitoris.
>
> FATHER: I'm sorry.
>
> SON: No, I'm sorry.
>
> FATHER: Jim, I'd like to just leave these magazines here for you to peruse at your pleasure. OK, that was good. See you at dinner.

There are several possible explanations for a difference in parent and adolescent reports about whether a sex talk has occurred. Parents may overreport these conversations because they want to appear to be competent, caring parents. Parents may consider some topics to be sexual, such as puberty, kissing, and relationships, while teens may not count conversations about these topics as sex talks. Older adolescents may forget about talks that occurred when they were children. Last, the talk may be subtle or ambiguous, and the adolescent may not perceive it as a sex talk, whereas a parent may feel that he or she made an important point about sex.

Do Parents Talk to Preteens and Emerging Adults about Sex?

Many preteens are interested in sexuality and a growing number have engaged in precoital activities, such as kissing, sexual touching, and oral sex (Centers for Disease Control and Prevention, 2009), so discussions about sex are appropriate before adolescence. In one study of African American mothers, a majority of mothers of 6- to 10-year-old children report that they have talked to their children about HIV/AIDS, pubertal development, reproduction, names for sexual body parts, gender roles, sexual orientation, and sexual abuse (Pluhar, Jennings, & Diiorio, 2006). In another study of mothers of 11-year-old children, most mothers report that they have talked to their children about HIV/AIDS and to their daughters about the human papillomavirus vaccine (McRee, Reiter, Gottlieb, & Brewer, 2011; Sly et al., 1995).

Parents become less important sources of sex information during emerging adulthood. In one study of who college students turn to when they have questions about sex, mothers are ranked seventh by young men and sixth by young women, while fathers are ranked eighth by young men and eleventh by young women (Sprecher, Harris, & Meyers, 2008). These emerging adults do not perceive their parents to be especially important sources of information about sex relative to knowledge they receive from friends, dating partners, and the media, all of which rank considerably higher than parents.

When Do Parents Talk to Their Teens about Sex?

What leads to the first parent–child talk about sex? Parent–child communication about sex is not highly related to the onset of puberty for boys (Koo et al., 2012), which is somewhat surprising given that puberty marks the beginning of development of adult sexuality, presumably a time when adolescents are interested in sex and most in need of basic information about sexuality. Talk about sex is more likely to occur when boys begin to date or engage in risky behaviors such as drinking alcohol and experimenting with drugs. One response to dating and to the risky behavior of sons is for parents to initiate a conversation about sex, perhaps in an attempt to prevent early sex and an unplanned pregnancy.

In one study of African American and Latino mothers of adolescent daughters, conversations about sex were related to puberty. Talk about sex generally occurred for one of three reasons (O'Sullivan, Meyer-Bahlburg, & Watkins,

2001). First, the girls began menstruating, which was a signal to the mother that the daughter was ready for a talk about sex and needed to have that conversation. Second, daughters showed an interest in boys by wearing makeup or sexy clothing or by spending more time with boys in person or on the phone. Third, daughters began to show an interest in sex.

■ PARENTAL MESSAGES ABOUT SEX

Why Don't More Parents Talk to Their Teens about Sex?

When asked why they do not talk to their teens about sex, parents mention several barriers to conversation (Malacane & Beckmeyer, 2016). First, many parents are unsure that they have enough knowledge about certain topics to have a good conversation about those issues (Jerman & Constantine, 2010; Swain, Ackerman, & Acherman, 2006). Second, some parents report that they cannot find the right time to talk to their teens about sex (Rosenthal, Feldman, & Edwards, 1998). Third, some parents report that they think their children, especially their preadolescent children, are too young and not ready to talk about sex (Wilson et al., 2010). Fourth, many parents report that they feel uneasy and embarrassed talking about sex with their children (Byers & Sears, 2012). A fifth barrier to talking about sex is that many parents do not think their adolescents are sexually active and not at risk of contracting an STI or becoming pregnant (Elliott, 2012).

A sixth reason some parents are reluctant to discuss sex with their children is that they are afraid the conversation will lead to sexual activity. One study of parents and adolescents living in Mexico revealed that many parents believe that discussing contraceptive methods with their teens encourages the teens to become sexually active (Rouvier, Campero, Walker, & Caballero, 2011). As one mother remarked, "I believe that once one talks to them and teaches them, 'look son, use a condom just in case,' . . . in spite of myself, yes, I think one is giving them permission" (Rouvier et al., 2011, p. 182).

One of the most important predictors of whether a mother talks to her adolescent about sex is the mother's intention to have a conversation with her teen about sex. A mother who intends to talk to her adolescent about sex is more likely to have that conversation than a mother who does not have that intention. Further, a mother who intends to talk to her teen about sex is a mother who believes it is important to have this type of conversation with her adolescent and thinks she has the skills to effectively talk about sexuality (Byers, Sears, & Hughes, 2017).

Why Don't Teens Talk to Their Parents about Sex?

It is not just the parents who shy away from talks with their adolescents about sex, but many teens are reluctant to ask their parents questions about sex (Wang, 2016). Teens say they would be embarrassed, their parent might ask too many personal questions, and talking about sex could make the parent suspicious of the teen's sexual behavior. Many confidently add that they do not need to talk to their parents about sex because they already know all they need to know (Jaccard, Dittus, & Gordon, 2000).

One reason teens do not talk to their parents about sex is because teens believe their parents will give them a lecture instead of talking to them. Researchers in one observational study examined the type of conversations parents had with their teens about sex and showed that many parents do lecture their adolescents about sex rather than converse with them. Parents who lecture have adolescents who are more likely to rate their conversations with their parents as poor. Further, parents who lecture have adolescents who are more likely to engage in sexual intercourse than adolescents with parents who do not lecture (Rogers, Ha, Stormshak, & Dishion, 2015). One explanation for this finding is that teens are less likely to internalize messages about sexual behavior that are delivered in an authoritarian style. Another interpretation is that parents are more likely to lecture adolescents who are already sexually active. In the Rogers et al. study, it is not possible to determine whether lecturing leads to sexual activity or if sexual activity leads to lecturing, but the findings do show that parent lecturing is not an effective form of parent–teen communication about sex.

In addition, some adolescents are reluctant to talk to their parents about sex because they see their parents as judgmental and closed-minded (Pistella & Bonati, 1999). As one girl put it: "I feel if parents could be more open-minded and try to be friends to their child, sometimes things such as birth control and sex topics would go over easier" (Pistella & Bonati, 1999, p. 312).

An additional reason some teens do not talk to their parents about sex is that the teens perceive their relationship with their parents to be somewhat cold and distant. When parents and teens have a close, trusting relationship, in

---

Many preteens find it difficult and uncomfortable to talk to a parent about sex, as the following story told by a young woman illustrates.

IN THEIR OWN WORDS

When I was 10 years old my mother said that dreaded phrase: "We need to talk." Earlier in the week I had refused to go to the fifth-grade class after-school talk about "down there." After trying to convince me to go, my mom called the teacher and said she would read me a book instead. She had an *American Girl* book in her hands that was about puberty and the like. We sat down and began to go through the book. It talked about the changes in your body, periods, hair growth, etc. I remember feeling very uncomfortable and blushing a lot. Then we got to the chapter entitled "Sex" and I practically had a heart attack. I jumped up and said, "That is enough for tonight." My mom continued to say that we could read that chapter another time but if I ever had any questions or concerns she was always there to talk.

The following story by a young woman about a "cool mom" is an example of an open, honest, comfortable talk about sex.

IN THEIR OWN WORDS

One of my friends had "the cool mom." One day after school I was at my friend's house and we were in her basement talking about some girl who KISSED A BOY! Apparently, her mom overheard us giggling about it and listened in. Then she decided it was time for an intervention. But she didn't do it the usual mom way; she was very stealthy about it. We came upstairs because she was making cookies and we wanted to help and she asked us what we were talking about. We told her that a girl at school kissed a boy with her tongue and we were grossed out. She laughed and said, "You didn't know people do that?" but she said it in a way that made us curious to what else we didn't know. We said no and she said, "well, tell me what you DO know." So instead of lecturing us about sex it was more of a story and tell. It was just three girls chatting about sex and things that we thought were true that really weren't. (Who knew you couldn't get pregnant by looking at it?!) She filled in the blanks and corrected our errors when we thought something was true that wasn't.

which teens can talk openly and honestly to their parents about personal issues, then talks about sex are more common and more comfortable for both parents and adolescents (Kotva & Schneider, 1990).

Although many adolescents do not talk to their parents about sex, some talk to extended family members, including siblings and cousins, and these conversations are especially likely to occur among teens who are sexually active (Grossman, Tracy, Richer, & Erkut, 2015). Many sexually active adolescents report that they are more comfortable talking to members of their extended families than to their parents, who they fear will respond negatively to their sexual activity.

What Do Parents Tell Their Adolescents about Sex?

In general, when parents talk to their adolescents about sex, they tend to focus on three issues: reproduction, abstinence, and safe sex (Grossman, Charmaraman, & Erkut, 2016).

In addition, the values and attitudes parents have about sex come across loud and clear in most conversations parents have with their adolescents about sex. One qualitative study examined what messages about sex college students remember getting from their parents when they were adolescents (Kauffman, Orbe, Johnson, & Cooke-Jackson, 2013). According to these emerging adults, sex was generally portrayed as a dangerous activity with potentially negative consequences, so it was important for the adolescent to either abstain or practice safe sex. Parents also cautioned their adolescents about engaging in casual sex and emphasized the importance of waiting until the right person came along.

The following story by a young female college student illustrates what some mothers say to their daughters about sex and also shows how conversations about sex can change as daughters get older.

IN THEIR OWN WORDS

When I was a lot younger, probably around middle school age, my mom's message about sex was clear: don't have sex before you're married. Her reason? Because it's a sin, and you'll go to hell. I found that very odd coming from her, considering I had never seen her step foot inside a church and that both my younger brother and I were born out of wedlock. I was smart enough to understand that this was just her scare tactic. Because of how forbidding she was about sex (even though I was just a child), I found it to be a lot harder and much more uncomfortable to ask questions. As I got older and into my high school years, her message seemed to change; it wasn't so much about forbidding any sexual act until I was married. It was more about waiting for the right person, until I'm in love, and until I'm completely ready (though she still stressed the fact that waiting until after marriage would be ideal). It was at this point that I felt a lot more comfortable talking to her about things like friends, dating, and even sex, though rarely still. Now that I look back, I see that she wasn't trying to scare me away from sex just for no reason; she didn't want me to make the same mistakes that she did.

In another study of African American and Latino mothers and daughters living in New York City, mothers reported that they spoke about three issues with their daughters (O'Sullivan et al., 2001). First, mothers emphasized the dire consequences associated with sex, especially pain, shame, and humiliation. They spoke about the possibility of getting pregnant, and the subsequent abandonment by the young man, and they talked about the expense and loss of educational opportunities associated with a pregnancy. Second, mothers stressed the importance of controlling interactions with boys in order to avoid sex altogether. The mothers described boys as sexual opportunists who would say anything to have sex with any willing girl, so girls always needed to be on guard. One Latino girl explained, "My mom said that I should never let a boy touch me. If a boy touches me, I should defend myself, kick him with anything I can" (O'Sullivan et al., 2001, p. 283). Third, mothers wanted reassurance from their daughters that they would avoid sexual relations at least until they finished high school, even though some of the girls were already sexually active.

Are There Gender Differences in What Parents Say to Their Sons and Daughters about Sex?

There are strong gender differences in how often parents talk to their sons and daughters about sex, and in what is said. Parents, especially mothers, are more likely to talk to their daughters about sex than to their sons, and they talk more frequently to their daughters (Kapungu et al., 2010; Widman, Choukas-Bradley, Helms, Golin, & Prinstein, 2014), which suggests that parents are more concerned about the sexual behavior of their daughters than their sons.

One large-scale study of Australian 16-year-olds examined the percentage of teens who had discussed 20 topics with their parents (Rosenthal & Feldman, 1999). Neither mothers nor fathers spoke about many of the topics with their sons, and when a parent did talk to a son, it was most likely the mother talking about physical development and dating. The situation was decidedly different for daughters, with mothers discussing many issues having to do with physical development, but also talking about pregnancy, abortion, and safe sex. Few fathers spoke about any of the 20 topics with their daughters.

Parent–adolescent discussions about sex, especially between parents and daughters, often focus on abstinence and on the importance of using effective methods of birth control for girls who are sexually active (Donaldson, Lindberg, Ellen, & Marcell, 2013). Two other themes common in conversations between parents and daughters about sex are learning how to avoid sexual situations, and developing the social skills to exert some control over male sexuality (Diiorio et al., 2003). Parents often present male and female gender roles as adversarial, with males pushing for sex, and the need for females to resist male sexual desires, descriptions based on reality, but furthering a double standard at the same time.

Other research on Latino emerging adults reiterates the negative messages parents send to their adolescents, especially their daughters, about premarital sex. Latino young women report receiving two strong messages from their parents about sex: daughters should wait until they are married before they have sex, and sex is appropriate only when the two people are in love. Many young men also heard these messages about waiting and love, but more young men than young women were given the message that sex was for pleasure, reflecting a parental double standard (Manago, Ward, & Aldana, 2015).

The following story by a young Latino woman illustrates the messages she received about sex from her mother, and how she responded to those messages.

IN THEIR OWN WORDS

When I was about 15, my mom started talking to me about the consequences of sex and her beliefs about it. It was not one big talk, but just a lot of little talks at least once a week. She explained that boys just want to have sex and that no matter what protection I used I would probably get pregnant. These warnings were stronger when my boyfriend and I started to get more serious. Our Latino culture probably played a role in the values she held when it came to sex. She stated that she was not against premarital sex, but she wanted me to wait until I was 19 to have sex. When I turned 19, she wanted me to wait until I was 21. I, of course, never told her that I started having sex when I was 16.

Who Do Teens Most Often Talk to about Sex, Their Mothers or Their Fathers?

Youth of both genders and all ages are more likely to talk to their mothers about sex than to their fathers (Martino, Elliott, Corona, Kanouse, & Schuster, 2008; Sprecher et al., 2008). Mothers most often talk to their daughters about sex, followed by their sons. Fathers rarely talk about sex to their children, but when they do they most likely talk to their sons and seldom talk to their daughters. (I recall a funny story told to me by a college student that illustrates the point that boys will talk to their mothers rather than their fathers even about the most intimate aspects of their lives. According to the student, the first time he needed a jockstrap was in his freshman year of high school in order to try out for the baseball team. He didn't have one, so whom did he go to see about buying him this most personal undergarment? Not his father, but his mother, who asked him what size she should buy, and the boy, not knowing anything about jockstrap sizes or his own relative size, answered boastfully, "Large!")

Several explanations have been offered for why fathers are less likely to be sources of sex information for their children than mothers (Turnbull, van Wersch, & van Schaik, 2008). First, fathers are more disengaged from family activities than mothers, making fathers less available to their children (Goldman & Bradley, 2001). Second, most fathers did not receive much sex education from their own fathers, and this lack of modeling and personal experience lands fathers in uncharted territory when it comes to sexually socializing their own children. Some evidence for this lack of experience is the finding that fathers who are most likely to talk to their children about sex are fathers who talked to their own fathers about sex when they were young (Lehr, Demi, Diiorio, & Facteau, 2005). Third, men have a general problem with the expression of intimacy that extends beyond talking about sex with their children, and includes discussion of personal matters and feelings in general (Marsiglio & Roy, 2013). Fourth, many fathers believe that the sex education of children is the responsibility of their wives, who they think are better equipped to handle this highly personal issue (Kirkman, Rosenthal, & Feldman, 2002).

Many fathers feel uncomfortable talking to their children about sex and expect their wives to have these conversations. As one father of three said:

> "My wife, she does a lot of talking . . . about life, sexuality. All sorts of things, all the time. Whereas I'm exactly the opposite. Not that I find—do I find it difficult? I don't know. I've never had to talk to my children . . . about these issues, because . . . my wife's already done it . . . I feel almost guilty for not partaking. The other thing, of course, is I don't know how—it's not an excuse, it's a fact. I don't know how comfortable they would be, me trying to talk to them about these topics. . . . So I guess it's a bit of a coward's way out, to save embarrassment by both parties, that I'll just leave it to my wife." (Kirkman et al., 2002, p. 60)

Father–son talks about sex can be uncomfortable, even for fathers who have a close relationship with their sons, as the following story told to me by a single father illustrates. According to the father, his 16-year-old son approached him one evening and said, "Dad I don't think I'll ever be able to have intercourse." The father asked why and the son told him it was because he had a bent penis. The father reassured his son that it was common for men to have a slightly curved penis and his son should not worry about it, but the son insisted that his penis was *really* bent, which if true, is called Peyronie's disease, a condition that can lead to painful erections and difficulty having intercourse. Now this modern father was having a very mixed reaction about this conversation—on the one hand pleased that he and his son were able to talk about this very personal issue, but on the other hand he told me that all he could think about was "Please let this conversation stop, please let this conversation stop, please let this conversation stop. . . ." He told me, "Ray, I was terrified that J. was going to whip out his penis and show it to me." The father made an appointment for his son to be examined by a doctor who reassured the boy that he and his penis were fine, bringing an embarrassing incident to a satisfying conclusion.

Are Mother–Adolescent Talks about Sex Different from Father–Adolescent Talks?

When fathers do talk to their children about sex, especially their sons, they tend to focus on practical matters such as obtaining and using condoms, while mothers are more likely to talk about relationship issues (Feldman & Rosenthal, 2000).

The following is an example of one father's last desperate attempt to instruct his son in the importance of using a condom when he has sex before the son heads off into the unsupervised world of college. Do you think a father would talk to his daughter in this way?

IN THEIR OWN WORDS

The day I was moving out and going to college was the day my dad decided to have a sex talk with me. While we were moving all of my things into the truck to take to school he stopped and told me to walk over to the truck and to open the door. After I opened the door, my dad opened the center console and threw a pack of condoms at me and said, "Do you know what those are?"

"Yeah, I know what they are." He then said, "When you have sex for the first time make sure you 'strap up' because you don't want any babies yet, that's how your sister got here." I laughed and told him that he was about 3 years late and that I have been "strapping up." He looked at me with a grin and said, "Well, then I want that entire box (24 pack) gone by Thanksgiving break!" I was like "I'm on it!!" while laughing even harder. We then got into the truck and went off to college and listened to the radio the whole way down.

The following story by a gay college student illustrates the difficulty adolescents with an uncertain sexual identity can have talking to their fathers about sex.

IN THEIR OWN WORDS

There were a few times in my life where one of my brothers or I would be out in our dad's workshop and he would ask if we had a girlfriend. I never dated in high school. . . . This question would often be answered by my middle brother, as he always had a girl with other girls waiting on the side to date him. My dad would in turn ask about how pretty she was . . . and tell my brother that he needed to use protection if he's going to fool around, but that he should not be messing around until marriage.

He did this to me once when I responded to the question, "I don't need to worry about that, as I have no interest in dating or girls at this time." My dad responded with, "One day you'll see her and go 'whoa' and do something stupid, because girls make you stupid." I disagreed and he shirked it off. Now that I'm on my own, I feel that this lack of direct communication from my parents, specifically my dad, has made communication harder for both of us. Though I was right in saying that I had no interest in girls, as once I came to college I discovered that I'm gay. Now, not only do I not pay attention to the lesson my father was trying to teach about messing around with girls, I'm having trouble telling him about my true identity as he's not one to try to understand, as he thinks that we need to listen to him because he is the father figure and that should be enough.

Another difference between fathers and mothers is that fathers are more concerned about the sexual orientation of their children, especially their sons, and implicitly and explicitly try to foster and encourage a heterosexual orientation (Kane, 2006; Solebello & Elliott, 2011). When asked whether he had ever talked with his two sons about sexual orientation, one father exclaimed, "Oh yeah. Definitely. Yeah, we want them to be as heterosexual as possible" (Solebello & Elliott, 2011, p. 301).

Conversations with mothers about sex are almost always evaluated more positively than talks with fathers, not only by the teens but also by the parents, with mothers rating themselves more positively than fathers rate themselves. Dads seem to know that they are not very good at talking about sex and they are willing to admit it. In comparison to their dads, teens describe their moms as more open, understanding, accepting, easier to talk to, less judgmental, and less likely to attempt to impose their own values about sex on them (Noller & Callan, 1991).

■ PARENT–ADOLESCENT TALKS ABOUT SEX AND ADOLESCENT SEXUALITY

The need for parents to talk to their teens about sex is an idea universally endorsed by parents, teachers, therapists, doctors, and anyone concerned about the sexual development of children and adolescents. It is an idea that is heralded by every child development expert and proclaimed as gospel in every self-help article, advice book, and website with recommendations to parents about how they should deal with the sexual development of their children. Talking about sex is viewed as a strategy parents can employ to delay the onset of sexual activity by their teenage children and to prevent the spread of sexually transmitted diseases and the occurrence of an unintended pregnancy. For example, a report released by the U.S. Department of Health and Human Services entitled *Healthy People 2010* illustrates the currently accepted wisdom: "[Parents] can encourage adolescent sexual health by providing accurate information and education about sexuality," and concludes, "Discussions between parents and their children about sexuality . . . are crucial" (U.S. Department of Health and Human Services, 2010, pp. 9, 28).

Are these discussions really crucial? Must parents and teens talk about sex? They should, if these talks affect teens' behavior in a positive way by reducing the incidence of STIs and unintended pregnancies, and lowering the frequency of risky sexual behavior. But what if talk about sex does none of the above, or even worse, what if it in some ways encourages risky sexual behavior? If all this talk is unrelated to responsible adolescent sexual behavior or is counterproductive, then perhaps we need to alter or fine-tune our messages to parents about parent–teen communication about sex.

A FOCUS ON RESEARCH

Typically, researchers interested in the relationship between parent–teen talks about sex and adolescent sexual behavior simply compare the sexual behavior of adolescents who indicate that they have talked to their parents about sex with those who have not talked to their parents about sex. This approach is plagued by a variety of shortcomings that are difficult, if not impossible, to remedy. First, researchers have no control over when the talk occurs, which can be before or after the adolescent becomes sexually active. Second, there is no consistency in the age of the child when the talk occurred. A third problem is that there is no commonality in the length of the talk, which could vary from minutes to hours. Fourth, there is no control over how many talks parents and adolescents have. Fifth, researchers have no control over what is said. For example, some parents may present adolescent sexual activity as morally wrong, while others may take a more practical approach and discuss the importance of using condoms in order to avoid contracting an STI or becoming pregnant. A sixth problem is that researchers have no control over the emotional tone of the conversations, which could range from anger that the teen is sexually active, to a neutral discussion about birth control, or even to happiness that the parent and adolescent can talk about this difficult, emotional topic.

It is not realistic to randomly assign a sex talk to one group of parents and teens and no sex talk to another group of parents and adolescents, in order to compare the sexual behavior of adolescents who received a sex talk with teens who did not get a sex talk. Because of this impossibility, it is possible to draw conclusions only about a correlation between parent–adolescent talks about sex and teen sexual behavior, but conclusions about whether parent–teen sex talks have a causal influence on teen behavior are invalid.

What Is the Relationship between Parent–Teen Talks about Sex and Teen Sexual Behavior?

Given the multiple problems associated with assessing the relationship between parent–teen talks about sex and adolescent sexual behavior, it is still possible to draw at least four tentative conclusions about this relationship (Aspy et al., 2007).

First, merely presenting facts about sex typically has little or no association with adolescent sexual activity and, under some circumstances, may be related to risky teen sexual behavior (Ayalew, Mengistie, & Semahegn, 2014; Deutsch & Crockett, 2016; Gillmore, Chen, Haas, Kopak, & Robillard, 2011). One explanation for these findings is that fact-based, value-neutral discussions about sex do not provide adolescents with guidance about how they should behave, and may lead some adolescents to think that their parents accept teen sexuality, even when they do not, unintentionally encouraging adolescent sexual behavior.

A second generalization is that mothers who urge their daughters to be sexually cautious tend to have daughters who are less likely to engage in risky sexual behavior, while mother–son talks about sex are less strongly related to the sexual behavior of sons (Khurana & Cooksey, 2012; Romo et al., 2002; Widman, Choukas-Bradley, Noar, Nesi, & Garrett, 2016). Daughters typically have a closer relationship with their mothers than sons and are more influenced by them. Less is known about the association between father–teen talks about sex and adolescent sexual activity because so few fathers talk to their teens about sex.

The following story about a father–daughter talk shows that some fathers do talk to their adolescents about sex, and that those conversations can have an effect on the behavior of adolescents, at least according to this girl.

IN THEIR OWN WORDS

So, I'm in the car and I'm telling my dad about the rumors of girls being pregnant or being on the pill. And, I tell my dad, "that as soon as I start having periods, I would like to be put on the pill. So I don't have to worry about getting pregnant." My dad then told me a very important piece of information. He said that I didn't have to have sex just because other people were having sex. That I should wait until I was old enough and responsible enough to take on the consequences of sex. Also, that I could say "no" to anyone and if they didn't respect my choice, then they aren't the right person to be with.

Even though our discussion was limited it still had quite an effect on me and my behavior. My father and I have always been very close and I've always appreciated and trusted his advice. It may not have been my mother who I had a conversation with, but because of our close relationship, my father was able to affect my behavior by showing his disapproval of sex at an early age and taught me a very important lesson of saying "no."

Consider the following story by a young college female in which her brother's sexual behavior was followed by a sex talk about birth control. In this story, the sex talk did not have, and could not have had, an impact on the son's sexual behavior.

IN THEIR OWN WORDS

I was riding in the car with my mom and brother, K., on one particular spring day. Out of nowhere, my brother said, "Mom, I have to tell you something." My mom kept her eyes on the road, but I could tell that she was just as intrigued as I was. Then, he came out and said it: "I had sex." I sat in the backseat with my jaw dropped as my mom just about swerved the car off the road. She slammed on her brakes and looked at him. "Did you use a condom?" she said. He replied, "Of course." We sat there for a moment so she could digest what she just heard and after a while she said, "Well, just make sure you don't hurt that little girl," and started driving. That was the end of that conversation, and now, five years later, he claims that they have never had a "sex talk" again.

Third, discussions about sex and birth control may be a *response* to adolescent sexual behavior rather than an influence on sexual behavior (Clawson & Reese-Weber, 2003; de Looze, Constantine, Jerman, Vermeulen-Smit, & ter Bogt, 2015). It is tempting to assume that what parents do affects adolescents, such that the knowledge, values, beliefs, and expectations about sex parents convey to their adolescents have an impact on adolescent behavior. But another possibility is that adolescents socialize parents, so that parents begin to talk to their adolescents when teens become sexually active or are on the verge of sexual activity (Cederbaum, Rodriguez, Sullivan, & Gray, 2017). Of course, these two possibilities are not mutually exclusive, and the true relationship between parent talk and adolescent behavior may be reciprocal.

Fourth, the relationship between parent–adolescent talk about sex and teen sexual behavior is small to modest (Diiorio et al., 2003; Widman,

Consider the following account by a young man that could be counted as an instance of a father–teen talk about sex. What prediction would you make about the impact this brief sex talk would have on this boy's sexual behavior? Considering all the other powerful forces acting on this teen, would you expect this brief, superficial talk to have any effect whatsoever?

IN THEIR OWN WORDS

The first memory I have of a sex talk was with my father. Dad and I were on a drive to my uncle's for the afternoon when I looked at him and asked, "Dad, where do babies come from?" He was completely shocked by the question and just kind of laughed initially. Then he looked at me smiling and said, "Sex." He didn't really know what else to say about it and found the whole situation amusing. But I think I did, too, even though the rest of the car ride was very awkward. I do remember a couple of the points he made such as "It is one of the funnest things you will ever do." He told me that if I thought roller coasters were fun, wait until I had sex. I don't remember another sex talk with my dad. . . .

Choukas-Bradley, Noar, et al., 2016). Of all the influences on adolescent sexual behavior, conversations between parents and their teens about sex are not highly related to adolescent sexual behavior in comparison to other factors such as biology, parenting style, monitoring, parent–adolescent closeness, peers, and adolescent personality. The low to modest association between one conversation about sex, or even several talks, and teen sexual behavior should not be surprising since sexual behavior is complex and multiply caused.

■ TEACHING PARENTS TO TALK TO THEIR ADOLESCENTS ABOUT SEX

Many parents find it difficult to talk to their adolescents about sex, even though most parents believe that these conversations are important. Few parents voluntarily abdicate their responsibility to socialize their children about sexuality but, instead, reluctantly relinquish that parental duty about this most personal and intimate of subjects for a variety of reasons, including embarrassment, discomfort, fear, and uncertainty. Is there anything that can be done to help parents overcome these emotions so that they can have the talk they want to have? In addition, are improvements in parent–adolescent communication about sex linked to a reduction of adolescent risky sexual behavior?

What Can Be Done to Make It Easier for Parents to Talk to Their Adolescents about Sex?

In 2007, the U.S. Department of Health and Human Services launched the *Parents Speak Up National Campaign* (PSUNC) designed to encourage parents to talk to their children about sex, especially about delaying sexual debut. The PSUNC uses television, radio, print, outdoor advertisements, and a government website to urge parents to talk to their children about sex "early and often." In one study, almost 60% of U.S. parents with children between ages 10 and 14 years were aware of PSUNC (Davis, Evans, & Kamyab, 2012). The campaign is designed to help parents improve their ability to talk to their children about sex in order to reduce adolescent risky sexual behavior. There is a positive relationship between exposure to PSUNC and parent reports of parent–child communication about sex, especially reports by mothers. Overall, PSUNC is a successful media intervention that promotes more extensive parent–child communication about sex (Evans, Davis, Ashley, & Khan, 2012).

One intervention program demonstrates the effectiveness of using a computer program to teach parents to effectively communicate with adolescents about STIs and unintended pregnancies (Villarruel, Loveland-Cherry, & Ronis, 2010). Latino parents living in Detroit, Michigan, were the target group for one intervention, called Cuidalos, consisting of two 60-minute computer sessions. A 3-month follow-up revealed an increase in parent–teen talks about sex as reported by parents and improvement in parent comfort discussing sex in comparison to parents who did not receive the intervention. The findings demonstrate the effectiveness of even a short-term computer-based intervention with an underserved population, and show that it is possible to teach parents the skills they need to talk to their adolescents about sex.

Other research has shown that in-person interventions can improve parent communication skills about sex according to parents and assessed by behavioral observations (Hadley et al., 2018). One promising program for parents entitled Talking Parents, Healthy Teens is run at the parents' worksite during eight lunch hours, and includes free lunches. The program uses role-playing, videotaped interactions, games, and discussions to help parents learn how to better communicate with their teens about sex (Schuster et al., 2008). There are after-school homework assignments for the parents to perform with their teens. Examples of skills taught during the sessions include active listening, paying attention to what their teens are saying without interrupting, and strategies for initiating conversations about sex, such as watching for teaching moments and overcoming roadblocks to talking about sex. Parents who complete the program, in comparison to a control group of parents not in the program, report more discussions about sexual topics and more openness discussing sex-related topics. These differences were maintained until the final measurement period 9 months after the completion of the program (Ladapo et al., 2013).

Research on Turkish parents of adolescents who are intellectually disabled reveals that after a 5-week intervention, parents gain a better understanding of the sexual development of their adolescents and more confidence in their ability to talk to their adolescents about their sexuality (Kok & Akyuz, 2015). Intervention programs for parents of children with special needs may be especially welcome by the parents, many of whom do not know how to cope with the sexual development of children with disabilities.

In general, parents who complete intervention programs designed to enhance communication with adolescents about sexual issues report improvements in all areas of communication, including frequency of communication, number of topics discussed, self-efficacy for talking about sexual topics, and comfort with communicating (Akers, Holland, & Bost, 2011; Santa Maria, Markham, Bluethmann, & Mullen, 2015). Two important limitations exist in most programs designed to improve parent communication about sex, however. First, interventions usually are not tailored to parents with children of different ages. This is an important shortcoming since the ability to talk to a 15-year-old about STIs and contraceptives requires different skills that are more sophisticated from those needed to talk to a 10-year-old about reproduction. A second limitation of interventions designed to improve parent communication about sex is that the large majority of participants in these programs are mothers. Interventions designed to improve paternal communication about sex need to be developed for fathers, along with techniques for recruiting fathers into the programs, in order to specifically address the difficulties fathers have talking about relationships, emotions, and sex.

Do Interventions Designed to Teach Parents How to Talk to Their Teens about Sex Affect Adolescent Sexual Behavior?

Examining the impact of parent communication programs on the ability of parents to talk to their adolescents about sex is an important issue, but one question stands above the rest as the most significant question that needs to be answered: Does teaching parents how to more effectively talk to their teens about sex have an impact of adolescent sexuality?

Wight and Fullerton (2013) evaluated the impact of 44 programs intended to improve the sexual health of children and adolescents by enhancing parent–child communication about sex. Most programs were designed to increase parental knowledge about sex and to teach parents how to talk to their teens about the dangers of risky sex. By and large, there was improvement in parent communication skills, an improvement associated with some reduction of adolescent risky sexual behavior. Results were especially promising for three programs that targeted African American parents, and included at least 14 hours of intensive training for the parents. All three programs were associated with a delay of sexual debut and an increase in condom use for those teens who were sexually active. In general, most of the programs improve parent–teen communication about sex and increase adolescents' knowledge about sex, and a few intensive programs even lead to some decrease in adolescent risky sexual behavior.

Research on the impact of parent communication interventions on adolescent sexual behavior is just beginning, but preliminary evidence suggests that parents can be taught the skills to improve their ability to talk to their adolescents about sex, an improvement associated with an increase in adolescent sexual knowledge and a decrease in risky sexual behavior (Santa Maria et al., 2015).

SUMMARY

■ PARENTS AND ADOLESCENTS TALKING ABOUT SEX

The percentage of parents and teens who talk about sex is modest, especially if the estimate is based on adolescent reports. The incidence of parent–adolescent talk about sex is substantially higher in the United States than in countries with more traditional belief systems, however. Parents generally report more parent–teen talks about sex than the teens report.

Talk about sex begins at a variety of ages. Puberty in boys is not related to the occurrence of talk about sex between parents and sons, but menarche in girls is often the cue parents use to have a sex talk with their daughters. Parent–adolescent sex talks are also likely to occur when teens begin to date and become involved in risky behavior. As adolescents enter emerging adulthood, the importance of parents as sources of information about sex declines, and emerging adults rely more on friends, dating partners, and the media when questions about sex arise.

◼ PARENTAL MESSAGES ABOUT SEX

There are several reasons why parents find it difficult to talk to their children about sex: parents are not sure they have the knowledge, they are afraid the conversations will lead to adolescent sexual activity, and many parents do not think their adolescents are sexually active and are not in need of information about sex. In addition, many parents are embarrassed about discussing sex. Many adolescents are also reluctant to talk to their parents about this very personal part of their lives. In general, parents and teens with a close relationship find it easier to talk about sex than parents and teens who are not close.

When most parents talk about sex they focus on reproduction, abstinence, and the importance of safe sex. Talk about the dangers of sexual activity are common, especially between parents and daughters.

Parents are more likely to talk to their daughters about sex than their sons. Talks with both daughters and sons tend to emphasize abstinence and the negative consequences of sex, but parents of sons are somewhat more likely to talk about the positive aspects of sex.

Sons and daughters of all ages are more likely to talk to their mothers about sex than their fathers. The difficulty fathers have discussing sex may reflect the more task-oriented male gender role and the personal histories of fathers, which often do not include any discussions with their own fathers about sex. When fathers do talk about sex they tend to focus on practical matters such as condoms. Mothers, more than fathers, are somewhat more comfortable talking to their children about sex.

◼ PARENT–ADOLESCENT TALKS ABOUT SEX AND ADOLESCENT SEXUALITY

It is not possible to confidently assess the impact of parent–adolescent talks about sex on teens' sexual behavior because researchers cannot randomly assign parents and teens to a sex talk group or a nonsex talk group. Simply talking about sexual facts is not highly related to responsible sexual behavior, especially when those conversations do not include discussions about values. Talks are related to lower teen risky sexual behavior when the conversations focus on the reasons why it is important to act responsibly, and the discussions occur between parents and teens who have a close relationship.

◼ TEACHING PARENTS TO TALK TO THEIR ADOLESCENTS ABOUT SEX

In general, parents who complete interventions designed to improve their ability to effectively communicate with their adolescents about sex show some improvement in sexual communication.

Most programs designed to enhance parent communication skills about sex have not assessed the impact of the programs on adolescent sexual behavior.

Results from several promising programs do indicate that interventions designed to improve parent communication skills about sex are related to a delay in sexual debut and an increase in condom use. Teaching parents to talk effectively to their adolescents about sex may be one approach to reduce adolescent risky sexual behavior.

SUGGESTIONS FOR FURTHER READING

Aspy, C. B., Vesely, S. K., Oman, R. F., Rodine, S., Marshall, L., & McLeroy, K. (2007). Parental communication and youth sexual behaviour. *Journal of Adolescence, 30,* 449–466.

Kapungu, C. T., Baptiste, D., Holmbeck, G., McBride, C., Robinson-Brown, M., Sturdivant, A., et al. (2010). Beyond the "birds and the bees": Gender differences in sex-related communication among urban African-American adolescents. *Family Process, 49,* 251–264.

Khurana, A., & Cooksey, E. C. (2012). Examining the effect of maternal sexual communication and adolescents' perceptions of maternal disapproval on adolescent risky sexual involvement. *Journal of Adolescent Health, 51,* 557–565.

Widman, L., Choukas-Bradley, S., Noar, S. M., Nesi, J., & Garrett, K. (2016). Parent–adolescent sexual communication and adolescent safer sex behavior: A meta-analysis. *Journal of the American Medical Association Pediatrics, 170,* 52–61.

Wight, D., & Fullerton, D. (2013). A review of interventions with parents to promote the sexual health of their children. *Journal of Adolescent Health, 52,* 4–27.

CHAPTER 5

Peers and
Adolescent Sexuality

Do friends, peers, and classmates have an influence on the sexual behavior of adolescents? The quick and straightforward answer to that deceptively simple question is a resounding *Yes*! But there is more to the question and the answer than at first meets the eye, and an army of social scientists has published numerous studies examining the intricacies of the relationship between peers and adolescent sexuality. This chapter examines that research, focusing on the complexities and subtleties of the answers to what turns out to be a complicated question.

In 1998, Judith Rich Harris published a provocative book entitled *The Nurture Assumption: Why Children Turn Out the Way They Do* that caused a sensation in the popular press and generated considerable debate among researchers. Harris reviewed the literature on parent and peer influence on children and adolescents and concluded that peers have a considerably greater impact on the development of youth than do parents. It is a debatable proposition, but what is not at issue is the conclusion that peers matter and, further, that peer influence and peer conformity are especially strong during adolescence. There are at least four reasons why peers might have a stronger and more pervasive influence on adolescents than on children, or in comparison to parents. First, adolescents spend more time with peers than they did when they were younger, time that was once spent with parents, and more time with peers translates into greater influence (Berndt, 1996). Second, adolescents share more common interests and experiences with their peers than they do with their parents, which leads to close bonds of friendship and a convergence of attitudes and values among friends. Third, adolescents understand that the world of their peers is their future, and to function and be successful in that world they must broadly fit in and embrace the values of its members (Harris, 1998). Fourth, the formation of an independent identity apart from parents elevates the importance of peers to center stage as adolescents strive for autonomy from parents (Crosnoe & McNeely, 2008). For all of these reasons, adolescents begin to internalize the attitudes and values of their peers and place a high premium on maintaining positive relations with peers, which leads to an increase in peer conformity and to difficulty resisting peer influence.

■ ADOLESCENTS TALKING TO ADOLESCENTS ABOUT SEX

Who Do Teens Talk to When They Talk about Sex?

Few in the United States would be surprised to discover that adolescents of both genders report they learn more about sex from their peers than they do from any other source, including parents, teachers, and the media. In one recent survey of a random sample of U.S. adolescents, a large majority of white youth report that they learn more about sex from their peers than they do from any other group. However, the media is nominated by African American, Latino, and Asian American adolescents along with peers as an important source of information about sex (Kaiser Family Foundation, 2003), perhaps revealing the beginning of a growing trend among adolescents of searching the Internet for answers to questions about sex (Suzuki & Calzo, 2004).

An important addendum to the finding that adolescents learn more about sex from peers than from their parents emerges from another national survey of teens and parents. Both teens and parents report that they think parents are more influential than peers when it comes to teens' sexual behavior. Together, these findings suggest that teens say they learn more about sex from peers, but teens and parents believe that parents have a greater influence on teens' sexual behavior (Albert, 2012).

The importance of peers over parents as sources of sex information is highly consistent across time. Peers have been significant sources of sexual knowledge for as far back as this issue has been examined, extending back to at least the 1940s in the United States (Ramsey, 1943), into the late 1970s (Thornburg, 1981), persisting until today. Although adolescents today continue to be more likely to turn to peers instead of their parents when they have questions about sex, parents may be gaining in importance, perhaps because parents and adolescents today have a relationship that is more open and egalitarian than parents and adolescents had in the past (Secor-Turner, Sieving, Eisenberg, & Skay, 2011; Widman, Choukas-Bradley, et al., 2014).

Peers are not the primary source of sex information for adolescents in every country. Many 12- to 14-year-olds in four sub-Saharan African countries report that teacher/school and mass media are more important sources of sex information than friends or family, including parents (Bankole, Biddlecom, Guiella, & Singh, 2007). One can only speculate on these cross-cultural differences, but peers may be important sources of sex information for adolescents in the United States, which has a well-defined youth culture and an emphasis on adolescent autonomy from parents. In more traditional societies, such as Africa, where there is less emphasis on achieving independence from parents, and which has a high incidence of HIV/AIDS, talk about STIs and contraception is emphasized more in social institutions, such as school and in the mass media, than among parents or friends.

What Do Teens Talk about When They Talk to Peers about Sex?

The finding that U.S. adolescents learn more about sex from peers than from their parents is an interesting factoid, but of what importance is this difference for adolescents? Does the primary source of sex information have an impact on adolescent sexuality? Results from one study indicate that talking to peers about sex is related to the belief that having sex leads to positive consequences for the self and one's partner (Holman & Kellas, 2015). In contrast, talking to parents about sex is associated with more negative beliefs about having sex, such as getting an STI or experiencing a pregnancy (Bleakley, Hennessy, Fishbein, & Jordan, 2009; Ragsdale et al., 2014). It is not possible to know whether who one talks to precedes one's beliefs, or whether beliefs precede talk. Whatever the relationship between sources of sex information and beliefs about sex, talking to peers about sex is related to beliefs that may increase the likelihood of having sex, while talking to parents about sex is associated with beliefs likely to delay sex.

In one study of the conversations young men have about sex with their parents and with peers, researchers reported that parents stress the importance of love, promote safe sex, and encourage their sons to save sex for marriage or a serious romantic relationship (Epstein & Ward, 2008). In contrast, male peers portray sex as positive, desirable, and natural, encourage sexual freedom and exploration, and approve of casual sex. Young men also share sexual experiences with one another, and trade stories. In general, parents emphasize the seriousness of sexual activity, while male peers depict sex as fun and positive, and encourage young men to have casual sex as a natural expression of their masculinity.

Sex talk among male peers may emphasize recreation and conquest, but that is a broad characterization of what young men talk about and it does not capture the variety of conversations young men have with their peers about sex. Sex talk among adolescent males may portray sex as cool and exciting, but talk about sex can also have a religious foundation to it, or may focus on the desirability of sex within a relationship (Bell, Rosenberger, & Ott, 2015). All three of these orientations are supported by some adolescent males who gravitate toward others with similar orientations, reinforcing already existing attitudes (Baams, Overbeek, van de Bongardt, et al., 2015).

What Is the Relationship between Talking to Peers about Sex and Adolescent Sexuality?

Adolescents who often talk to peers about sex expect to have sex and are more sexually active than adolescents who rarely talk to peers about sex (Busse, Fishbein, Bleakley, & Hennessy, 2010; Ragsdale et al., 2014). One reason for this association is that peers have more liberal attitudes about sex than do parents (Charmaraman & McKamey, 2011), attitudes that get translated into talk that disinhibits the sexual behavior of teens by presenting sex as cool, exciting, and pleasurable.

One might think that adolescents would be more likely to talk to a sexual partner than to a peer about sex, but it turns out that the opposite is true—adolescents are less likely to talk to a sexual partner about sex than to a peer. In one study, only a minority of sexually active adolescents discussed sex with their sexual partner, while a majority talked to friends about sex (Widman, Choukas-Bradley, et al., 2014). The lack of conversations about sex with a sexual partner, especially talks about condom use, can lead to problems, since sexually active adolescents who do not talk to their partners about condom use are less likely to use condoms, and more likely to use them inconsistently than adolescents who talk to their partners. One implication of these findings is that any program designed to increase condom use among adolescents should include information about how to talk to a partner about this sensitive and awkward topic.

Why Do Adolescents Prefer to Talk to Peers about Sex Instead of Their Parents?

Answers to the question about why adolescents prefer peers over parents as sources of sex information emerges from a study of Turkish university students (Gelbal, Duyan, & Öztürk, 2008). Students reported two reasons why they discuss sexual matters with peers instead of parents. First, the students perceive parents to have more conservative views about sexual behavior than peers, who are perceived to be more liberal and open-minded. Second, students have more trust that peers will keep personal discussions about sexual issues private and confidential, while they worry that parents might share information with others in and outside the family.

There is nothing inherently wrong about relying on peers for information about sex if the information adolescents receive from peers is accurate. Is information about sex learned from peers as accurate as information learned from parents? It turns out that adolescents who talk to their peers about sex are as knowledgeable about sex as youth who talk to their parents (Handelsman, Cabral, & Weisfeld, 1987). What is disheartening about the results from this mid-1980s study is that both groups of adolescents only got about 66% of the sexual knowledge questions correct, a letter grade of D on a standard scale, indicating that neither parents nor peers did an especially good job teaching adolescents about sex. Adolescents today know more about the basics of sexual reproduction, but many adolescents, especially younger teens, continue to be poorly informed about contraception and STIs, two topics teens rarely discuss with their peers (Kaye, Suellentrop, & Sloup, 2009).

Whom Do LGBTQ Adolescents Talk to about Sex?

Researchers who study sources of sexual information almost exclusively focus on the majority of adolescents who are heterosexual, but leave LGBTQ adolescents largely unstudied. How do LGBTQ adolescents find answers to the questions of importance to them? Most sex education courses are silent about LGBTQ issues, talking to parents may be off limits, and the majority of heterosexual peers do not have the answers to the questions of interest to sexual-minority youth, and may even be hostile toward adolescents who raise these issues. LGBTQ adolescents may be teased by their peers if their questions even hint at the possibility that the teens may be uncertain about their sexual orientation, and ostracized, or even worse, if those adolescents who are LGBTQ reveal their true sexual identity. Given such a situation, it is not surprising that many LGBTQ adolescents turn to the Internet for answers to questions they have about sex (Arrington-Sanders et al., 2015; Bond, 2015).

In one study of young men who have sex with men (YMSM), researchers found that the primary sources of sex information for YMSM are the Internet, pornography, and older men (Kubicek, Beyer, Weiss, Iverson, & Kipke, 2010). Information learned from peers focuses on heterosexual sex because as one young man explained, he could not ask about anal sex or homosexuality when he was a teen since "Nobody was gonna be out there at that age" (Kubicek et al., 2010, p. 253). Eventually, most YMSM in this study found friends who were gay, with whom they could ask questions about sex and what it means to be gay. For many YMSM, gay friends are the primary source of information about sex and about the meaning of a same-sex attraction. As one man reported, it was in his junior year of high school that he met a gay friend who "helped me discover who I am and what I am" (Kubicek et al., 2010, p. 253). Some young men report that they had gay mentors, generally young men a few years older, who were sometimes called a "gay big brother," who helped them explore gay issues.

■ PEER INFLUENCE AND ADOLESCENT SEXUALITY

What Is Peer Influence?

Researchers who study peer relations often use the terms *peer pressure* and *peer influence* interchangeably. The two phrases are not quite the same, however. Peer pressure, commonly used by parents and writers of self-help books for parents of adolescents, has the connotation that an individual is coerced or cajoled into doing something against his or her will. The phrase *peer influence* not only includes the idea of pressure but also the idea of less compelling, but no less powerful influences, such as persuasion, suggestion, and conformity to group norms.

Peer influence, especially peer pressure, is often viewed as a negative influence on teens associated with violating a personal belief. An example might be a girl who reluctantly has sex with her boyfriend after months of persistent pressure by him to do so, even though she believes that premarital sex is wrong. But peer influence can also be positive, such as when one girl reassures another that she is doing the right thing by holding on to her personal standards about sexual behavior in the face of pressure to do otherwise by an indefatigable boyfriend.

How Important Is Peer Influence to Have Sex, According to Parents and Adolescents?

Parents and youth believe that peer influence has a powerful effect on teens to have sex, and to have it at an early age (Suleiman & Deardorff, 2015). In one qualitative study, parents of adolescents reported that they thought peer pressure and the media are the main reasons adolescents have sex (Wilson et al., 2010). The parents go on to say that they think peer pressure is greater today than it used to be. As one father explained:

> "When I was in junior high school, the kids that were sexually active were few and far between, and now it seems that the ones who *aren't* sexually active are the ones who are few and far between. So there's a lot more pressure." (Wilson et al., 2010, p. 58)

The perception that peer pressure is a significant influence on adolescent sexual behavior is not a uniquely American idea. Adolescents living in Singapore believe that peer pressure is the main reason teens have sex. The adolescents think that teens who are unable to resist peer pressure are more likely to be sexually active than youth who are able to resist peer pressure (Wong et al., 2009).

Older adolescents feel more pressure to have sex than younger adolescents (Kaiser Family Foundation, 2003), which is not surprising since there are more sexually active older adolescents who model and reinforce sexual activity (Centers for Disease Control and Prevention, 2011). As more adolescents become sexually active, a new, more liberal norm becomes the standard by which adolescents judge themselves and others, which leads to an increase in sexual activity.

In contrast to the belief many have that peer pressure has a significant influence on adolescent behavior, Ungar (2000) argues that the importance of peer pressure is overblown. In his own work, Unger found that teen participation in many social behaviors, such as cigarette smoking, substance use, and sexual activity, is not the result of peer pressure but is a conscious choice made by some adolescents based on their identity and designed to enhance their social status.

Teens make an intriguing distinction between the pressure they think others experience to have sex and the pressure they themselves experience. A majority of adolescents believe that teens in general experience a lot of pressure to have sex, but only a minority report personally experiencing pressure to have sex (Kaiser Family Foundation, 2003). One possible explanation for this discrepancy is that people in general believe their own behavior is the result of personal choice, while the behavior of others is highly influenced by situational factors and other people (Pronin & Kugler, 2010).

The perception adolescents have that peer pressure is a powerful influence on sexual behavior points to the need to include information in sex education courses on resisting peer pressure. Girls need to learn how to deal with a persistent boyfriend who continues to push for sex, but boys also need to know how to respond to the implicit, or explicit, pressure from other boys and the media to have sex as an expression of their masculinity.

Is All Peer Influence the Same?

Peer pressure to have sex can take many forms and emanate from a partner or friends (Maxwell, 2006). In one study of English adolescents, many females describe direct pressure from their boyfriends to have sex. Many of these girls feel obliged to have sex when their boyfriend wants sex, and feel guilty for not wanting to satisfy their boyfriend's desires. Some young males feel pressure from friends to have sex, and indicate that they are ridiculed by their friends if they are virgins, so they have sex because they want to be accepted and to have a reputation as a boy with a long list of sexual conquests (Maxwell & Chase, 2008).

Hyde, Drennan, Howlett, and Brady (2008) studied the sexual behavior of Irish adolescents who described two types of peer influence to have sex. *Interpersonal coercion* is the direct pressure by one individual to influence another to have sex, usually by talk. Girls, but not boys, reported many instances of interpersonal coercion that usually takes the form of verbal persuasion, as well as unwelcome physical advances. A common theme that emerged from the interviews with girls is male sexual pushiness, especially when the male is intoxicated.

A second type of peer influence is *social coercion,* defined as pressure to adhere to the sexual norms of a group (Hyde et al., 2008). Hyde and colleagues found that both sexes reported experiencing social coercion, which is revealed in the following account given by a 16-year-old girl:

> INTERVIEWER: Do you think that . . . girls or boys in a way feel pressured to perform oral sex?
>
> GIRL: Yeah.

INTERVIEWER: Can you spell it out a little bit?

GIRL: Yeah, if your friends are doing it with their boyfriends you feel pressurized. And if your boyfriend was in a relationship before that and did it, you'd want to do it, wouldn't you? (Hyde et al., 2008, p. 485)

Note that this girl does not indicate that her boyfriend is pressuring her to have oral sex, but instead insinuates that her motivation for oral sex is a desire

---

The following account of an unwanted sexual experience illustrates the unrelenting interpersonal coercion one boy put on a girl to have sex with him.

IN THEIR OWN WORDS

When my best friend and I were freshmen in high school, she was in a relationship with another female. One day I was at her house to spend the night. Her mom had left and we were sitting at home, bored. Her girlfriend called and asked if we wanted to go to the movies, like on a double date. We agreed and she asked her cousin, a male, to come with us as my date. We then got ready to leave and waited for them to pick us up. I was immediately attracted to her cousin and couldn't wait to talk to him.

When we got into the car, the music was playing loud. He turned it down and then we all discussed what movie we wanted to see. Once we arrived to the movies, we got out of the car and the guy told me how cute he thought I was. When we were inside the theater and sitting down, he laid his hand on my thigh. I didn't really mind at first, I just wondered why he did that so quickly. Instead of watching the movie, the whole time he was talking to me. Making advances. He then asked me if I was a virgin and I told him yes. He told me that there was no way that I was a virgin and that he didn't believe me. About halfway through the movie, he asked if I was ready to leave and I told him that I wasn't leaving without my friend.

We left the movies and began driving around town getting food and just hanging out. We decided to stop behind a school to sit, talk, and listen to music. My friend and her girlfriend got out of the car and started walking around. The guy kept talking to me and laid his hand on my thigh again. I don't remember how he asked me, but he wanted to have sex. I told him no, I couldn't because I was a virgin.

We were sitting in the front seat and he began to unbuckle my belt and stick his hand in my pants. I was OK with the touching and didn't want to do anymore at first. He kept asking me for more. He told me to come closer to him. Before I knew it, he had pulled his penis out and was waiting for me to agree. He then pulled out a condom and insisted that I do it to him. Eventually I gave in and let him penetrate me.

Afterward I felt awful. I just wanted to run away, so I got out of the car. He began to run after me to ask me what was wrong. I was confused, ashamed, and felt a little guilty. My friend knew what I had done and looked at me with a face of disappointment. During the drive back home I was silent. I was having mixed feelings. I was torn between "OMG, what did I do?" and "That was a good feeling."

Once my friend and I got back into the house, she barely talked to me. I knew she was disappointed but didn't want to tell me. In a weird way I felt like I had let her down. I also felt like I had let myself down and I felt like I had entered a whole new world. I had taken the word *sex* to another level. I was no longer a virgin and I didn't know how to deal with it.

to live up to the normative standards set by her friends and by a previous girl-friend.

In a similar way, boys feel social coercion to have sex in order to fit in with their friends and to feel normal, implying that there is something abnormal about a boy who has not had sex when all his friends have, as the following excerpt illustrates:

INTERVIEWER: How would the pressure come about then?

BOY 1: Just your friends like. They are doing it, they have talked about it and you want to know what it's like, so you feel pressured into doing it.

BOY 2: It would be you yourself that feels pressured 'cos if all your friends have done it, you must think that there is something wrong with you that you haven't. (Hyde et al., 2008, p. 488)

In addition, reports of the sexual behavior from some young men reveal a male-specific form of social coercion, fear of being labeled homosexual, as the following excerpt illustrates:

BOY 1: If you said "No" [to heterosexual intercourse] and all your friends find out . . . they'd say "Oh, you're queer" or something.

INTERVIEWER: Is that what you'd say to each other?

GENERAL: Yeah.

BOY 2: They'd say you're a faggot or something. (Hyde et al., 2008, p. 489)

The pressure to have sex can be different for boys and girls. Girls feel pressure from their boyfriends, but many boys say they do not want to be teased by their friends for being a virgin. The pressure on girls is more personal and involves interpersonal coercion. The pressure on boys may be equally as strong, but it often takes the form of social coercion, in which boys feel pressure to live up to the sexual norms of their group, and may be mocked and taunted if they are a virgin.

■ PEER ASSOCIATION AND ADOLESCENT SEXUALITY

Adolescents and their friends are likely to share the same attitudes about sex and to be similar in their sexual behavior. This similarity is especially strong for younger adolescents who are in the process of forming their ideas about sexuality (Buhi & Goodson, 2007; Nagamatsu, Yamawaki, Sato, Nakagawa, & Saito, 2013). The finding that the sexual attitudes and behavior of adolescents who are friends are alike is not surprising, but the reason for the resemblance is anything but obvious. Explanations for this similarity can be grouped into two categories (Brechwald & Prinstein, 2011). *Selection theories* propose that similarities in the attitudes and behavior of friends are due to the tendency of like-minded adolescents to select friends who are like themselves. Birds of a feather flock together, and individuals are attracted to and prefer to associate with other individuals like themselves, a tendency called *homophily*. *Socialization theories* suggest that group members exert an influence on one another and on new group members to act or think in a certain way. These two forces are not mutually exclusive, and in the real world they may act together; teens select friends who are like themselves, and teens put pressure on each other to think and act in a certain way.

Do Peers Affect Adolescent Sexuality?

There is a concordance between the sexual attitudes and behavior of adolescents and their friends. Adolescents who are sexual risk takers—for example, those who have many partners or are inconsistent condom users—are more likely to have sexual risk-taking friends than adolescents who are more responsible (Bachanas et al., 2002; Black, Ricardo, & Stanton, 1997; Harrison et al., 2012).

The following story illustrates the effect of both peer selection and peer socialization on the sexual behavior of one adolescent young man.

IN THEIR OWN WORDS

My close group of friends throughout high school had somewhat conservative views on sex. That is, they felt more like you should wait for someone who was somewhat special. Not necessarily marriage, but at least a girl who you were exclusively dating for an extended period of time. And my early behaviors reflected this. It wasn't until my sophomore year when I first received oral sex, and my attitudes at the time led me to believe that this was crossing some sort of a line seeing as how I had only been dating this girl for a few weeks.

However, my other group of peers held much more liberal views on sex. This group I didn't necessarily choose to be around, but rather, I was forced to interact with them on a daily basis. I'm talking, of course, about my football peers. I never interacted with the guys in this group very heavily outside of football. Up until high school, football wasn't that involved, so my relationship with these guys wasn't very strong. However, once we were all playing varsity, things changed. I was around them a lot more and, therefore, was more exposed to their sexual attitudes. After one season of playing varsity with these guys, my views on sex had drastically changed. At the end of my junior year, I ended up having sex with this girl that I had just met about a month prior. Plus, at the time of intercourse, she was dating another guy. Before that football season, I would never even consider sleeping with a girl who I wasn't planning on marrying, let alone one who was dating another guy for so long. My close group of peers were all still virgins at the time, and they still held the same relatively conservative views on sex that they had always held. However, due to football, I spent far less time with my close group of friends than I did with my football peers.

Friends also have similar attitudes and behavior about healthy sexuality (Kapadia et al., 2012). In one study of French adolescents, those teens who think that their friends usually use condoms are more likely to use condoms themselves than teens who think that condom use is rare among their friends (Potard, Courtois, & Rusch, 2008). Further, adolescents who have friends who believe in the importance of postponing sex are, themselves, more likely to hold similar attitudes and to delay sexual activity for a longer period of time than teens with friends who do not believe in the importance of postponing sex (Carvajal et al., 1999).

It is tempting to conclude from this research that friends influence what adolescents do, but the same research can also be thought of as demonstrating that adolescents choose friends who are like themselves. Which is it? The answer is that both explanations are true. The evidence from several longitudinal studies indicates that both selection and socialization processes are at work (Henry, Schoeny, Deptula, & Slavick, 2007). Pathways of influence between adolescents and their friends are bidirectional rather than unidirectional; adolescents select friends who are consistent with and supportive of their own sexual attitudes and behavior but, once selected, teens are influenced by what their friends think and do (Henry et al., 2007; van de Bongardt, Reitz, Sandfort, & Deković, 2015).

The following story is an illustration of the influence of the social environment, including one's friends, on one young woman's decision to remain abstinent.

IN THEIR OWN WORDS

Growing up, I was constantly surrounded by conservative, Christian people. Whether it was my family, church, or school, Christianity was always placed in front of my face and heavily weighed on my decision making. Coming from a Christian family, I was taught beliefs and standards to which I was expected to live by. From the way I dressed to the type of friends I chose to hang out, Christianity dictated my decisions. Once I turned 7, my family moved from T. to D. Naturally, my parents enrolled me in a private Christian school where I attended second to twelfth grade. My class never had more than 25 students, so needless to say, we were all very close and knew each other a little too well. Sexuality of any kind before marriage was considered a huge sin and was always discouraged. Rumors would spread sometimes though of two people who had hooked up the past weekend. With it being such a small school, these rumors spread like wildfire and before the day was over, everyone knew. These people were either looked at as promiscuous or slutty. I cannot recall one time where the students encouraged other students to have sex or oral sex or even approved if they did.

Now that I am a senior in college, it is interesting to hear that most students experienced the exact opposite in high school. Students would normally pressure one another to have sex or hook up. It was rarer that sexuality was discouraged. One of the things I am thankful for attending a Christian high school is never having to experience the pressure to hook up and have sex. I am glad I was able to make that decision on my own and not do it because I felt the need to, in order to fit in with my peers.

Longitudinal studies of peer influence on sexual activity reveal that in general, girls are more resistant to peer influence to become sexually active than boys (Widman, Choukas-Bradley, Helms, & Prinstein, 2016). Further, when friends do have an influence on sexual behavior, that influence acts in opposite directions for boys and girls. Boys with friends who are sexually active are more likely to be sexually active themselves than boys with friends who are not sexually active (Kinsman, Romer, Furstenberg, & Schwarz, 1998). In contrast, girls are more likely to be abstinent if they have friends who are sexually abstinent (Sieving, Eisenberg, Pettingell, & Skay, 2006). Thus, it is easier for friends to influence boys to become sexually active than to remain abstinent, while it is easier for friends to influence girls to remain abstinent than to become sexually active, perhaps reinforcing gender-specific norms about sexual activity.

How Do Peers Affect Adolescent Sexuality?

How do peers promote or inhibit adolescent sexuality? Several theories have been proposed to explain the influence of peers on adolescents, with two of the most important being social learning theory and social norm theory. *Social learning theory* includes two salient mechanisms of influence: peer modeling and peer reinforcement. Peers are exemplars of sexual behavior, and adolescents may model their own behavior on the behavior of others in their group, especially high-status others whose friendship and esteem the adolescent highly values. A second social learning mechanism is peer reinforcement, which is when adolescents socially reward other adolescents with attention, praise, and approval when they behave in a certain way.

According to *social norm theory,* people have a general tendency to act in accordance with norms they perceive to be shared by people who are valued and admired (Caldini & Trost, 1998). The motivation to conform to social norms comes from a desire to appear "normal" and to be accepted, avoiding the appearance of abnormality and the risk of rejection. These two theories are not mutually exclusive and both operate together to affect an adolescent's sexual behavior.

How Strong Is Peer Influence on Adolescent Sexuality?

Peers have an influence on adolescent sexuality, but how much of an influence do they have? Results from several studies reveal that peers have a measurable effect on sexual behavior, but the effect is small to moderate (Ali & Dwyer, 2011; Jaccard, Blanton, & Dodge, 2005), a finding that should please many parents who worry about what they perceive to be a strong, negative effect of peer pressure on their adolescents. Peers have a considerable influence on a wide range of adolescent activities such as tastes in music, clothes, and movies, but when it comes to attitudes and behaviors more central to one's self-concept such as sexuality, the influence of friends is less pervasive and less powerful.

Further, peer influence is especially powerful when the influence is in the direction the adolescent already is leaning, rather than in an opposing direction (Padilla-Walker & Carlo, 2007). For example, adolescents who hope to have sex will be more easily influenced by peer pressure to have sex than adolescents who are trying to remain abstinent.

Although peer influence can affect teen behavior, adolescents are not lemmings who unthinkingly follow the lead of their friends. They are conscious actors with beliefs and values of their own, which they can put into practice even in the face of strong pressure to violate a personal value. One study of sixth-grade Latino girls found that these girls had already developed several strategies to resist peer pressure to engage in sexual behavior. Four strategies were especially common: assertively saying "No," stating a reason not to

A FOCUS ON RESEARCH

Researchers interested in studying the similarity of sexual behavior among friends typically ask adolescents to report on their own sexual behavior and on the sexual behavior of their friends. Thus, what is actually being assessed is the relationship between reports of one's own behavior and the *perceptions* of the sexual behavior of friends. Ideally, adolescents would report on their behavior and friends would report on their own behavior and the reports would be compared. This approach is rarely taken.

Reasons for comparing self-reports with perceptions of friends' behavior instead of friends' reports stem from the methodological and ethical problems of matching self-reports of sexual behavior with friends' reports of their own sexual behavior. Comparing self-reports with other reports requires adolescents to identify themselves in order to match up the responses of the adolescents with their friends, revealing the identities of the respondents. Researchers are reluctant to ask adolescents to put their names on reports of their own sexual behavior for several reasons. First, researchers assume that adolescents are more likely to tell the truth about their sexual behavior when their reports are anonymous. Second, many adolescents may not participate in a sexual behavior survey if they have to reveal their true identities. Third, many

parents may not allow their adolescents to take part in a study of sexual behavior if sexual behavior can be tied to specific adolescents. Fourth, institutional review boards, charged with protecting the rights of research participants, may not allow researchers to ask minors to report on behavior as personal and sensitive as their own sexual activity unless the reports are anonymous.

The perceptions of adolescents about their friends' sexual behavior are rarely compared to the friends' own reports of their sexual behavior to assess the accuracy of the perceptions. One study of the similarity of health risk behaviors among friends found that perceptions of friends' behavior were significantly correlated with friends' reports of their own behavior, but those correlations were far from perfect (average r = .50; Prinstein & Wang, 2005). Adolescents' perceptions of the sexual behavior of their friends tell us something about the actual sexual behavior of the friends, but those perceptions can be influenced by cognitive distortions, such as the *false consensus belief*, which is the belief that people are like ourselves. The false consensus belief leads to an overestimation of the actual similarity between friends in their attitudes and behavior. Thus, the actual similarity of sexual attitudes and behavior among friends may be less than what adolescents think it is.

participate, actively avoiding the pressure, and leaving the situation (Norris et al., 2015). Any intervention program designed to reduce early adolescent sexual behavior should help teens develop personal strategies to avoid risky sex.

■ POPULARITY AND ADOLESCENT SEXUALITY

Do Popular Teens Have More Sex Than Other Teens?

Popular teens are more sexually active than other teens (De Bruyn, Cillessen, & Weisfeld, 2012; Feldman, Rosenthal, Brown, & Canning, 1995). Further, popularity precedes sexual activity for both boys and girls, since high popularity provides opportunities for sexual behavior. For boys, popularity is also a consequence of sexual behavior (Mayeux, Sandstrom, & Cillessen, 2008). Sexual activity does not raise the social status of girls, however, and can even damage the reputations of girls with many sexual partners (Prinstein, Choukas-Bradley, Helms, Brechwald, & Rancourt, 2011).

The relationship between popularity and number of sexual partners for boys is alarming because it indicates that popular boys are a risk group for sex with many partners. Traditionally, popular adolescents have been portrayed as socially adept and well-adjusted, but this sunny depiction reveals only one side of the story. Many boys who are highly successful in the adolescent society also engage in risky behaviors such as early sex and sex with multiple partners.

Do Jocks Have More Sex?

Anyone who has attended an American high school can attest to the fact that schools do not have a homogeneous peer culture with sexual norms that apply equally to all students. Instead, schools are segregated into distinct *crowds,* which are groups of students perceived as being similar in some defining way. The five most common crowds in U.S. high schools are jocks, brains, burnouts, populars, and nonconformists—crowd names that should conjure up common distinct images, at least among U.S. readers. Most students are not concerned about being popular in general, but they are concerned about being popular in their crowd, so in order to understand the relationship between popularity and adolescent sexual behavior one has to know who the referent crowd is, and what are the sexual norms of that crowd. Little is known about the linkage between crowd membership and sexual activity, but one study did examine the connection between crowds and health risk behaviors, including risky sex (La Greca, Prinstein, & Fetter, 2001). Large differences are found for the percentage of students in each crowd who are sexually active: nonconformists are followed by jocks, burnouts, average students, populars, and brains. Burnouts have the most number of sexual partners and the highest rate of unprotected sex, while brains have the fewest number of partners. These data indicate that

In the following story, one young woman describes her experiences in high school of dating and having sex with a boy who was not a member of her crowd, who she pursued precisely because he did not know her very well.

IN THEIR OWN WORDS

I am from a suburb of C. where a small high school consists of 580 students per class. You knew everyone in your grade and typically the grades right above and below you. The group of friends you spent time with was important but not necessarily for popularity reasons. The most important part of your social status was just that you belonged to a group. If you did not have a group of friends to call your own or could not be categorized, you were considered an outcast. It didn't matter what type of friends you had, everyone belonged somewhere. Growing up, I was the overweight girl in a group of girls where one was prettier than the next. Needless to say I had competition when it came to boys, even competition to get a boy to pay attention to me period. Eventually I went through puberty, my baby fat fell off, but the boys I grew up with still wouldn't give me a chance. Even today, many years later, the boys I went to elementary school with still will not talk to me if I see them when I'm home. As a freshman, I found myself in high school where the options of boys seemed endless and where many of them didn't know I used to be overweight. Consequently, I found myself venturing toward guys in different groups of friends who wouldn't judge me for my past and would give me a chance based on who I was now. Not only did I lose weight, but I blossomed into a person who was finally comfortable with myself and finally comfortable talking to people.

Most of the students [in my high school] only had sex within groups of friends (and I will add that most sexual intercourse only happened between two people that were in a relationship). First off, it was really hard to hang out with someone who wasn't in your approved group of friends. No one would dare show up by themselves somewhere they may not be wanted. Therefore, it was always an orchestrated event of asking (or begging) a friend or two to come with you to see the boy you had a crush on.

efforts to deal with peer influence to have sex should take into account the sexual norms associated with different crowds, and the unique pressures to have sex within each type of crowd.

■ THE SEXUAL DOUBLE STANDARD

The *sexual double standard* refers to the idea that there are different norms and expectations for the sexual behavior of males and females. More specifically, females are expected to show more sexual restraint than males (Crawford & Popp, 2003). According to the sexual double standard, males are praised and rewarded for the same behavior that stigmatizes females.

Traditional Western norms about premarital sexual behavior strongly emphasize the importance of female virginity. Going as far back as pre-Christian Greece, there was a framework of social law in which females were expected to remain virgin until they married (Blank, 2007), while males were

In the following story, one young woman describes her feelings about a girl who had sex with many boys, and how those feelings changed now that she is older.

IN THEIR OWN WORDS

One of my good friends in high school, a friend I have to this day, engaged in a lot of sexual activity. At least, that was what she told us. Her sexual experiences, while she had several steady boyfriends throughout school, were often outside the contexts of a steady, monogamous relationship. The rest of us girls weren't always sure whether to believe what she told us, but we certainly judged her as dirty.

What I now realize is that I never thought about the behavior of the boys she was with. I didn't think of it as a negative or positive thing; it simply never entered my train of thought. If nothing else, we often felt bad for the guys she dated because we thought she would eventually cheat on them. And it certainly never occurred to me that my friend enjoyed sex and did it for her own pleasure. My friends and I thought she only behaved this way to get attention from boys (she had daddy issues too, naturally).

What was interesting, at least in my experience, was that none of us ever really asked her more about her behavior. We weren't interested in the details, like how it felt, what was good technique, how he tasted. And we definitely never asked her about her motives for being "easy." Perhaps we didn't feel that her opinions or explanations were "real" because how could someone who behaves in this "bad" way ever have something valuable to offer.

Ten years later, as a proud feminist and advocate of sex-positive attitudes, I'm regretful that I judged my friend negatively. Whatever her motives for having a lot of sex (both oral and intercourse), whether she had genuine desire, wanted to be liked, or was trying to fill the void left by her abusive father—all are valid and she deserved support. I imagine being a "slut" in high school, while having the attention of the partner for a limited time, is probably incredibly lonely. I also certainly never considered that she had ever been coerced or forced to have sex.

granted more sexual freedom. There is little evidence that adolescents today expect females to remain virgin until they marry, at least among most youth in Western societies. Remnants of this traditional standard continue to exist in some cultures, however, such as in India (Saraswathi & Pai, 1997) and among some traditional Latino (Bouris et al., 2012) and African American (Fasula, Miller, & Wiener, 2007) parents and adolescents in the United States.

Do Adolescents and Emerging Adults Subscribe to the Sexual Double Standard?

Do adolescents and emerging adults have different standards of sexual conduct for boys and girls? Age matters, and the sexual double standard is more common among teens, especially younger teens than among emerging adults.

For example, evidence for a sexual double standard was found among early and middle adolescents who become sexually active. Peer acceptance increases for boys who become sexually active, while sexual initiation among girls is asso-ciated with a decrease in peer acceptance (Kreager, Staff, Gauthier, Lefkowitz, & Feinberg, 2016). Data for this study come from two rural communities in the United States, which may have more traditional gender role standards than nonrural settings, raising the possibility that a sexual double standard may be more common in conservative communities than in more liberal settings, espe-cially among young adolescents.

In another study, researchers uncovered evidence of a double standard for teens with many sexual partners (Kreager & Staff, 2009). In this study of ado-lescents in grades 7–12, girls with many partners have lower social status among both girls and boys than girls with a few number of partners. In contrast, a boy's social status is higher among other boys, but not among girls, for boys with many sexual partners. At the other end of the scale, virgin girls have higher status than virgin boys. Thus, having many sexual partners jeopardizes a girl's popularity, but enhances a boy's popularity, at least among other boys.

Evidence from one middle school indicates that negative terms such as *sluts, bitches,* and *whores* are common for girls who initiate sex (Eder, 1995). Many adolescents still use the term *easy* to describe a girl who has many sex partners. There is no parallel term for boys, who are often considered "studs" for the same behaviors used to stigmatize girls.

In 1996, Martin argued that many aspects of the traditional sexual double standard are disappearing, especially among U.S. emerging adults. According to Martin, young women are no longer labeled "sluts" simply for having sex. Recent quantitative research on emerging adults validates the idea that merely having sex does not damage the reputation of a young woman, but young women who have sex with many partners do put their reputations at risk (Alli-son & Risman, 2013).

There has been a historical decline, but not a complete disappearance, of the double standard among American college students when it is measured as the attitudes students have about the sexual behavior of others. The majority of both males and females do not endorse a traditional sexual double standard that allows males to have sex, but discourages females from having sex (Allison & Risman, 2013; Marks & Fraley, 2005). Some remnants of the double standard continue to exist, however, especially about casual sex (Sakaluk & Milhausen, 2012). College students of both genders report that it is equally acceptable for men and women to have sex in a committed relationship, but students are more accepting of male casual sex than female casual sex (Sprecher, Treger, & Sakaluk, 2013). Thus, although contemporary emerging adults generally reject a traditional double standard, they do expect females to be more sexually restrained than males and to have fewer casual sex partners.

In general, sexual standards are no different for male and female emerg-ing adults in romantic relationships, where sexual intercourse is as accepted for young women as for young men. A double standard continues to exist for young women who have casual sex, sex with many partners, and initiate sex, all of which are associated with a higher negative evaluation of young women in comparison to young men (Bordini & Sperb, 2013; Crawford & Popp, 2003).

Who Endorses the Sexual Double Standard?

Not all adolescents espouse a sexual double standard. What are some of the characteristics of adolescents who support and accept the idea that males should be allowed more sexual freedom than females? Gender matters, and boys are more likely to believe in a traditional double standard than girls, perhaps because boys reap the most benefit from the double standard, which accepts and even encourages sexual exploration among boys (Emmerink, Vanwesenbeeck, van den Eijnden, & ter Bogt, 2016). In addition, religious adolescents are more likely to endorse a sexual double standard than nonreligious youth, and this is especially true for religious boys. In general, a sexual double standard is part of a larger religious belief structure that endorses traditional gender roles and prescribes modesty and sexual restraint for females. Last, adolescents who have traditional gender role beliefs are likely to endorse a sexual double standard as part of those beliefs (Lyons, Giordano, Manning, & Longmore, 2011).

■ DEVIANT PEER GROUPS AND RISKY SEXUAL BEHAVIOR

What Is the Relationship between Membership in a Deviant Peer Group and Risky Sexual Behavior?

There is a type of peer group that deserves special mention because of its strong and pervasive association with many adolescent norm-breaking behaviors. That group is referred to as a *deviant peer group,* which comprises adolescents who engage in illegal and unhealthy behaviors, such as juvenile delinquency, alcohol and drug use, and risky sex that includes sex at an early age, multiple partners, and inconsistent contraceptive use (Crockett, Bingham, Chopak, & Vicary, 1996; Tubman, Windle, & Windle, 1996). Results from studies of adolescents in deviant peer groups support *problem behavior theory* (Jessor, 2014), which posits that delinquency, substance use, and risky sexual activity form a triad of problem behaviors such that the presence of one often indicates the presence of the other two, especially during early adolescence.

The relationship between membership in a deviant peer group and risky adolescent sexual behavior is not only present in the United States but is also found in other countries, such as South Africa where deviant peer groups have been studied (Brook, Morojele, Zhang, & Brook, 2006). Members of deviant peer groups in South Africa, as in the United States, are rebellious, impulsive, delinquent, and involved in risky sexual activity, which consists of having a high number of sexual partners, frequently having sex with a partner who is drunk or high, and inconsistently using condoms.

Some girls rebel against cultural norms by pushing the limit of sexual activity and substance use, as the following story reveals.

IN THEIR OWN WORDS

In my high school, although we had a very solid health education program, the students were more promiscuous than most. Breaking news about who had just hooked up with who were very common, and the pregnancy rate of girls was quite high, especially in my grade. Something that stuck out to me, however, was the importance of the number of sex partners. I remember having this discussion with several of my friends, and we always had our numbers ready and waiting to be judged. My best friend at the time had a very clear system for judging people based on their number. Between zero and two was permissible for freshmen and sophomores, but was too low for juniors or seniors. A number higher than five was most acceptable. This system spread to the members of our peer group, who also started to use the system. Also, at least with most members of my peer group, higher numbers were judged as better. I believe the reason for this is because my peer group prided itself on being "above the curve" in terms of having participated in a variety of deviant behavior, from drinking and drug use to music genres. Everyone wanted to be able to brag about having tried different deviant or unique behaviors before others. The goal was to not fit in with normal society. This probably drives up the competition to want to have a higher number.

Why Is Membership in a Deviant Peer Group Related to Risky Sexual Behavior?

Well-functioning youth do not suddenly become members of deviant peer groups during adolescence and begin engaging in risky sexual behavior. Membership in a deviant peer group along with risky sexual behavior is the result of a pattern of deviant behavior that first appears in early childhood. The path toward risky sexual behavior can begin with conduct problems in early childhood, followed by deficient parental socialization that leads to inadequate impulse control and poor school performance. These difficult-to-manage middle school children often are rejected by nondeviant peers who find one another and form deviant peer groups in which antisocial behavior and early substance use is common. With the awakening of the sexual drive at puberty, these norm-breaking young adolescents are drawn into risky sexual activity, which often leads to an early pregnancy or contracting an STI (Boislard, Poulin, Kiesner, & Dishion, 2009; Capaldi et al., 2002; Dishion et al., 2012).

The authors of one study of Mexican-origin students attending school in Phoenix, Arizona, identified an important characteristic of teens who become members of gangs and who engage in risky sex. Gangs and deviant peer groups are similar in many ways, but gangs have a more formal structure. The researchers examined what they referred to as the *compensation hypothesis*, which is that adolescents with distant, unloving parents look to peers for the support and closeness they do not get at home (Killoren, Updegraff, Christopher, &

Umaña-Taylor, 2011). The authors report that adolescents with cold, distant parents are especially susceptible to peer overtures to become members of gangs that give adolescents the sense of belonging they do not receive at home. Gang membership is related to problematic behavior, including risky sex (Goldstein, Davis-Kean, & Eccles, 2005).

Being a member of a deviant peer group not only is related to risky sexual behavior during adolescence but is also a predictor of risky sexual behavior in emerging adulthood (Lansford, Dodge, Fontaine, Bates, & Pettit, 2014). Risky sexual behavior expressed and reinforced by peers in deviant peer groups during adolescence often endure into emerging adulthood and can lead to an STI or an early pregnancy (Dishion et al., 2012).

What Can Be Done to Decrease the Power of Deviant Peers on Teen Sex?

Research on deviant peer groups shows that risky sex during adolescence rarely occurs in isolation from other unhealthy behaviors, but is part of a constellation of problem behaviors that includes substance use and delinquency. Effective sexuality education programs for high-risk children and teens, especially those living in dangerous neighborhoods with many deviant peers, not only need to focus on delaying the onset of sexual behavior and increasing compliance with safe-sex procedures but also on decreasing involvement with deviant peers. Programs that help high-risk children and teens learn to control their emotions, focus on the future, and resist peer pressure may lead to a decrease in deviant peer group membership, which is the key to lowering rates of risky sexual behavior, substance use, and delinquency. In addition, programs for parents need to help parents maintain a close, supportive relationship with their teens. Further, parent interventions need to teach parents how to better supervise and monitor their teens as a way of discouraging their adolescents from spending time with deviant friends, while at the same time encouraging teens to become friends with nondeviant teens. In an ideal world, prevention programs designed to decrease risky sexual behavior among high-risk adolescents would be broad-based interventions that include techniques to resist peer pressure, improve social skills, and enhance school performance, along with helping parents improve their parenting skills.

SUMMARY

■ ADOLESCENTS TALKING TO ADOLESCENTS ABOUT SEX

Adolescents in the United States indicate that they learn more about sex from peers than from parents, but they also think that parents have a stronger influence on them than do peers, making a crucial distinction between knowledge and behavior. Two reasons why adolescents talk to peers rather than their parents about sex include the following: they view peers as more liberal and open-minded, and they believe peers are more trustworthy. Adolescents who typically talk to peers about sex have more liberal attitudes about sex than adolescents who more usually talk to parents. One group for whom peers may not be a major source of information about sex is LGBTQ adolescents, who get more information about sex from the Internet, pornography, and older adults.

■ PEER INFLUENCE AND ADOLESCENT SEXUALITY

Many adolescents report that they think the sexual behavior of their peers is influenced by peer pressure, although they do not think peer pressure has a major effect on their own sexual behavior. Peer influence certainly exists, but people overestimate its power, and view it as stronger than it actually is. Adolescents are more likely to succumb to peer influence if they are already leaning in the direction of engaging in the behavior.

■ PEER ASSOCIATION AND ADOLESCENT SEXUALITY

Two reasons why peers share similar attitudes about sex include the following: adolescents select other adolescents as friends based on similarity of attitudes, and peers socialize each other toward similar beliefs. Social learning theory suggests that peers model certain attitudes and behaviors and reinforce each other for those attitudes and behaviors. Social norm theory is based on the idea that adolescents want to be accepted by their peers, which leads to conformity to peer standards.

■ POPULARITY AND SEXUAL BEHAVIOR

Popular adolescents are more sexually active than other adolescents. Popularity precedes sexual activity for boys and girls. Sexual activity increases the social status of boys, especially among other boys, but it does not lead to an increase in popularity among girls. Crowds are groups of students perceived to be similar in some defining way. Sexual activity is more common in some crowds than in others.

■ THE SEXUAL DOUBLE STANDARD

According to the double standard, males are given more sexual freedom than females. In the United States, a girl's reputation is not ruined if she has sex, especially in a romantic relationship, but boys are allowed to have more casual sexual partners than females. Adolescents who are most likely to endorse a double standard are boys, religious adolescents, and youth who have traditional gender role beliefs.

■ DEVIANT PEER GROUPS AND RISKY SEXUAL BEHAVIOR

Deviant peer groups comprise adolescents who engage in illegal and unhealthy behaviors. Being in a deviant peer group is related to involvement in risky sex that includes early sexual activity, many partners, and inconsistent contraceptive use. Risky sex often is part of a cluster of problem behaviors that include substance use and delinquency, a finding that supports problem behavior theory, which predicts that these three problem behaviors often occur together. Membership in a deviant peer group is predictive of problem behavior in general, and of risky sexual activity in particular.

SUGGESTIONS FOR FURTHER READING

Allison, R., & Risman, B. J. (2013). A double standard for "hooking up": How far have we come toward gender equality? *Social Science Research, 42,* 1191–1206.

Buhi, E. R., & Goodson, P. (2007). Predictors of adolescent sexual behavior and intention: A theory-guided systematic review. *Journal of Adolescent Health, 40,* 4–21.

Dishion, T. J., Ha, T., & Véronneau, M. H. (2012). An ecological analysis of the effects of deviant peer clustering on sexual promiscuity, problem behavior, and childbearing from early adolescence to adulthood: An enhancement of the life history framework. *Developmental Psychology, 48,* 703–717.

Henry, D. B., Schoeny, M. E., Deptula, D. P., & Slavick, J. T. (2007). Peer selection and socialization effects on adolescent intercourse without a condom and attitudes about the costs of sex. *Child Development, 78,* 825–838.

Sieving, R. E., Eisenberg, M. E., Pettingell, S., & Skay, C. (2006). Friends' influence on adolescents' first sexual intercourse. *Perspectives on Sexual and Reproductive Health, 38,* 13–19.

CHAPTER 6

Dating, Romance, and Hooking Up

D o adolescents still date, or has dating disappeared into the recesses of the 1950s and earlier? Dating during adolescence is common, but terms such as *hanging out,* or *going out with someone* have replaced the term *dating* for most adolescents (Collins et al., 2009). Although the term *dating* may be falling into disuse among adolescents, the functions of dating remain, even among the digital generation for whom Facebook, Texting, Instagram, and Snapchat have become important forms of social interaction (Eaton, Rose, Interligi, Fernandez, & McHugh, 2016).

■ DATING AMONG ADOLESCENTS AND EMERGING ADULTS

What Has Happened to Dating?

Dating serves many different functions, including romance, recreation, companionship, raising one's social status, improving relationship skills, sexual behavior, and courtship. A dating relationship is an opportunity for adolescents to spend time with a potential or current romantic partner and, at least among heterosexuals, is a developmental turning point in relations with peers of the opposite sex (O'Sullivan, Cheng, Harris, & Brooks-Gunn, 2007). A boy–girl friendship during childhood may turn into a dating relationship and eventually into a romantic relationship during adolescence.

Parents always have been apprehensive about the dating behavior of their adolescents: nervous about teens pairing up too soon in a steady relationship and worried that dating may lead to sex (Weigel, 2016). Parent admonitions about the dangers of dating and their advice to avoid a steady, exclusive relationship have been common parent warnings to their adolescents for as long as teens have been going out together. Long before today's concerns about the hookup culture, parents were worried about teenage "parking" and "petting parties," legitimate concerns during a time when teen pregnancies and teen marriages were much more common than they are today.

Older adolescents are more likely to date than younger adolescents, although a substantial percentage of teens have never dated, ranging from about 60% of 8th graders to about 40% of 12th graders (Child Trends, 2015b). Surprisingly, the percentage of 12th graders who have not gone on a date has been increasing since the early 1980s. Some of this historical difference may be due to changing definitions of the term *dating,* but adolescents today are less likely to pair up in a dating relationship than in times past, and more likely to engage in group dating and casual relationships.

There is much cultural variation in heterosexual dating among U.S. adolescents. For example, African American youth are less likely to date than white and Hispanic adolescents. Further, many Asian American parents view adolescents' developing interest in the opposite sex as inappropriate, and believe

---

In the following story, one young woman describes the progression of a relationship from first meeting, to "talking," to "Facebook official," to seduction and breakup.

IN THEIR OWN WORDS

During high school, I dated a boy named Y. for about 2 years. We met through some mutual friends and started texting soon after that. Then came the awkward "we're talking" period. This meant we were more than friends, but not dating yet. However, we weren't seeing other people at the time. We would hang out with large groups of people or meet up at parties. Very rarely would we go on a date as just a couple. The whole idea sounds incredibly stupid, but in high school, it was what you did.

Anyways, we started officially dating very quickly after "talking." This meant we were Facebook official and everyone would know we were together. At this time I was very excited, considering this was the first real relationship I had had. Now we started going out alone much more frequently. We would go to movies, dinner, or each other's house.

Entering the relationship, I was a virgin and he was not. Initially, I thought he may be the one who I'd first have sex with, but quickly changed my mind after becoming bored with the relationship. Y. would ask if/when we were going to do it and I simply kept replying, "I'm just not ready." After some time he started to try more smoothly. His favorite attempt was "Let's watch a movie in the basement on the big screen." I'd agree and we would go downstairs. After about 10 minutes he'd complain of the glare on the TV and turn off the lights. Next thing I'd know I was getting a back rub and kisses on my neck. After a couple of minutes I'd thank him and then say some bullshit line such as "My legs are sore from soccer, I need to stretch out more," and then I'd go sprawl out on the opposite couch. Similar events went on for a good while until I finally ended the relationship because I had found someone else.

that dating during adolescence leads to sex and early marriage. Many Asian American adolescents, especially girls, are forbidden to date (Brotto, Chik, Ryder, Gorzalka, & Seal, 2005). Academic excellence is emphasized and dating is seen as a distraction (Kim & Ward, 2007). According to one 16-year-old Asian American boy:

> "You are allowed to have friends that are girls, but you are not allowed to go out until you graduate college or until you are from 25 to 30ish. You cannot talk to any girls. I mean you can talk to girls, they can be your friends, but they can never be more than that." (Lau, Markham, Lin, Flores, & Chacko, 2009, p. 104)

What Do We Know about Youth Who Start to Date at an Early Age?

Early maturation sets the stage for early dating, which is even more likely to occur if the adolescents are risk takers and extraverted (Ivanova, Veenstra, & Mills, 2012). In addition, adolescents who are early daters are more likely to have parents who are divorced, whom adolescents perceive as rejecting, and who are poor monitors (Ivanova, Mills, & Veenstra, 2011). Last, early daters have friends who are also dating and who tend to be involved in delinquent activities, including early sexual behavior (Friedlander, Connolly, Pepler, & Craig, 2007). In general, the early development of secondary sexual characteristics among adolescents who are risk takers, have poor relations with their parents, and have friends who engage in unconventional behavior puts adolescents on a path that includes early dating and early sexual debut (Zimmer-Gembeck & Collins, 2008).

What Is the Relation between Dating and Sex?

Sexual intercourse is considerably more common between adolescents who are dating than between teens who are not dating, and even more common if the adolescents are in some type of steady, exclusive relationship (Cooksey, Mott, & Neubauer, 2002; Zimmer-Gembeck, Siebenbruner, & Collins, 2004). Sexual activity among adolescents often occurs in an exclusive, romantic relationship, not only in the United States but also in other countries as well, such as Mexico, where premarital sex is rare (Espinosa-Hernández & Vasilenko, 2015).

What Predicts Early Sexual Activity among Dating Adolescents?

Two of the strongest predictors of whether adolescents in a dating relationship will have sexual intercourse are when both adolescents are nonvirgins at the beginning of the relationship and when both adolescents want to have sex (Cleveland, 2003). In addition, two adolescents are more likely to have sexual intercourse if the female drinks alcohol and has a history of rebellious behavior.

Further, the association between each characteristic and sexual intercourse is especially strong when both partners possess the same sexual risk characteristic (e.g., when both partners are nonvirgins or both drink alcohol).

Another factor related to whether two adolescents in a dating relationship have sexual intercourse is the gap in ages between the two youth. It is more common for girls who date boys much older than themselves to have sex than girls who date boys close to their own age (Morrison-Beedy, Xia, & Passmore, 2013; Oudekerk, Guarnera, & Reppucci, 2014). It may be that girls who date older boys are more likely to be drawn into an older peer group where sex is expected and more common. Older boys, more than younger boys, are also more likely to be nonvirgins who expect a dating relationship to be sexual. The

In the following story, one young woman describes the relationship she had with an older boyfriend and the effect it had on her. Note that his older friends became her friends, exposing her to an older peer group and the behaviors that exist in that type of group.

IN THEIR OWN WORDS

Living in a single-parent household, money was tight, so when we were struggling financially, I applied as a cashier at our local grocery store to help with the bills. I hated it. The uniforms were ugly, the customers were annoying, and my boss was rude. I made friends with a few people who made work more enjoyable but I noticed this one boy was always staring at me. In high school, I was friends with many guys but that was it—we were friends. So when this guy kept staring at me I was intrigued. As I continued to get more comfortable with my new job, I stopped being shy and learned more about this boy. Turns out he is 22, a senior at the university, and plays soccer. I mean he could not be a better match for me! We somehow exchanged cell phone numbers and I literally had my phone attached to my hip at all times texting him. We went out on numerous dates, but I was so hesitant to make it official. I knew he was more experienced in the dating world than I was. I was intimidated. I mean he was 3 years older than me! At first I thought it was weird he was interested in a high school senior. Why wasn't he interested in girls his own age? But I could not blame him; my senior year was such a great year.

I may have been seen as valuable catch to him. However, at the same time, the fact that a 22-year-old liked a high school senior made me feel special.

In the summer going into my freshman year at the university, we finally became an official couple. My boyfriend had already gone through the freshman partying stage and he was of drinking age so I was influenced to go out more than usual. He exposed me to new situations I would have never put myself into before. But with my older boyfriend, who already went through this stage of his life, I trusted him that I would be safe. During my freshman year of college, my friends were his older friends. I rarely met anyone my own age.

He was my first serious boyfriend. Being 3 years older, he was obviously more sexually experienced then I was and that scared me to death. I often compared myself to his ex-girlfriends and I became obsessed with trying to impress him. Many of my first sexual experiences were with him and I think it is due to the fact I felt pressured not to seem as young as I was. I had to keep up with him and at the same time fit in with his older peers. I had to be seen as older.

wider the age gap, the more likely it is that sex will occur, and the less likely it is that the pair will use some form of protection against pregnancy and STIs (Swartzendruber et al., 2013). In addition, girls in a dating relationship are more likely to be victimized—emotionally, physically, and sexually—by older boys than by boys close to their own age. Further, girls with older male partners are more likely to be depressed and involved in risky behaviors such as drinking alcohol, using drugs, and delinquency, all of which are related to early sexual activity (Young & d'Arcy, 2005).

■ ROMANTIC RELATIONSHIPS

What Is a Romantic Relationship?

Researchers have defined *romantic relationships* and measured them in several different ways. Building on the work of Robert Sternberg (2004), Connolly and her colleagues found that young adolescents defined a romantic relationship as including three components—intimacy, passion, and commitment (Connolly, Craig, Goldberg, & Pepler, 1999). Intimacy includes feelings of attachment, closeness, and connectedness; passion encompasses sexual attraction; and commitment includes a decision to remain together.

Some researchers studying adolescent romantic relationships use definitions of romantic relationships that are based on behavior. For example, in the National Longitudinal Study of Adolescent Health (Add Health), researchers use a behavioral definition of a romantic relationship that includes the following four behaviors in the past 18 months: held hands with someone who is not a member of your family, kissed someone on the mouth who is not a member of your family, told someone who is not a member of your family that you liked or loved them and did these things with the same person (e.g., Meier & Allen, 2009).

Other researchers emphasize the idea that a true romantic relationship is a mutual relationship in which both people agree that a romantic relationship exists (Collins & van Dulmen, 2014). A discrepancy between two people about whether they are in a romantic relationship is called *relational asymmetry,* which is common among teens, since many adolescent relationships are short-lived and characterized by volatile feelings that can change quickly (Giordano, Manning, & Longmore, 2014).

Another perspective on romantic relationships is to differentiate them from friendships. Giordano and colleagues (2014) describe three features that differentiate adolescent romantic relationships from friendships. First, romantic relationships during adolescence often include social and communication *awkwardness,* in comparison to friendships. Second, romantic relationships have heightened *emotionality* attached to feelings such as love and jealousy. Third, *exclusivity* is more common in romantic relationships than in friendships; one can have many friends, but only one romantic relationship.

All of these definitional approaches are useful attempts to define what is a fuzzy concept, but which includes a core idea of a special emotional connection to another person. None of these definitions mention gender, since romantic relationships are as much a part of LGBTQ communities as they are of the heterosexual community.

How Common Are Romantic Relationships among Adolescents?

The percentage of adolescents who report that they had a romantic relationship in the past 18 months increases from about 27% among 12-year-olds to about 73% among 18-year-olds (Carver, Joyner, & Udry, 2003). Asian Americans are considerably less likely to have a romantic relationship than adolescents of other races and ethnicities. About 2% of boys and 4% of girls report a same-sex romantic relationship.

The duration of heterosexual romantic relationships is dependent on the age of the adolescents, lasting about 5 months for adolescents under the age of 14 years and about 21 months among adolescents over the age of 16 years. Although African American adolescents are less likely to be in a romantic relationship than white adolescents, romantic relationships between African American adolescents are more stable than romantic relationships for other races and ethnicities, lasting over 24 months.

What Effect Does Timing of First Sexual Intercourse Have on Romantic Relationships?

Is it better for two people to get to know each other before they have sex or to have sex early in a relationship in order to test for sexual compatibility? Emerging adults who have sex before they begin dating or early in their relationship are less satisfied with their relationships, have poorer communication, and have less stable relationships than couples that wait longer to have sex (Harden, 2012; Willoughby, Carroll, & Busby, 2014). The findings support the idea of *sexual restraint,* which is that couples that delay sexual involvement until they really get to know each other are more likely to have more satisfying relationships, including better sexual relations, than couples that have sex early in their relationship (Busby, Carroll, & Willoughby, 2010).

It is not clear why a delay in sexual activity is associated with a good relationship. One possibility is that couples that have sex early in their relationship may later discover that they are personally and socially incompatible with their partner, a discovery that leads to relationship problems and eventual breakup. Another possibility is that individuals who wait to have sex possess characteristics such as emotional self-regulation that have a positive effect on general relationship quality (Shulman, Seiffge-Krenke, & Walsh, 2017). Whatever the explanation for the value of sexual delay, waiting to have sex is an advantage for adolescents and emerging adults in romantic relationships.

Do Parents Have an Effect on Romantic Relationships?

Parents have a major influence on the ages when adolescents first start to date, form a romantic relationship, and have sexual intercourse. Parents who approve of early dating have adolescents who reach each of these relationship milestones earlier than adolescents with parents who do not approve of early dating (Bouris et al., 2012).

Positive parent–child relations are associated with a delay in the ages when adolescents begin to date, form a romantic relationship, and have sex, while negative relations with parents are linked to an earlier achievement of each of these relationship events (de Graaf et al., 2011; Walper & Wendt, 2015). In particular, when the emotional bond between parents and adolescents is weak, referred to as low *family cohesion,* adolescents often begin dating, enter into romantic relations, and have sex earlier than when family cohesion is strong. When parent–adolescent cohesion is weak, adolescents may seek the closeness they do not get at home from a romantic partner, leading to an intense emotional connection and early sexual relations. This scenario is especially true for early adolescent females, but less true for older females and males of all ages for whom parents have less of an influence on dating, romance, and sex (de Graaf, van de Schoot, Woertman, Hawk, & Meeus, 2012).

Family stress is another family factor related to the early formation of romantic relations and to early sexual intercourse. Among young girls, family

Even if parents are strict, two teens who want to have sex will find a place to have sex, as the following story told by a young woman demonstrates.

IN THEIR OWN WORDS

When I was 17, my parents had moved to Z. and I remained in our hometown in W. to finish out the school year. I was living at a friend's house and rules were much stricter there than I had ever experienced before, but it wouldn't have been a big problem if I hadn't just started dating my new boyfriend. His parents were also very strict so we had a really difficult time engaging in any sort of sexual behavior. Determined to be together, we would lie to the adults in charge of us (usually telling them we were at the town library) and go to an old graveyard that was on top of a hill and surrounded by trees. No one ever came there, especially not at 3 in the afternoon on a weekday, so we thought we were alone. We thought we were so clever. At least twice a week we would sneak off and have sex. One day we were

there and one of us, I can't remember who, realized that there was a car pulling into the graveyard. We got up immediately, pulled all our clothes back on, and got in my boyfriend's car. As we drove away, we saw the car pull up to the same gravestone we'd just been up against and an elderly couple get out and put flowers at it. Based on the date on the gravestone, it probably belonged to that couple's son, who likely died in the first Gulf War.

Thinking about this story now, I'm absolutely horrified at my actions, even though I know my boyfriend and I laughed about it at the time. It is still a bit funny to think about how desperate my boyfriend and I were to have sex and the lengths we went to in order to do so.

stress is associated with feelings of low self-worth, social isolation, low positive affect, and high negative affect, all characteristics of depression, which predicts early involvement in a romantic relationship and early sexual activity (Davila et al., 2009). These findings are consistent with the idea that some adolescents, especially girls, attempt to cope with depression caused by family stress by seeking support and validation from a romantic partner, which often leads to early sexual intercourse. Taken together, these results suggest that low family emotional support and high family stress are associated with the formation of romantic relations and early sexual debut, especially for females.

■ DATING AND ROMANCE AMONG LGBTQ ADOLESCENTS

More than 20 years ago, Ritch Savin-Williams (1994), a psychologist at Cornell University, wrote a chapter about dating and romantic relationships among lesbian, gay, and bisexual adolescents, provocatively entitled "Dating Those You Can't Love and Loving Those You Can't Date." The point of the title and the purpose of the chapter was to describe the dilemma many LGBTQ adolescents face as they navigate through the complicated social scene of most U.S. middle schools and high schools. In most U.S. schools, LGBTQ adolescents have two realistic social options: date adolescents of the opposite sex or not date at all. Although LGBTQ youth are more visible and accepted by the straight community today than ever before, victimization, prejudice, and social harassment remain problems for many LGBTQ youth, problems that discourage same-sex dating (Diamond, Savin-Williams, & Dubé, 1999). In fact, few adolescents who are attracted to same-sex individuals have romantic relationships during adolescence, which typically do not emerge until after graduation from high school (Hu, Xu, & Tornello, 2016). The proliferation of school-based gay support groups such as gay–straight alliances, have improved social relations for many LGBTQ students, but problems remain, especially for students in small schools, rural areas, and conservative communities. As a result of realistic fears of bullying and retribution, not only from schoolmates but also from friends and family, many LGBTQ adolescents conceal their true feelings for someone of the same sex and form friendships with individuals of the opposite sex, which may lead to pretend dating and to the appearance of "normality."

What Are Some Characteristics of LGBTQ Romantic Relationships?

LGBTQ dating and romantic relationships do not suddenly appear with the onset of puberty and passage into early adolescence. Instead, same-sex sexual and romantic behaviors emerge gradually throughout adolescence into emerging adulthood. In one study of *sexual milestones,* which are the first time a romantic or sexual behavior appears, two sequences were identified: one for young men who had sexual experiences only with females, and one for young men who had sexual experiences only with males (Smiler, Frankel, & Savin-Williams, 2011). The sequence of sexual milestones for female-exclusive men and the ages when they typically occurred was kissing (13.8 years), sexual touching (15.9 years), and intercourse (17.8 years); while the sequence for male-exclusive men and the average ages was sexual touching (15.9 years), intercourse (16.1 years), and kissing (16.6 years). Note that male-exclusive men experienced first intercourse before female-exclusive men, but first kiss was almost 3 years later than female-exclusive men. The authors speculate that the sexual behavior of female-exclusive men often follows the establishment of a romantic relationship, while the sexual behavior of male-exclusive men frequently precedes the establishment of a romantic relationship. This difference may reflect the strong sexual interests of two males in a male–male relationship, while male–female relationships reveal more of a balance between male sexual yearning and female desire for a relationship.

Several characteristics of romantic relationships were identified in another study of mainly gay white males (Savin-Williams, 1998b). First, it is rare for a friendship to turn into a romantic relationship, which more typically occurs with a new acquaintance or with someone the adolescent has just met. Second, some kind of sexual behavior often occurs on the first or second date. Third, gay males report that their first romantic relationship occurs about the time they turn 18 years of age. Fourth, most romantic relationships last less than 3 months.

Gay couples often cite infidelity as a problem in gay romantic relationships, which can lead one partner to become highly possessive of the other partner (Eyre, Milbrath, & Peacock, 2007). As one young African American gay adolescent recounted:

> "My most serious boyfriend would have to be the first person I was with sexually for two years, and it was good. . . . But he cheated on me. . . . One day when I got [home], he was in bed with somebody. I couldn't even speak . . . I saw them kissing and everything. . . . My first reaction was to run to the kitchen. I picked up a knife. I was just trying to cut somebody." (Eyre et al., 2007, p. 124)

In another study, about half of gay, adult African American men reported that they had an agreement with their partner to remain monogamous, although two-thirds reported that they had affairs since the beginning of the current relationship (Peplau, Cochran, & Mays, 1997).

What Are Some Sexual Risks for LGBTQ Adolescents in Romantic Relationships?

In which type of situation are YMSM more likely to acquire a new HIV infection: sex between two young men who have just met, or sex between two young men in a romantic relationship? The surprising answer is that sex between men in a romantic relationship has more risk than sex between new acquaintances

(Sullivan, Salazar, Buchbinder, & Sanchez, 2009). The main reason for the difference is that YMSM in romantic relationships are less likely to use a condom when they have anal intercourse than two new acquaintances (Newcomb & Mustanski, 2016). In fact, the probability of using a condom decreases as the length of the relationship increases (Newcomb, Ryan, Garofalo, & Mustanski, 2014).

There are several reasons why YMSM stop using condoms once they enter into a serious, long-term relationship: first, one partner may perceive condom use by the other partner as an expression of a lack of trust (Mustanski, Newcomb, & Clerkin, 2011); second, condoms reduce pleasure (Mustanski, DuBois, Prescott, & Ybarra, 2014); and third, the perception of the two partners that a monogamous relationship protects the partners from contracting an STI (Greene, Andrews, Kuper, & Mustanski, 2014). Unfortunately, many HIV-infected YMSM are unaware they are infected and unknowingly put their partner at risk (Centers for Disease Control and Prevention, 2013).

■ CASUAL SEX, HOOKUPS, AND FRIENDS WITH BENEFITS

Have college students today gone wild, living in a world of alcohol-infused parties and sexual nights with people whose names the students may not know and with people they may never see again? This is certainly the view some have of the college scene from mass media reports of modern campus life (Taylor, 2013). But how true is it?

Casual sex has been around since time immemorial. People, especially the young, have been pairing off at bars and parties to have one-night stands for a long time. Casual sex did not suddenly appear in the 2000s (Garcia, Reiber, Massey, & Merriwether, 2012; Monto & Carey, 2014). The claim by some commentators and researchers, however, is that a seismic shift has occurred in relations between young men and women (Adshade, 2013; Bogle, 2008). As stated by Kalish and Kimmel (2011), "Today, American campus culture is not about dating to find an appropriate mate; it's more about mating to find an appropriate date!" (p. 139).

According to some reporters, hooking up has replaced traditional dating as the typical setting in which young men and women meet and initiate sex. Whereas in the past people would meet, date, begin a romantic relationship, and then possibly have sex, today, according to some, the traditional sequence has been reversed and now follows a pattern of meeting, having sex, possibly dating, and occasionally becoming romantically involved.

Several perspectives exist about the sex lives of contemporary emerging adults, especially college students. On the one hand, there are those who see a moral breakdown among college students who are part of a hookup culture fueled by alcohol in which sex takes place between people who know little about each other and may not even know each other's names (Rosin, 2012).

A FOCUS ON RESEARCH

Studying hookups brings to the forefront a fundamental issue that all social science researchers must address in their research, which is to clearly define the variables being investigated. In order to study the occurrence of hookups, for example, a researcher must define *hookup* clearly, precisely, and in a way that validly captures the meaning of the term as it is generally used. Males and females, students of different ages, and students who attend different universities all must share the same definition of hookup, otherwise results from studies cannot be compared. Asking college students a question such as "Have you had a hookup experience in the past month?" on a questionnaire may appear to be a straightforward question, but it is not if hooking up means sexual intercourse to one group of students, while passionate kissing qualifies as a hookup for another group. Ambiguity about the meaning of the term *hookup* may partly explain gender differences in reports of hookups.

Defining variables can be a problem in any area of social science research, and it is clearly a problem in the study of adolescent sexuality. Consider the following examples: What does *date* mean in the question "Have you been on a date in the past month?"; What does it mean to ask a question such as "Have you ever been in a romantic relationship?" Even a question as apparently straightforward as "Have you ever had sexual intercourse?" may have multiple meanings for people, especially middle school children who may not fully understand the phrase *sexual intercourse*. Clearly defining variables is a critical first step in any research study, especially when a variable may be ambiguous or have multiple meanings. How variables are defined and how they are understood by respondents can have a major effect on study results.

Then there are those who believe that the hookup culture is a victory for promiscuous male sexuality over female relational sex, to the detriment of females who are abandoned to a walk of shame after a night of hot, no-strings-attached sex (Regnerus & Uecker, 2011). On the other hand, there are those who view the new sexuality as an indication of how far women have come, who are now focused on their education and careers, uninterested in the complicated confusion of a relationship, but who enjoy the physical pleasure of temporary sexual connection (Kalish & Kimmel, 2011). Which perspective, if any, is accurate?

What Does It Mean to Hook Up?

Hooking up is a slang term that came into existence in the early 2000s. The phrase is not clearly defined, even by the people who use it. Hooking up generally refers to having sexual intercourse with someone you just met and may never see again, but it can also mean something less than intercourse, such as kissing, or "fooling around," which includes sexual touching, or oral sex (Garcia et al., 2012). A group of friends may have a shared meaning of what hooking up means in their group, but that definition may be different for emerging adults in another group.

One reason why the definition of a hookup is vague is that it serves different meanings for men and women. Many men who say they hooked up with someone may want the listener to infer that sexual intercourse occurred, as a way of inflating their self-concepts and increasing their social status among their peers. On the other hand, some women who say they hooked up with someone may want to protect their reputations by having their listeners think that something less than sexual intercourse occurred (Bogle, 2008). Thus, the ambiguous phrase "I hooked up" has a gendered meaning that serves to enhance or preserve the self-concepts and reputations of the young men and women who use it (Allison & Risman, 2013).

One feature of hooking up that is near-universally understood to be true is that a hookup does not mean that a commitment exists between the two people who hooked up. A hookup may be the beginning of a relationship, and two people may decide to see each other again, but most college students report that a hookup usually means a one-time-only erotic encounter with no emotional entanglements. Students may exchange phone numbers or email addresses, or make a date to see each other again, but most do not expect a hookup to lead to a romantic relationship (Bogle, 2008).

Although emerging adults understand that a hookup is a no-strings-attached encounter, a majority of young men and an even larger majority of young women who have hooked up indicate that they would rather be in a traditional romantic relationship than have uncommitted sex (Garcia et al., 2012). Many of these students report that they made an attempt to discuss the possibility of beginning a romantic relationship with a hookup partner even though they know most hookups do not lead to a romantic relationship (Owen & Fincham, 2011).

The following young woman describes her strong need for sex, which, to her, feels like a biological imperative that can only be satisfied with multiple sex partners. She is not interested in one-night stands, however, but has had many friends with benefits whom she calls "casual sex buddies."

IN THEIR OWN WORDS

. . . I was having sex and messing around because it felt good to me and improved my lifestyle. I had sexual tension that I needed to relieve with another person and masturbation did not cut it. . . . I was able to find casual sex buddies who I would hook up with "no strings attached." The idea of consistent sex buddies excited me, because I felt I was not sleeping around with completely random people. It felt more justifiable than just one-night stands. But on the contrary, I had multiple sex buddies at one time.

. . . I am now at the point in my life though where I am ready for a steady relationship, but it is proving difficult. I have never been successful in finding a guy who doesn't take advantage of the fact that I love sex. They do not seem to understand that sex is a need for me, and not a recreation. As long as we are open about it, I do not mind "adding" another sex buddy to my tally of partners. I am fully committed to the belief that sex and emotions are separate. Only in special instances are they combined to create something magical. I want magic in my life and I hope to soon find a guy who feels the same way and accepts me and looks past my sexual history.

Hookups are different from *friends with benefits,* a phrase that refers to a long-term sexual relationship with someone without being emotionally involved with that person (Furman & Shaffer, 2011; Jonason, Li, & Richardson, 2011). In one small-scale study, 60% of 125 undergraduate students reported that they had a friends-with-benefits relationship at some point in their lives (Bisson & Levine, 2009). These are complicated relationships that sometimes endure, often do not, and rarely evolve into a romantic relationship (Lehmiller, Vander-Drift, & Kelly, 2014; Manning, Giordano, & Longmore, 2006).

How Common Is Hooking Up?

Estimating the prevalence of hookups on college campuses is difficult because the estimate depends on the definition of a hookup and the characteristics of the sample surveyed. The results of three large studies indicate that about 70% of college students report that they have hooked up at least once, with about 30% of those hookups including sexual intercourse (Armstrong, England, & Fogarty, 2012; Kalish & Kimmel, 2011; Paul, McManus, & Hayes, 2000). As expected, males report a higher incidence of sexual intercourse than females, a difference that makes it impossible to determine how often intercourse actually occurs. By their senior year in college, students report that they have hooked up between three and 11 times.

Mass media reports indicate that the hookup culture is relatively recent, widespread, and has replaced traditional dating on college campuses (Freitas, 2013). Monto and Carey (2014) evaluated the claim that hookups are a recent phenomenon by using data from the General Social Survey, which is a nationally representative sample of U.S. emerging adults between ages 18 and 25 years. Comparisons were made for data collected between 1988 and 1996 and 2004 and 2012 in order to examine historical trends. Emerging adults from the recent era were more likely to report that they had sex with a close friend or a "casual date/pickup" than emerging adults from the previous era. This finding does indicate that hooking up is more common today than in the past, although emerging adults in the recent cohort did not report more total number of sexual partners, more partners during the past year, or more frequent sex during the previous year. The researchers conclude that emerging adults today are having more casual sex than before, but in other ways, their sexual behavior is similar to the sexual behavior of emerging adults from the previous generation. Many would be surprised to discover that the sexual behavior of emerging adults today is not very different from the sexual behavior of parents when they were emerging adults, with the important difference that emerging adults today have more casual sexual partners than before.

Who Hooks Up?

One study investigated the relationship between hookups and problem behavior among middle school and high school students. A hookup was broadly defined as anything from kissing to sexual intercourse with a stranger, brief acquaintance, or friend. About 18% of middle school students and 34% of high school students reported that they had engaged in a hookup. For all students, hooking up was associated with smoking cigarettes, drinking alcohol, using illicit drugs, gambling, and skipping school (Fortunato, Young, Boyd, & Fons, 2010). The results suggest that hooking up in middle school and high school is not a normative experience, but is part of a problem behavior syndrome that includes a variety of risky behaviors. We do not know whether these specific findings hold true for college students, but they do indicate that young adolescents who hook up are more likely to be unconventional risk takers.

What do we know about the college students who hook up in comparison to students who do not hook up? In general, college students who hook up are more unconventional, higher risk takers, and more impulsive than students who do not hook up (Lyons, Manning, Longmore, & Giordano, 2014). Two other characteristics of students who hook up are a desire for sexual pleasure and a higher level of substance use (Lyons, Manning, Longmore, & Giordano, 2015). In addition, students who hook up have positive attitudes about hooking up (Owen, Rhoades, Stanley, & Fincham, 2010) and think their close friends approve of hooking up (Napper, Kenney, & LaBrie, 2015).

Also, college students who hook up have a passionate or erotic approach to relationships, and place a greater emphasis on the physical attractiveness of their partners than on their personal characteristics. Further, students who hook up have greater fears of relationship intimacy. In contrast, students who do not hook up are more likely to want intimacy in a romantic relationship, and have little interest in superficial relationships (Paul et al., 2000).

What Is the Relationship between Drinking Alcohol and Hooking Up?

The majority of hookups are preceded by drinking alcohol, sometimes a prodigious amount of it (LaBrie, Hummer, Ghaidarov, Lac, & Kenney, 2014). A large percentage of college students are drunk at the time they hook up (Johnson & Chen, 2015). In one study, men averaged almost five drinks per hookup, women nearly three (Kalish & Kimmel, 2011). In addition to binge drinking, many hookups are preceded by marijuana use, which, along with drinking alcohol, is associated with an increase in the risk of unprotected sex (Kuperberg & Padgett, 2017).

Given that many hookups are partly fueled by excessive drinking, it is not surprising that some students, especially young women, later report that the hookup was not consensual (Livingston, Testa, Windle, & Bay-Cheng, 2015). Many young women report that they engaged in a hookup at least once when they were drunk, and perceived the sex as unwanted (Flack et al., 2007). Many women are unwilling to label such encounters assault or rape, however, and, instead, blame themselves for what occurred (Stinson, 2010).

How Do Young People Feel after Hooking Up?

Hookups are not emotionally inconsequential. Most emerging adults have ambivalent to positive reactions to a hookup. In one study of U.S. college students, nearly 70% of men and 56% of women reported more positive than negative feelings after a hookup (Strokoff, Owen, & Fincham, 2015). Students typically report feeling happy, excited, and desirable, but they also feel awkward around the person they hooked up with (Glenn & Marquardt, 2001; Lewis, Granato, Blayney, Lostutter, & Kilmer, 2012). Students who are well functioning to begin with, and who have a strong friendship network, are more likely to enjoy their hookup experience than students who have psychological difficulties and few friends (Owen, Quirk, & Fincham, 2014; Snapp, Ryu, & Kerr, 2015). Most students who hook up report that they have a positive experience even when they do not think the hookup will lead to a future romantic relationship.

Even though hooking up is a positive experience for most emerging adults, some students, especially females, have negative reactions to their hookups, which include feeling used, empty, confused, and disappointed (Owen et al., 2010). Emerging adults who are distressed and lonely to begin with are more likely to experience negative emotions after hooking up (Owen et al., 2014; Snapp et al., 2015). Many of these students engage in a hookup thinking it will lead to a romantic relationship and feel betrayed when their romantic hopes are not reciprocated. Negative reactions such as regret, guilt, shame, and anger are more common following a hookup among students who have been drinking alcohol before and during the hookup, and this is especially true for young women (LaBrie et al., 2014; Paul et al., 2000). Regret is also associated with sex that is unfulfilling, a reaction that may intensify any ambivalent emotions that were present before hooking up (Fisher, Worth, Garcia, & Meredith, 2012). Negative emotions, especially for young women, are more likely to occur when the hookup includes sexual intercourse, in contrast to oral sex, sexual touching, or kissing, suggesting that many young women believe that sexual intercourse should be reserved for a romantic relationship (Eshbaugh & Gute, 2008).

Do Hookups Lead to Mental Health Problems?

Feeling regret and disappointment after a hookup is different from having more serious mental health problems, such as depression and suicidal ideation following a hookup. Are hookups associated with serious, long-term psychological disturbances? Research on a possible relation between casual sex and the poor mental health of both men and women is inconclusive. The majority of research indicates that engaging in casual sex is associated with poorer psychological well-being, including more anxiety and depression, and lower self-esteem among male and female emerging adults (e.g., Anatale & Kelly, 2015; Fielder, Walsh, Carey, & Carey, 2014; Mendle, Ferrero, Moore, & Harden, 2013). One study examined the mental health correlates of casual sex in a large national sample of U.S. college students and found that casual sex was correlated with psychological distress and diminished well-being for both young men and young women (Bersamin et al., 2014). Although the correlations were low (ranging from $r = .06$ to $r = .26$), casual sex was related to lower self-esteem, higher depression and anxiety, and lower psychological well-being.

Two researchers at The Ohio State University attempted to untangle the relationship between casual sex and mental health problems in a longitudinal study of a national sample of over 11,000 U.S. emerging adults (Sandberg-Thoma & Duch, 2014). Findings revealed that both depressive symptoms and suicidal ideation predicted engagement in casual sex, while casual sex predicted thoughts about suicide, associations that were true for males and females. The authors speculate that individuals with a history of poor mental health may be drawn to casual sex because they cannot successfully enter into or maintain a long-lasting romantic relationship. Further, casual sex among individuals who are already depressed may lead to thoughts of suicide when these casual encounters do not turn into a romantic relationship. Thus, casual sex may not cause mental health problems, but casual sex may exacerbate already existing problems.

Other research has not found a relationship between casual sex and poor psychological well-being (Eisenberg, Ackard, Resnick, & Neumark-Sztainer, 2009). In one longitudinal study, casual sex did not predict later depression or suicidal thoughts, nor did depression or suicidal thoughts predict later casual sex (Deutsch & Slutske, 2015). In conclusion, the relationship between casual sex and poor psychological well-being is inconsistent, and when that relationship is present, it is weak.

Another factor that may influence the relationship between casual sex and mental health problems is the ages of the individuals who hook up. The relationship between casual sex and depression or low self-esteem is stronger among young adolescents than among emerging adults (Vrangalova, 2015a). Casual sex is not a norm for teens, and those youth who do engage in casual sex are more likely to engage in other problem behaviors, such as drinking alcohol, using drugs, delinquency, and poor academic performance. These same adolescents are also more likely to be depressed and have low self-esteem. In contrast, casual sex is more normative among emerging adults and, therefore, less linked to problem behaviors or to mental health problems.

One's motivation for hooking up is another reason some people who hook up may experience psychological distress (Vrangalova, 2015b). Hooking up is not related to depression, anxiety, physical complaints, or low self-esteem for students who freely choose to hook up. Well-being is lower among male and female college students who are pressured to engage in a hookup or who hook up out of a desire to please the other person. It is not clear whether feeling pressure to hook up leads to psychological distress, or if psychological distress leads to the feeling that one was pressured to hook up.

All in all, the results from studies of the relationship between hooking up and emotional distress indicate that it is an oversimplification to say that hookups are related to short-term distress or long-term mental health problems. Emerging adults, especially females, are more likely to experience short-term distress after a hookup when the hookup includes sexual intercourse, the sexual experience is unfulfilling, the individual is already distressed and lonely, and the individual has been drinking. Hoping for a meaningful relationship from a hookup is also associated with distress when such a relationship does not materialize. In addition, youth are more likely to experience long-term mental health problems after hooking up if they are young, have preexisting mental health problems, and feel pressure to engage in the hookup.

Are Young Women More Likely to Have Negative Reactions to Hooking Up Than Young Men?

Many social commentators and researchers have voiced concerns about the possible negative short- and long-term effects of casual sex on the psychological well-being of young women. Some argue that short-term mating is evolutionarily costlier for women than for men (Buss, 2016), less in tune with a woman's natural desire to pair up (Townsend & Wasserman, 2011), and comes with more social costs because of the existence of a sexual double standard (Allison & Risman, 2013; Kreager & Staff, 2009).

Research does not strongly confirm theoretical ideas that casual sex is psychologically costlier for women than for men. Men report engaging in more casual sex than women (Owen, Fincham, & Moore, 2011; Townsend & Wasserman, 2011), but the evidence that women have more long-lasting negative reactions to casual sex than do men is inconsistent. Some researchers do find that hooking up is associated with higher distress in women than in men, especially when the hookup includes sexual intercourse (Bersamin et al., 2014; Fielder & Carey, 2010), but other researchers report no gender differences in depression or suicidal ideation (Deutsch & Slutske, 2015; Mendle et al., 2013; Sandberg-Thoma & Duch, 2014). These inconsistent findings are difficult to explain, but they indicate that casual sex is not inevitably related to more mental health problems among women than among men.

For most young women, the typical hookup is unlikely to lead to serious, long-term mental health problems, such as depression or suicidal thoughts, although casual sex can be associated with negative, short-term emotional reactions. Townsend and Wasserman (2011) suggest that women, more than men, are likely to feel unfulfilled and have stronger negative reactions shortly after a casual sexual experience, but these feelings do not necessarily translate into full-blown depression or suicidal ideation for most women.

SUMMARY

◼ DATING AMONG ADOLESCENTS AND EMERGING ADULTS

Adolescents today continue to pair up and go out with each other, although many youth do not use the term *date* to describe their relationship. The term remains a useful word to describe a certain kind of relationship, however.

Dating increases as adolescents get older. The percentage of youth who have gone out on a date has declined over the past several years, perhaps replaced by group dating or more casual relationships. Some adolescents begin to date at an early age, which is associated with early sex, and those adolescents tend to be early maturers who are also risk takers and outgoing. Early daters are also more likely to live in single-parent households or with parents who are not good monitors.

Sexual intercourse is more likely to occur between two adolescents who are dating than between two adolescents who are casual acquaintances or friends. Intercourse is especially likely to occur if the two teens are nonvirgins at the start of their relationship, and if both adolescents desire to have sex. A large age difference between the two dating teens also predicts early sexual behavior.

ROMANTIC RELATIONSHIPS

A romantic relationship can be defined in several ways, but at its core it means having a special connection to another person. Romantic relationships are common during adolescence, although a substantial minority of adolescents have not been in one. Positive relations between parents and teens are associated with a delay in the formation of a romantic relationship and with a delay in the onset of sexual behavior.

DATING AND ROMANCE AMONG LGBTQ ADOLESCENTS

LGBTQ youth in middle school and high school face unique challenges as they attempt to find other LGBTQ youth to date and with whom they can form romantic relationships. Many LGBTQ teens have to conceal their identities and true desires for connection out of fear of victimization and discrimination. For many gay young men, sexual behavior precedes the formation of a romantic relationship, the reverse of which is more common among heterosexual adolescents. Sex between gay youth frequently occurs early in a relationship, as soon as the first or second date, a situation less common among heterosexual youth. One risk associated with sex between young gay men in a romantic relationship is that they are less likely to use a condom when they have sex than when they have sex with a stranger or new acquaintance.

CASUAL SEX, HOOKUPS, AND FRIENDS WITH BENEFITS

Casual sex is increasingly common among emerging adults. *Hooking up* is the phrase generally used to describe a casual sexual encounter between two people, but it is difficult to know what people mean when they say they have hooked up with someone. It may mean that sexual intercourse has occurred, but it may not. About 70% of college students report that they have hooked up with someone, and about one-third of those hookups include sexual intercourse. Hookups are increasingly common among college students, although in other ways, college students today have sex lives that are not very different from the sex lives of college students in the recent past. Students who hook up tend to be unconventional, risk takers, and more impulsive than students who do not hook up. Alcohol plays an important role in the initiation of hookups, a situation that can lead to nonconsensual sex and even rape.

Most emerging adults report that they have positive feelings after hooking up, although some feel regret and disappointment. Young women have more short-term negative reactions to hooking up than young men, but the evidence that women have more long-term mental health problems after hooking up than men is inconclusive. Negative feelings are more common among youth who feel pressure to hook up. Although casual sex is correlated with depression, it appears that depression often is present before the hookup, rather than an outcome of the hookup.

SUGGESTIONS FOR FURTHER READING

Collins, W. A., & van Dulmen, M. (2014). "The course of true love(s) . . .": Origins and pathways in the development of romantic relationships. In A. C. Crouter & A. Booth (Eds.), *Romance and sex in adolescence and emerging adulthood: Risks and opportunities* (pp. 63–86). New York: Psychology Press.

de Graaf, H., Vanwesenbeeck, I., Woertman, L., & Meeus, W. (2011). Parenting and psychosexual development in adolescence: A literature review. *European Psychologist, 16,* 21–31.

Diamond, L. M., Savin-Williams, R. C., & Dubé, E. M. (1999). Sex, dating, passionate friendships, and romance: Intimate peer relations among lesbian, gay, and bisexual adolescents. In W. Furman, B. B. Brown, & C. Feiring (Eds.), *The development of romantic relationships in adolescence* (pp. 175–210). New York: Cambridge University Press.

Garcia, J. R., Reiber, C., Massey, S. G., & Merriwether, A. M. (2012). Sexual hookup culture: A review. *Review of General Psychology, 16,* 161–176.

Monto, M. A., & Carey, A. G. (2014). A new standard of sexual behavior?: Are claims associated with the "hookup culture" supported by General Social Survey data? *Journal of Sex Research, 51,* 605–615.

Mustanski, B., Newcomb, M. E., & Clerkin, E. M. (2011). Relationship characteristics and sexual risk-taking in young men who have sex with men. *Health Psychology, 30,* 597–605.

CHAPTER 7

Adolescents, Sex, and the Media

The popular MTV reality series *16 and Pregnant* follows a pregnant teenage girl over a period of months as she copes with the reality of her pregnancy and early motherhood. Episodes focus on the interactions the teen mother has with her baby, her boyfriend or father of the baby, and other significant people in her life. The unscripted episodes neither glamorize teen pregnancy nor preach about the evils of early motherhood.

Comments about the show are mixed. Some view the series favorably and focus on the realism of the episodes. Others think that a highly polished hour-long show that "stars" a pregnant, teenage girl glorifies and implicitly endorses teen pregnancy and presents an unrealistic view of the lives of teen mothers. Few of the episodes explicitly focus on some of the darker issues that are all too often associated with a teenage pregnancy, such as drug and alcohol use, delinquency, abuse, and sexual assault. A further concern about the negative effect *16 and Pregnant* might have on teen girls is that some of the young mothers and fathers on the show become mini-celebrities among MTV viewers and readers of tabloids, and even have fan pages on Facebook, glorifying what is definitely not an attractive situation for teen mothers or fathers.

What should one think about the possible impact on teens of shows such as *16 and Pregnant* and its spinoff, *Teen Mom*? Are the shows part of the problem of teenage pregnancy leading to further teen pregnancies, or part of the solution? Two recent evaluations suggest that the programs are associated with a decrease in risky sexual behavior (Wright, Randall, & Arroyo, 2013) and with a decline in teen pregnancy (Kearney & Levine, 2014). What about other portrayals of sexuality in other media, such as the Internet, television, movies, and music? Do these sexual images and words have any impact on adolescent sexuality, or are they too weak and infrequent to influence attitudes and behaviors deeply rooted in core values and in one's personal identity? These are some of the questions examined in this chapter. The issues are subtle and complicated, and do not have simple answers.

■ MEDIA SEX

What Do Experts Say about Sex in the Media?

In the minds of many, there are serious psychological and social costs of exposure to sex in the media for children and adolescents. Many experts believe that sex in the media has a negative effect on adolescent sexual behavior, leading teens to early sexual activity and risky sexual behavior (Heins, 2007). An additional worry is that the portrayal of sex in the media influences the formation of sexual attitudes and values among young impressionable adolescents that too often lead to negative stereotypes of females as sexual objects (Mattebo, Larsson, Tydén, & Häggström-Nordin, 2013).

Can Sex in the Media Be a Good Thing?

Several writers and researchers have made a point not often made about sex in the media, which is that the media can be an opportunity to disseminate accurate information about sexuality and to promote responsible sexual behavior (Keller & Brown, 2002; Levine, 2002). Some potential benefits of portraying sex in the media not often discussed include educating youth about AIDS and STIs, portraying sexually responsible females, providing healthy models of gay and lesbian relationships, and fostering open and honest conversations about taboo topics (Watson & McKee, 2013).

The Internet, social networking sites, and text messaging are opportunities to provide information, support, and guidance about sexual issues to the young, who naturally use technology to explore personal issues (Selkie, Benson, & Moreno, 2011). The Internet is already widely used by adolescents to get answers about sex-related questions. In one study of Spanish teens, almost 70% indicated they had received information about sex online (González-Ortega, Vicario-Molina, Martinez, & Orgaz, 2015). The majority of the Spanish adolescents who had obtained information about sex online also indicated that they were sexually active, revealing a positive association between searching for information about sex on the Internet and sexual behavior.

The Internet is an ideal venue for adolescents to ask difficult questions about sensitive topics and receive accurate information and advice. Several sex education sites exist specifically designed for teenagers, such as *https://sexetc.org, www.iwannaknow.org,* and *www.advocatesforyouth.org.* The Internet already provides information about sexual issues to millions of adolescents and emerging adults (Lightfoot, 2012). One problem is that there is plenty of material about sex on the Internet, but no way for adolescents to distinguish high-quality from low-quality information (Buhi et al., 2010).

■ SEX IN THE MEDIA

How Common Is Sex on the Internet?

Nudity and sexual intercourse have been portrayed in painting and photographs for as long as there has been art and photography, but the Internet is the first medium in which sexually explicit pictures and videos are easily accessible and widely available. Indeed, in the past few years there has been an increase in the number of free, amateur sex sites, which opens the door to explicit videos of just about any sex act with any combination of people to anyone of any age with access to a computer (Forrester, 2016). People in general, and parents in particular, are especially concerned about the impact on the young of these graphic, sexually explicit images.

One Internet experience most people find irritating is the unintentional exposure to X-rated content through pop-up advertisements, spam email, or through links within websites. In one study, about 42% of adolescents reported that they had been exposed to online sex sites in the past year, and of that 42%, about two-thirds reported accidental exposure (Wolak, Mitchell, & Finkelhor,

---

Exposure to online sexually explicit images through the irritating practice of hard-to-remove pop-ups and deceptive labeling of websites is illustrated in the following story told by a female college student about her search for information on the Internet about bubble gum.

IN THEIR OWN WORDS

My first exposure to pornography was at the age of 11 when I was working on a project for school about inventors and I had chosen John B. Curtis, the inventor of bubble gum. I immediately got to work, and by that I mean I put it off for a bit. When I finally got around to googling bubble gum I was not expecting the results I got, porn. Every link I seemed to click had pornography on it. I tried all kinds of different web searches but I seemed to get the same result every time I tried. My next attempt was to maybe just image search bubble gum since I needed a picture for my report anyways, this was also a mistake. I was young so I had no idea what it was or what any of it meant, I eventually ran to my mom because I was afraid I was going to get into trouble because of the results that I was getting, not because of the content they had, but because they didn't contain information on bubble gum and I needed to do my project. It never really seemed like that big of a deal to me, it definitely didn't seem normal or something that I should be looking at, but it wasn't some huge scarring moment in my life. My mom seemed shocked at the results, and at the time I thought she too couldn't believe that there was no information on bubble gum, I mean how is a girl supposed to get any work done? Even though we had intensive parental filtering, somehow those results were still able to get through. We never really had a discussion about what I had seen other than that it wasn't a good thing and I could tell from my mom's tone that she was upset that I had seen it. I don't think she really remembers that situation very much but I do because I never really understood why she got so upset over what I had seen because I didn't really understand that there was things on the Internet that weren't meant to be seen by everyone.

2007). Most adolescents, especially girls, have negative reactions to unwanted online sexual content and often feel personally threatened by these images and messages (Ševčíková, Simon, Daneback, & Kvapilik, 2015).

How Much Sex Is on Television?

The 2000s saw the appearance of television streaming that, along with network and cable TV, dominates the media lives of most young Americans (Rideout, Foehr, & Roberts, 2010). Adolescents report that they watch about 4½ hours of TV per day, much of it on platforms other than a television, according to one extensive survey of a national sample of over 2,000 American youth conducted between 2008 and 2009 by the Kaiser Family Foundation (Rideout et al., 2010). The majority of TV viewing is done apart from parents, alone or with friends.

Considering the great amount of free time youth spend watching TV, it is not surprising that parents are deeply concerned about TV content and the potential impact that content may have on their children. In one national telephone survey of 1,001 parents of children between ages 2 and 17 years, two out of three parents said they are "very concerned" about exposure to children

Not all parents prohibit their adolescents from watching sexually graphic TV programs, and some even watch them with their adolescents, as the following story told by a college-age female illustrates.

IN THEIR OWN WORDS

Gigolos is a reality television show on Showtime, and like many shows on Showtime, it is graphic, perhaps too graphic—as it has been questioned for its legality of being shown on television. The show follows the lives of several men who work for a male escort service in Las Vegas. In short, their lives consist of drinking and being paid to have sex. The men are filmed going to their paid appointments and performing the sexual activities that occur during these appointments. Well, my best friend's father, who discovered this show flipping through channels, thought this was preposterous, and in a very innocent manner, wanted us to see how ridiculous these men's lives were. So, as a family (not your ideal "family time," right?), including my best friend, her father, stepmother, sister, boyfriend, and myself, we watched a few episodes of this ridiculous television show.

As I mentioned, it is extremely graphic and though it is not labeled porn, it certainly is watching these men have sex, in many different positions, with many different women.

Now, I can't imagine how any "normal" family would view or accept this. I say normal because most families aren't extremely open, if open at all, with sexuality and talking about sex. I would also like to reiterate that this is a reality television show—and all members of the family were over 18 and no one was forced to watch it. We weren't watching this show to gain pleasure or any other reason why people watch graphic sexual content—we simply found the idea of this reality show and the lives of these men entertaining. Yet, my experience hits a double whammy on porn and parent–teen communication.

of inappropriate content on entertainment media (Rideout, 2007). Parents are especially concerned about exposure to sexual content on television programs, even more than they are worried about their children viewing violent and aggressive behavior. This concern is motivated by the belief that exposure to sexual content on TV contributes to early sexual behavior.

As anyone who watches television knows, there is a profusion of sex on TV, most of it implied or talked about. During the 2001–2002 television season, nearly two out of three prime-time, network shows contained some sexual content, typically sex talk, and sexual behavior was portrayed in one-third of the shows (Kunkel, Eyal, Biely, Donnerstein, & Rideout, 2007). Recent content analyses of the sexual content of programs on U.S. and Israeli television reveals that talk about sex is endemic in both countries, but is especially widespread on U.S. television (Eyal, Raz, & Levi, 2014). The most common genres of shows that portray sexual content are soap operas, followed by movies, comedies, and dramas. Given the high average amount of time the young spend watching TV programing, adolescents are almost certainly likely to encounter sexual content on TV, even if they are not searching for it.

What Is Television Sex Like?

One characteristic of sexual content on television is that it is virtually free of negative consequences. Unwanted pregnancies, abortions, and STIs are rare occurrences. Related to the absence of sexual risks is the fact that sex is often presented in a humorous context in situation comedies, and serious emotional and physical consequences of sex are ignored. A humorous presentation of sexual intercourse may signal to young viewers that potential negative consequences are rare or inconsequential (Eyal, Kunkel, Biely, & Finnerty, 2007). Sexual abstinence and safe-sex messages are uncommon, and programs that include sexual content rarely raise issues about sexual patience, sexual precaution, and the negative consequences that may result from sexual intercourse.

One recent analysis of U.S. network shows found that explicit sexual behavior is virtually nonexistent on TV, but there is an abundance of sexuality even on programs produced for young adolescents. Surprisingly, flirting, intimate touching, and sexual talk are as common on adolescent programs as on adult programs (Malacane & Martins, 2017). The majority of episodes on programs for adolescents contain at least one instance of sexual behavior or one sexual comment. The real or soundtrack reactions of audiences to sexual behavior and sexual talk typically are laughing, cheering, and applauding, reinforcing these sexual activities for viewers. Portrayals of sexual risk are rare and, when they do occur, they are quick, casual references that have little to do with the plot.

A content analysis of portrayals of sexuality on Scottish TV programs aimed at young people largely replicates findings from research on U.S. television, revealing cross-cultural similarity in the messages youth receive about sex on TV (Batchelor, Kitzinger, & Burtney, 2004). Scenes of youth engaging in

A characteristic of sex on TV is that most adolescents are heterosexual, white, attractive, and do not have a disability. Portraying sexuality among nonmajority teens might be especially important to the many teens who do not fit a conventional mold, as the following story told by a college female illustrates.

IN THEIR OWN WORDS

I distinctly remember my first pornographic experience. It wasn't a video, but the erotic writings of the Internet were perfect for a 9-year-old. The story I was most interested in was a story about a lesbian's first experience with a girl. At the time, I didn't realize that I was interested in the same sex, but thinking back, my desire to read erotic writings about lesbians could have been an indication of my current identification as a lesbian. I remember thinking about looking up stories like this numerous times before, but I just didn't have the courage to do it, and I was really afraid that my parents would find out. Finally, one night, I woke up during the middle of the night and ventured down into the basement. I sat down at the computer desk and I remember feeling really excited and really nervous at the same time, but not nervous enough to stop. I searched the same phrase, *sex stories,* every single time I went looking for the sexual feelings I craved. The feelings that were evoked while reading this erotic writing were unbelievably satisfying and scary at the same time. My mouth would get dry, which was the complete opposite reaction I was feeling below the belt, and at times my hands would tremble with anticipation of what was to come next. If the story wasn't explicit enough, I didn't waste my time and moved on to a story that quenched the feelings I was after. As a 9-year-old, I was very much on my way to discovering what it is I desired sexually.

sexual intercourse are rare. Instead, the predominant portrayal of teenage sexuality on TV involves youth talking about sex, which includes discussions about the opposite sex, flirting, bragging, teasing, and sexual negotiation. There is virtually no reference to contraception. Females discuss their decision to have sex, while males typically boast about their sexual prowess. Boys are portrayed as sexual pursuers, and girls as the pursued.

How Much Sex Is in Movies?

About one-third of the most popular movies released between 1983 and 2003 depict sexual intercourse (Gunasekera, Chapman, & Campbell, 2005). Most of the intercourse scenes involve heterosexual intercourse between unmarried young adults. In over 80% of the scenes of intercourse, no birth control of any kind is used, and there are no consequences of unprotected sex. Further, in movies rated R because of excessive violence, the violent character is often portrayed as being sexually active, pairing violence with sex (Bleakley, Romer, & Jamieson, 2014).

Sexual content, including images and talk, is also common in movies targeted at teens. In one survey of movies popular with adolescents, 12% of scenes included sexual content (Pardun, L'Engle, & Brown, 2005). Sexual intercourse is rare, but about half of the sexual scenes involve partial or full nudity. Other common sexual scenes contain sexual innuendo, sexual touching, and passionate kissing. When sexual intercourse does occur, it typically occurs between unmarried individuals (Callister, Stern, Coyne, Robinson, & Bennion, 2011).

How Much Sex Is in Music and Music Videos for Adolescents?

Most of the music adolescents listened to in the late 1990s did not include references to sexuality, although themes of love and romance were common (Christenson & Roberts, 1998). Popular music has become more explicitly sexual since then. The increase in overt sexuality is almost entirely explained by the rise of hip-hop/rap music, which has a tradition of explicit lyrics not found in other genres of music (Hall, West, & Hill, 2012). References to sex in rap music often include degrading sex, typically a man with a large appetite for sexual intercourse, or oral sex with a physically attractive woman (Primack, Gold, Schwarz, & Dalton, 2008).

In 1981, MTV was launched, which began an era of 24-hours-a-day music television. More recently, music videos can now be seen on the web and on YouTube and purchased on iTunes and elsewhere, making music videos widely accessible and available. Content analyses of music videos show that sexual content is a staple of music videos, and that sexual behavior is often implied or endorsed (Vandenbosch, Vervloessem, & Eggermont, 2013).

■ SEX IN THE MEDIA AND ADOLESCENT SEXUAL ATTITUDES AND BELIEFS

One of the most important questions about the portrayal of sex in the media is Does media sex have an influence on adolescent sexuality? This is a tricky question for researchers to answer because of the key word *influence,* which implies that sex in the media might be a *cause* of adolescent sexual behavior, maybe not the *only* cause, maybe not even the *main* cause, but *one* cause of adolescent sexuality.

What Is the Relationship between Exposure to Sex in the Media and the Sexual Attitudes and Beliefs of Adolescents?

The results of research on the relationship between sexual content in the media and adolescent sexual attitudes and beliefs are highly consistent—the more teens report they have been exposed to sex on TV, the Internet, movies, music, and music videos, the more they have permissive attitudes and beliefs about sexual behavior (Braun-Courville & Rojas, 2009; Brown & L'Engle, 2009; Koletić, 2017). For example, male college students who watch many television

A FOCUS ON RESEARCH

Establishing a causal link between two variables is one of the most important and most difficult tasks for any scientific investigation. Strong statements about causality can only be obtained from experimental research that, in the social sciences, requires at least two groups of people who are alike in every way except that one group receives an experimental treatment and the other group does not. Any difference between the groups after the treatment has been administered must be due to the treatment, since that is the only difference between the two groups. In the social sciences, the only way to ensure that people in the two groups are alike before the treatment is administered is to randomly assign people to the two groups, thereby making the two groups equivalent. In order to show with a high degree of certainty that sex on TV, for example, has an impact on adolescent sexual attitudes and behavior, it is necessary to randomly assign adolescents to two groups: a treatment group that receives a steady diet of sexual TV and a control group that is not allowed to watch programs with any sexual content. Such a real-world experiment is neither practical nor ethical. So researchers find themselves in the less-than-satisfactory situation of searching for an *association* between sex in the media and adolescent sexuality and trying to make the case through theory or the use of sophisticated statistical techniques that media sex is a cause of sexual behavior. Unfortunately, even if a correlation is found between media sex and real-world sexual behavior, at least three interpretations are possible for that correlation. First, media sex may be a cause of sexual behavior. Second, adolescents who are sexually

active may seek out and enjoy media sex. Third, some third variable may be responsible for the correlation between media sex and sexual behavior. For example, it might be that males with high testosterone both watch programs with high sexual content and are sexually active. In this case, the relationship between media sex and sexual behavior is *spurious,* an apparently causal relationship that is in fact not causal. The inability to perform real-world experiments on the relationship between media sex and sexual behavior means that even a strong correlation is not evidence of a cause.

Since a true experiment designed to study the effect of media sex on teen sexual behavior cannot be performed, researchers have resorted to a different strategy, which is to measure exposure to media sex and sexual behavior at two points in time. A *longitudinal research design* is one in which two variables are measured at two points in time. The assumption is that if variable A has an influence on variable B, then variation in variable A at Time 1 should be related to variation in variable B at Time 2. For example, if exposure to sex on TV is related to sexual behavior, then adolescents who frequently watch sexual TV at Time 1 should be more sexually active at Time 2 in comparison to adolescents who are infrequent viewers of sexual TV programs at Time 1. Although a longitudinal research design does not allow us to make strong, unequivocal statements about causality since there is no random assignment of subjects to conditions, research from longitudinal studies can provide evidence of a temporal relationship between two variables showing that one variable predicts another variable.

programs with high sexual content expect to have sex with many sexual partners, while females exposed to high sexual content programs expect to have
sex at an early stage in their relationships (Aubrey, Harrison, Kramer, & Yellin,
2003). In addition, preference for rap music is associated with permissive sexual
attitudes and gender stereotypes that view men as sex driven and tough, and
women as sex objects (ter Bogt, Engels, Bogers, & Kloosterman, 2010). The
correlations between exposure to media sex and adolescent sexual attitudes
and beliefs are low, however, indicating that other factors, such as parenting
and peer norms, are more strongly associated with sexual attitudes and beliefs
(Ragsdale et al., 2014).

Not all portrayals of sex in the media are the same, and the way sex is
portrayed is related to the sexual attitudes and beliefs of adolescents. Some portrayals are meant to be true to life, others unrealistic, often played for laughs.
Realism matters, and realistic portrayals of sex in the media are more strongly
related to permissive sexual attitudes and beliefs of adolescents than unrealistic portrayals (Baams, Overbeek, Dubas, et al., 2015; Taylor, 2005). Unfortunately, the more adolescents view sex in the media, the more they perceive it to
be realistic (Peter & Valkenburg, 2006a). It is easy to see why sexually inexperienced adolescents may be especially vulnerable to believing that media sex is
realistic since they have little experience with actual sex, making the portrayal
appear authentic (Peter & Valkenburg, 2010). These results on the importance
of realism suggest that parents and teachers might lessen the development of
recreational attitudes toward sex among adolescents by emphasizing to teens
that most media sexual behavior is staged by actors for the entertainment of an
audience and is not meant to be realistic.

Besides realism, the consequences of sex to the characters in the media are
related to sexual attitudes and beliefs. If the consequences of casual sex in the
media are negative, adolescents are more likely to develop negative attitudes
about casual sex (Eyal & Kunkel, 2008). Media portrayals of sex rarely result
in negative consequences, however, so it is not surprising that adolescents who
often view sex in the media have positive attitudes about casual sex.

■ SEX IN THE MEDIA AND ADOLESCENT SEXUAL BEHAVIOR

The findings in the previous section show a positive relationship between
exposure to sex in the media and the sexual attitudes and beliefs of adolescents,
but the question of the relationship between exposure to sex in the media
and sexual behavior is not answered by investigations of sexual attitudes. The
relationship between attitudes and behavior is complicated, and there is not a
one-to-one correspondence between attitudes and behavior (Jones, Smith, &
Llewellyn, 2014). If one wants to understand behavior, then one needs to study
behavior, which is the focus in this section.

Does Exposure to Media Sex Lead to Teen Sex?

Dozens of studies have found a significant, positive correlation between exposure to sex in the media and adolescent risky sexual behavior, including having sex at an early age, sex with many partners, and teen pregnancy (Koletić, 2017; Ybarra, Strasburger, & Mitchell, 2014). The most sophisticated of these studies have employed a longitudinal design, and almost all of this research shows a positive relationship between exposure to sex in the media at Time 1 and sexual behavior at Time 2. Based on this relationship, most researchers argue that exposure to sex in the media is a possible cause of sexual behavior.

One of the best longitudinal studies of the relationship between sex in the media and adolescent sexual behavior is by Collins and colleagues (2004) at the RAND Corporation. They found that adolescents who watched the most TV with sexual content in 2001 are about twice as likely to be nonvirgin in 2002 as youth who watch the least television with sexual content. The authors go on to say that there is a plausible influence of TV sex on adolescent sexual behavior. Brown and L'Engle (2009) also found that adolescents who viewed sexually explicit images in the media in the seventh and eighth grades are more likely to sexually harass someone, engage in oral sex, and have sexual intercourse 2 years later. In both studies, the correlation between exposure to media sex and sexual behavior is low, indicating that other influences are more strongly associated with adolescent sexual behavior.

Further research by Brown and colleagues (2006) also examines the relationship between exposure to sex in the media and later sexual behavior. These researchers studied what they called a *sexual media diet,* which is the total amount of sexual content adolescents are exposed to from all media sources. Results reveal that students in middle school with a high sexual media diet are more likely to be sexually active in high school than students with a low sexual media diet (Brown et al., 2006). The relationship is true for white, but not for African American adolescents, however, indicating that media portrayals of sex are less predictive of the sexual behavior of African American adolescents than other influences.

One important study examined the relationship between viewing sexual content on television and a later adolescent pregnancy (Chandra et al., 2008). Chandra and colleagues at the RAND Corporation analyzed data from a national longitudinal study of youth collected between 2001 and 2004. The results reveal that teenagers who prefer to watch TV programs high in sexual content are significantly more likely to experience a pregnancy, as a mother or father, 2–4 years later. The authors point out that television sex is infrequently portrayed as a risky activity, and the use of contraception is rare, perhaps lulling adolescents into a false sense of security, putting them at risk for an early pregnancy.

Longitudinal research on the relationship between music videos, music, and adolescent sexuality reveals an important gender difference. Watching music videos predicts an increase in sexual activity for boys, but for girls, sexual activity predicts watching music videos (Frison, Vandenbosch, Trekels, &

Eggermont, 2015). The authors suggest that music videos may act as a peer influence on the sexual behavior of boys, while girls who are already sexually active seek out music videos that validate their sexual experiences. Other research reveals that listening to music high in sexual content is predictive of an earlier age of sexual initiation for both boys and girls (Coyne & Padilla-Walker, 2015). These two studies suggest that watching music videos and listening to music high in sexual content are both associated with an increase in risky sex for males, while the relationship between music videos, music, and risky sexual behavior is more complex for females.

What Is the Relationship between Exposure to Sex in the Media and Adolescent Sexual Behavior?

The relationship between exposure to sex in the media and adolescent sexual behavior appears to be reciprocal—exposure to media sex is predictive of more sexual activity, which in turn predicts further exposure to media sex (Bleakley, Hennessy, Fishbein, & Jordan, 2011).

One question raised by the finding of a feedback loop between sex in the media and adolescent sexual behavior is Why do sexually active adolescents seek out media with sexual themes? The obvious answer is that they are sexually aroused by portrayals of sex in the media. There are other reasons why adolescents who are sexually active might seek out sexual content, however. For example, they may think they will learn something about sex by observing it in the media, or sexual images in the media may reinforce and validate the self-concept of a sexually active youth. At this time, it is unclear what youth get out of observing sexual images or listening to music with a sexual theme, other than enjoyment and stimulation.

The finding that adolescents are interested in and seek out media content relevant to their interests is consistent with a theory called the *media practice model* (Steele, 1999). According to this theory, adolescents, like all of us, make media choices based on the personal salience of the programs. The content teens are drawn to reflects the stage of life they are in. Adolescents are beginning to have thoughts and feelings about sexuality, so it is not surprising that they show a keen interest in media sex. According to the media practice model, some adolescents select programs with sexual content in them because the teens are sexually active and interested in sexual issues, which leads to viewing and listening to more programs with sexual content, leading to more sexual activity, and so on. According to the media practice model, a reciprocal relationship exists between viewing sex in the media and adolescent sexual behavior.

Why Is Exposure to Sex in the Media Related to Adolescent Sexual Behavior?

Several explanations have been proposed for the relationship between exposure to sex in the media and adolescent sexual behavior. One is that sex in the media can lead to the acquisition of sexual scripts that are activated during romantic or sexual encounters (Wright, 2011). A *sexual script* is composed of ideas and images about how males and females are supposed to interact with each other in romantic or sexual situations. The script guides one's own behavior and leads to expectations about how the other person should behave. A sexual script is activated when a situation occurs in real life that is similar to a situation that has been observed in the media. For example, sexual intercourse in movies is rarely preceded by the man putting on a condom. According to script theory, the more often adolescents observe that script in movies, the more likely it will be acquired and later activated in real life when the opportunity arises.

A second pathway by which sex in the media might influence sexual behavior is through an increase in sexual sensation-seeking, which stimulates a desire for thrilling sexual experiences. Sensation-seeking is already high in adolescence, and the excitement that comes from watching sexual behavior on-screen may stimulate even further the development of sexual sensation-seeking in some adolescents, increasing a desire for sex.

A third pathway by which exposure to sex in the media might increase adolescent sexual behavior is by influencing beliefs about what other adolescents are doing (Bleakley, Hennessy, Fishbein, & Jordan, 2011). Specifically, the more adolescents are exposed to sex in the media, the more they come to believe that people like themselves are having sex (van Oosten, Peter, & Vandenbosch, 2017). These beliefs in what others are doing exert some pressure to act in accordance with the norms and behavior of others, leading to sexual behavior.

■ SEX IN THE MEDIA AND ADOLESCENT SEXUAL RISK-TAKING

What Is the Relationship between Exposure to Sex in the Media and Risky Sexual Behavior?

Several studies have shown a relationship between viewing sexually explicit Internet material (SEIM) and later risky sexual behaviors, such as engaging in sex at an early age, having many sexual partners, engaging in casual sex, and having sex without a condom (Braun-Courville & Rojas, 2009; Hald, Kuyper, Adam, & de Wit, 2013; O'Hara, Gibbons, Gerrard, Li, & Sargent, 2012). One study of Belgium teens found that frequent users of SEIM were five times more likely to initiate sexual intercourse than nonusers (Vandenbosch & Eggermont, 2013). In addition, more frequent viewing of SEIM is associated with more hooking up and with more hookup partners (Braithwaite, Coulson, Keddington, & Fincham, 2015).

One study of Dutch adolescents uncovered gender differences in the viewing of SEIM in the seventh grade and sexual attitudes and sexual risk in the tenth grade (Doornwaard, Bickham, Rich, ter Bogt, & van den Eijnden, 2015). Specifically, for boys, viewing SEIM increases over time, as do permissive sexual attitudes and risky sexual behavior. For boys, a plausible model of the relationship between viewing SEIM and risky sexual behavior is that viewing SEIM is related to an increase in permissive sexual attitudes, which are predictive of an increase in risky sexual behavior. In contrast, viewing SEIM among girls is low throughout adolescence and unrelated to developmental changes in permissive sexual attitudes and risky sexual behavior. For girls, the development of permissive sexual attitudes and an increase in risky sexual behavior are related to factors other than viewing SEIM.

One study of adolescent girls examined the relationship between watching X-rated films and risky sexual activity. Girls who view X-rated movies have sexual intercourse more often and with more partners than girls who do not view X-rated movies. In addition, girls who watch X-rated films have more negative attitudes about contraception use, are inconsistent contraceptive users, and have a stronger desire to conceive a child during adolescence (Wingood et al., 2001). These girls also are more likely to test positive for chlamydia. It is not possible to determine causality in this study, but the authors speculate that the limited sexual experience of young girls may make them vulnerable to the highly sexual images and risky sexual behavior they see in these movies, making it more likely that they will imitate those behaviors.

Exposure to sex in music and music videos is also related to risky sex. There is considerable concern about the themes and images in hip-hop/rap music and videos, which often glorify casual sex and degrade women. Results

---

The following story shows one young woman's attempt to come to grips with her exposure to pornography as a child and her later feelings of guilt and involvement in casual sex as an adult.

IN THEIR OWN WORDS

My older sister and I would sneak and watch soft-core pornography when we were little. We would watch these movies together, late at night on HBO. Many weekend nights we would stay up late and sleep on the pull-out bed and watch HBO or "sexy TV," as we called it.

Fast-forward about 15 or so years, I can say that at some points I still feel guilty and a little upset about watching the pornography with my older sister. I think it's more because we got caught by our parents more than anything, but I also remember feeling guilty for years when she chastised me for having some sort of sensation in my clitoris in response to the porn. Maybe too, the fact that we were girls and had a 5-year difference may have affected the amount of remorse I experienced.

Another reason as to why I might feel guilty now about watching the pornography in my childhood, adolescence, and now adulthood is that I am more sexually experienced than many of my female peers who never seemed to get into pornography. I've had more casual sexual experiences than I'd like to admit. I can't say that I started younger than some of my friends, but once I got started having sex, it became more about instant gratification rather than for love and significance. Being from a Christian home that is also liberal, I have been taught to cherish my body and not give it up so freely.

from one important longitudinal study indicate that students who frequently listen to rap music in seventh grade are more sexually active in ninth grade than students who do not listen to much rap music, suggesting that listening to rap music may play some role in the sexual behavior of young adolescents (Johnson-Baker, Markham, Baumier, Swain, & Emery, 2016). In addition, girls who report that they spend many hours watching rap music videos are more likely to have multiple sex partners, inconsistently use a condom, and acquire an STI than girls who do not watch many rap music videos (Robillard, 2012; Wingood et al., 2001).

■ SEXTING

What's Up with Sexting?

Over the past several years, considerable attention in the media and among parents and professionals has appeared about *sexting,* which involves sending sexual images of oneself to someone by means of a cell phone or a computer. Concerns have focused on sexting as inappropriate and wrong, possibly ruining one's reputation, jeopardizing one's future to potential employers, and violating the law by possessing and disseminating child pornography. Further, sending sexual images of oneself to someone can end up being upsetting to the adolescents who send the images, leading to distress, embarrassment, and even legal action. These concerns have been magnified by media reports that sexting is a widespread phenomena, involving millions of teens (Rosin, 2014).

The best prevalence estimate of sexting among adolescents is based on the Third Youth Internet Safety Survey (YISS-3) of a U.S. sample of 1,500 Internet users between the ages of 10 and 17 years (Mitchell, Finkelhor, Jones, & Wolak, 2012). A total of 2.5% of youth report appearing in or creating nude or nearly nude images of themselves, and 7.1% indicate they have received these types of images. Other studies of high school students find higher prevalence rates of sending a sext message (up to 19%), and receiving a sext message (up to 38%; Perkins, Becker, Tehee, & Mackelprang, 2014; Strassberg, Rullo, & Mackaronis, 2014). The percentage of college students who have sent a sext message is considerably higher than the percentage of high school students who have sent a sext message (Drouin, Vogel, Surbey, & Stills, 2013). Estimates from the YISS-3 may be at the low end of the actual rate, since sexting is narrowly defined as transmitting nude or seminude photos. Although the percentages are low, they translate to over a million adolescents who send a sexual image of themselves each year, an even larger number who receive these images, and a larger number still of adolescents and emerging adults who send and receive sexually explicit text messages.

Most of the adolescents who appear in these images are girls between 16 and 17 years of age who photograph themselves. Girls are slightly more likely to receive the images than boys (56% vs. 44%), indicating that it is common for girls to send images of themselves to other girls. Four typical reasons for creating and receiving a sext are that it is a joke or a playful activity between friends, a form of flirting, part of a romantic relationship, or a response to pressure from a partner (Cooper, Quayle, Jonsson, & Svedin, 2016; Drouin & Tobin, 2014). Most of the images are sent to friends or romantic partners. Few of these images are forwarded to anyone else.

Forwarding explicit images to others who are not the original recipients of the images does occur, which raises several difficult legal questions. Some people are concerned that young people are disseminating child pornography, while others believe that some youth are being charged with sex crimes and placed on sex offender registries for what amounts to teenage recklessness (Stillman, 2016). A relatively small number of cases come to the attention of law enforcement agencies, about 1,800 per year during the late 2000s (Wolak, Finkelhor, & Mitchell, 2012). About two-thirds of these incidents are considered serious, involving adults or youth engaged in blackmail or other criminal behavior. About one-third have no malicious intent and are better characterized as adolescent irresponsible behavior. It is important for the law to distinguish between these two categories of behavior so that some youth are not labeled juvenile sex offenders for what is better thought of as adolescent indiscretion. Parents and teachers should carefully explain the risks to adolescents, even students in middle school, many of whom are unaware of the possible social and legal consequences of sexting.

Is Sexting an Indicator of Sexual Risk-Taking?

Sexting can be a marker for adolescent sexual risk-taking (Brinkley, Ackerman, Ehrenreich, & Underwood, 2017; Cooper et al., 2016). Sexting is part of a cluster of sexual risk behaviors that include sex at an early age and inconsistent condom use (Ybarra & Mitchell, 2014). Adolescents who send sext messages or pictures are likely to be sexually active and to have engaged in a variety of sexual behaviors, including sexual touching, oral sex, and vaginal sex (Houck et al., 2014; Rice et al., 2012). Sexting often precedes sexual behavior and may serve as an indicator that one is interested in having sex or ready to take a relationship to the next level (Temple & Choi, 2014).

Adolescents who receive a sext message are more likely to be sexually active than adolescents who have not received a sext message. In one study, middle school students who have received a sext message are six times more likely to be sexually active than those who have not received a sext message (Rice et al., 2014). In addition, those adolescents who send a sext message are almost four times more likely to be sexually active. Sexting and sexual activity go hand in hand. The relationship between sexting and sexual behavior is reciprocal and sexting predicts future sexual behavior, but sexual activity also predicts future sexting (Strassberg, McKinnon, Sustaita, & Rullo, 2013).

References to sexual activity are also common on social networking sites such as Facebook. In several studies of Facebook content, about 25% of adolescents between the ages of 10 and 19 years in the United States and the Netherlands posted revealing photographs of themselves with descriptions of sexual behavior (Doornwaard, Moreno, van den Eijnden, Vanwesenbeeck, & ter Bogt, 2014; Moreno, Brockman, Wasserheit, & Christakis, 2012). Adolescents who post sexual displays are more sexually experienced and interested in having sex than nondisplayers, indicating that online displays reflect off-line behavior and interests. Posting sexy pictures on social media is related to participating in oral sex and sexual intercourse (Reitz et al., 2015; van Oosten, Peter, & Boot, 2015). Although only a minority of adolescents post sexual material about themselves on social networking sites, those who do broadcast to others that they are sexually active or ready to become sexually active.

■ ADOLESCENTS AND PORNOGRAPHY

What Is Pornography?

Researchers often use the phrase *sexually explicit images* to refer to images and videos that many would call pornographic. Sexually explicit images are clear, unambiguous, graphic pictures or videos of penile–vaginal sexual intercourse, oral sex, anal sex, masturbation, or other sexual acts that are not presented in a medical context or for purposes of education. Sexually explicit images and pornography are often used synonymously, but *sexually explicit images* is a more descriptive phrase. One problem with the term *pornography* is that it is virtually impossible to define. Supreme Court Justice Potter Stewart famously said in reference to *obscenity,* the legal term referring to pornography, he could not define it, "but I know it when I see it"—the larger point being that obscenity is in the eye of the beholder (Jacobellis v. Ohio, 1964). Although it is impossible to define *pornography,* the term continues to be used in everyday speech and even by some researchers.

Does Everyone View Pornography as Harmful?

Pornography is a part of the sexual world of many emerging adults who do not believe that looking at sexually explicit images is wrong or harmful (Carroll et al., 2008). For many emerging adults, especially males, looking at pornography is a stimulus for sexual arousal, a source of information about sex, and a social activity done with friends (Löfgren-Mårtenson & Månsson, 2010). Women are more ambivalent about pornography, some accepting it as harmless sexual entertainment, while others are critical of the sexist portrayal of women as sex objects. There has been an increase in the percentage of people in the United States who view pornography since the 1970s (Price, Patterson, Regnerus, & Walley, 2016), which may signal a cultural shift in attitudes about pornography, especially among the young who have integrated it into their sexual lives.

For one young man, pornography and masturbation are intimately connected. He fondly remembers the first time he saw pornographic images, as described in the following story.

IN THEIR OWN WORDS

Planning the what, where, and when of my first online porn segment was quite the event to me at the age of 14. This sort of personal experience took strategic planning and all the details were taken into careful consideration. I was always on the fence on whether or not to watch pornography while I masturbated. In my eyes, masturbation was enough sin for me to handle at that age. I obviously felt ashamed of masturbating, but watching pornography while I did it meant that there could not be the slightest chance that I was going to be caught (hence the planning). I waited one day until I was all alone at my mother's house while everyone else was busy away from home. I had a laptop at that point as a kid since I was going to be in high school soon and needed it to write papers and whatnot. My parents had website blockers on certain inappropriate sites, but I of course did my research leading up to this one day and found a free online porn website that I could get access to without any red flags. The main purpose of watching pornography for the first time was to satisfy my curiosity. The second was because my friends were always talking about random pornography videos and the sexy girls in them, so I figured that I might as well try it. Nevertheless, my curiosity was indeed satisfied. The entire experience was way more than I expected since I had only been exposed to regular movie sex scenes at this point (the online pornography video blew that way out of the water). Soon after, watching the free online pornography website while masturbating became a habit at the age of 14 and on, and to tell you the truth, I justified the pairing up of the two as normal for kids my age and that it was all just a developmental stage.

Why Is Pornography Mainly a Guy Thing?

One of the strongest findings in the area of research on human sexual behavior is that males of all ages, races, and nationalities are considerably more likely to look at images of sex in the media than are females (Petersen & Hyde, 2010). In one study of Australian adolescents, 38% of boys but only 2% of girls reported that they had deliberately looked at explicit sex sites on the Internet (Flood, 2007), while in a study of U.S. adolescents 40% of boys but only 13% of girls reported going to Internet porn sites (Bleakley, Hennessy, & Fishbein, 2011). The magnitude of these percentages match findings for adolescents in the Netherlands and Germany, suggesting that gender difference in interest in pornography is widespread (Peter & Valkenburg, 2006b; Weber, Quiring, & Daschmann, 2012).

Some scientists believe that this gender difference is biological, based on our evolutionary history. Evolutionary psychologists argue that males have much to gain from having sex with as many females as possible, increasing their number of offspring, while females benefit from being more selective. Thus, for males, having sex with many females is exciting, both in fantasy and reality, so men are turned on by images of people having sex.

Another explanation for the gender difference in involvement with pornography is that males have a stronger sex drive than women, which leads to

> *The following story shows that some women are interested in pornography, although as this young woman indicates, she is not sure why she is interested.*
>
> ## IN THEIR OWN WORDS
>
> I started watching porn when I discovered that it existed online, probably in early high school. It's not a habit or anything, but it's something entertaining to do and it relieves stress. I hope that one day I can be with a man who understands and respects that women can and do enjoy the same sexual pleasures that men do and who will be willing to watch porn with me. If I was a man, I would find any woman who is comfortable enough with her sexuality to admit to enjoying porn and masturbation to be very attractive because she would seem confident, courageous, and even exciting. There are women who enjoy all kinds of porn and who are being shamed into not admitting it.
>
> There have been times when I have looked back on myself and tried to assess why it is that I view and enjoy pornography at times. Perhaps I was trying to fit in with my mostly male friends, maybe I was just curious about what sex would be like before I actually became sexually active, or maybe I wanted to be educated and prepared for any sexual experiences I could have in the future. But I eventually came to the realization that I do not need to have an explanation or excuse for my sexual behavior and my desire to watch pornography. I watch pornography because I find it entertaining and interesting. I watch it because I can. And I am not ashamed to say so.

more frequent thoughts and fantasies about sex (Baumeister, Catanese, & Vohs, 2001). In one study of adolescents, early-maturing males were more likely to go to Internet sex sites than late-maturing males, suggesting that testosterone may affect interest in pornography. There is no relationship between pubertal status and viewing Internet sex sites for females (Peter & Valkenburg, 2006a).

Some suggest that there is a methodological issue that might account for some of the gender differences in involvement with pornography. Some females may be reluctant to admit that they look at pornography and enjoy it, because pornography is viewed as a male activity that is inappropriate for females.

Others argue that more females would like pornography if the porn industry would create female-friendly porn. The worldwide success of the book *Fifty Shades of Grey* (James, 2012) attests to the large audience of mainly women who are interested in a certain kind of written erotica. In fact, descriptions of sexual encounters ranging from passionate kissing to sexual intercourse are common in young adult novels, much of it read by females (Callister et al., 2012). Several Internet porn sites do exist that are targeted specifically at women, such as *www.sssh.com* and *www.forthegirls.com,* but these sites get very little traffic and even less business in comparison to porn sites catering to men.

Who Are the Frequent Viewers of Pornography?

For most young people who view pornography, including teenage males, looking at sexually explicit images is occasional and appears to be motivated by a desire for sexual stimulation and sexual curiosity emerging from age-related biological development and changes in interests that begin in early adolescence (Doornwaard, van den Eijnden, Overbeek, & ter Bogt, 2015). There are many personal accounts of people who are frequent viewers of pornography, who spend hours every day looking at it, however. There is no single definition of "frequent use," which usually implies viewing explicit sex almost every day. Frequent viewers of pornography are of special interest because their use pattern may be symptomatic of other risky behavior or of underlying psychological or social problems. Frequent viewing of pornography is associated with higher depressive feelings (Doornwaard, van den Eijnden, Baams, Vanwesenbeeck, & ter Bogt, 2016) and poor off-line social relations (Smahel, Brown, & Blinka, 2012). A habit of frequent use is associated with viewing more extreme images of sexual relations, including sex between more than two people, violent sex, and sex between an adult and a minor (Svedin, Åkerman, & Priebe, 2011). Presumably, people who frequently view pornography eventually become bored and satiated by portrayals of ordinary sex and seek out more unusual forms of sexual expression.

Frequent viewers of sexually explicit images also share some common social characteristics (Peter & Valkenburg, 2016). Frequent viewers are older adolescents and emerging adults, mainly males, who usually look at this material when they are alone. One of the most significant differences between frequent viewers and occasional viewers is that frequent viewers report that they often feel sexually aroused, suggesting a greater than average sex drive (Doornwaard, van den Eijnden, et al., 2015).

Frequent viewers are also more likely to have behavioral conduct problems and poor peer relations (Tsitsika et al., 2009). Frequently viewing sexually explicit images, especially on Internet sex sites, is correlated with delinquency and substance use among adolescents, suggesting that frequent viewing of pornography is part of a syndrome of antisocial behavior that may emerge from high risk-taking and sensation-seeking (Owens, Behun, Manning, & Reid, 2012). Adolescents who are frequent viewers of sexually explicit material have poor relations with their parents, who are poor monitors with few, if any, rules about computer use (Tomić, Burić, & Štulhofer, 2018). Not every frequent viewer fits this profile, but many young men who are frequent viewers exhibit problem behavior in several areas of their lives, including poor relations with parents, that set them apart from the majority of youth who occasionally check out these sites (Mattebo, Tydén, Häggstrom-Nördin, Nilsson, & Larsson, 2013).

One scenario to account for these findings is that some young males with weak bonds to parents and poor social skills gravitate toward other troubled boys with similar backgrounds and form deviant peer groups with a delinquent subculture that prizes hypermasculinity, misogyny, and the consumption of pornography. The findings from studies of frequent viewers have clinical implications and suggest that frequently viewing pornography during adolescence may be an indicator of disrupted relations with parents and involvement with deviant peers (Mesch, 2009).

The following deeply personal story by a college female shows that frequent pornography consumption can also be a problem for females who attempt to cope with depression through the sexual excitement that comes from pornography use.

IN THEIR OWN WORDS

The onset of my depression was about seventh grade. One of my symptoms was my relationship with porn and masturbation. I understand that these things are normal but watching porno after porno and masturbating climax after climax because you feel like you can't accomplish anything else in your life except self-pleasure is not normal. I would look at porn especially when I felt hopeless.

While watching porn you can't think about anything else but the very "eye-catching" scene in front of you. Not only did it concentrate my attention elsewhere, it was extremely pleasurable. It was a very successful distractor from my warped sense of reality that I do not amount to anything. Eventually I got the help of medication and therapy so I could fight back against my depression. The amount of porn I watched decreased and how long I would watch it for decreased also. I still enjoy porn to this day but I do not use porn as a crutch for my mental illness. There is a difference.

SUMMARY

■ MEDIA SEX

Many experts believe that exposure to sex in the media leads to early sexual activity and risky sexual behavior among adolescents. An additional concern is that exposure to sex in the media is related to the formation of negative stereotypes about females. Several writers have made another point, which is that the media can be an opportunity to promote positive sexual behavior. In fact, many adolescents report that they use the Internet to find answers to questions they have about sex.

■ SEX IN THE MEDIA

Many network and cable shows on television contain some sexual content, typically talk about sex. Depictions of sexual behavior on TV are uncommon. Sexual intercourse that is portrayed on television is usually free of negative consequences.

Sexual videos on the Internet are readily available to anyone who wants to see them, even to those not looking for them. Accidental exposure to sexual images through pop-ups or inadvertent links to X-rated websites are common.

Movies are another medium high in sexual content, even movies for teens. Music, especially hip-hop/rap music, and music videos contain many references to sexual behavior. Depictions of men and women in music and music videos typically are highly stereotyped.

■ SEX IN THE MEDIA AND ADOLESCENT SEXUAL ATTITUDES AND BELIEFS

There is a positive relationship between exposure to sex in the media and more permissive attitudes about sexuality among male and female adolescents (Escobar-Chaves et al., 2005; Ward, 2016; Wright, Malamuth, & Donnerstein, 2012). Media sex presented realistically is more strongly related to permissive sexual attitudes than unrealistic sexual scenes. Consequences to the sexual actor matter, especially when those consequences are negative, in which case adolescents are less likely to endorse positive attitudes about casual sex.

■ SEX IN THE MEDIA AND ADOLESCENT SEXUAL BEHAVIOR

Four conclusions emerge from research on the relationship between exposure to sex in the media and adolescent sexual behavior. First, a positive relationship exists between exposure to sex in the media and adolescent sexual behavior. Second, because a true experiment with random assignment of subjects to conditions cannot be conducted on the relationship between viewing sexual content in the media and adolescent sexual behavior, it is impossible to demonstrate beyond a reasonable doubt that sexual media content has an impact on adolescent behavior. Third, based on longitudinal research, many researchers argue that viewing sex in the media has some effect on adolescent sexual behavior. Fourth, the relationship that does exist between media sex and adolescent sexual behavior is small to modest. It appears that the sexual behavior of adolescents is more highly influenced by other factors, such as parents and peers, than it is by what teens see and hear in the media.

Several explanations have been offered to account for the relationship between media sex and sexual behavior. One is that adolescents learn sexual scripts from media sex, which they enact when the situation arises. A second explanation is that there is an increase in sexual sensation-seeking as a consequence of viewing and listening to media sex, which leads to a desire for sex. A third explanation is that sex in the media contributes to the belief that risky sex is common among young people, encouraging adolescents to conform to what they see as a norm.

■ SEX IN THE MEDIA AND ADOLESCENT SEXUAL RISK-TAKING

A positive relationship exists between exposure to sex in the media and risky sexual behavior, including sex at an early age, having many partners, and inconsistent condom use. SEIM is especially related to having risky sex.

◼ SEXTING

Only a minority of adolescents, especially high school students, have engaged in sexting, but many more youth have received a sexually explicit image. Sexting is associated with many sexual risk behaviors, including having sex at an early age and inconsistent condom use.

◼ ADOLESCENTS AND PORNOGRAPHY

Many experts view pornography as unhealthy, a view that is not shared by many emerging adults, especially young males. Males are more interested in pornography than females, and there are several explanations for this gender difference, including biological differences between the sexes, and because most pornography deliberately targets a male audience. Frequent viewing of explicit sex by adolescents is associated with delinquency and substance use, in addition to poor relations with parents and association with deviant peers.

SUGGESTIONS FOR FURTHER READING

Buhi, E. R., Daley, E. M., Oberne, A., Smith, S. A., Schneider, T., & Fuhrmann, H. J. (2010). Quality and accuracy of sexual health information web sites visited by young people. *Journal of Adolescent Health, 47,* 206–208.

Chandra, A., Martino, S. C., Collins, R. L., Elliott, M. N., Berry, S. H., Kanouse, D. E., et al., (2008). Does watching sex on television predict teen pregnancy? Findings from a national longitudinal survey of youth. *Pediatrics, 122,* 1047–1054.

Collins, R. L., Elliott, M. N., Berry, S. H., Kanouse, D. E., Kunkel, D., Hunter, S. B., et al. (2004). Watching sex on TV predicts adolescent initiation of sexual behavior. *Pediatrics, 114,* e280–e289.

Mitchell, K. J., Finkelhor, D., Jones, L. M., & Wolak, J. (2012). Prevalence and characteristics of youth sexting: A national study. *Pediatrics, 129,* 13–20.

Ward, L. M. (2003). Understanding the role of entertainment media in the sexual socialization of American youth: A review of empirical research. *Developmental Review, 23,* 347–388.

Ward, L. M. (2016). Media and sexualization: State of empirical research, 1995–2015. *Journal of Sex Research, 53,* 560–577.

Wright, P. J., Malamuth, N. M., & Donnerstein, E. (2012). Research on sex in the media: What do we know about effects on children and adolescents? In D. G. Singer & J. L. Singer (Eds.), *Handbook of children and the media* (pp. 273–302). Thousand Oaks, CA: SAGE.

Ybarra, M. L., Strasburger, V. C., & Mitchell, K. J. (2014). Sexual media exposure, sexual behavior, and sexual violence victimization in adolescence. *Clinical Pediatrics, 53,* 1239–1247.

CHAPTER 8

LGBTQ Adolescents in a Heterosexual World

Imagine filling out a questionnaire in which you are asked the question "Which of the following best describes your sexual orientation: heterosexual, gay male, lesbian female, bisexual, or other?" If you are like most adults, you would probably have an easy time answering that simple question. You know who you are and whether you are sexually attracted to people of the opposite sex, the same sex, or both sexes. Some adolescents who are still in the process of establishing their sexual orientation find the question difficult and have a hard time choosing an answer. The goal of this chapter is to examine issues related to one's sexual orientation during adolescence and emerging adulthood in order to better understand the development and expression of an LGBTQ identity.

■ DEFINING SEXUAL ORIENTATION

At the start, it is important to define sexual orientation, gender identity, and questioning. *Sexual orientation* refers to the gender of the people to whom one is sexually attracted. Most of this chapter focuses on individuals who are lesbian, gay, or bisexual (LGB). *Gender identity* refers to a personal sense that one is a male or a female. It is not a sexual orientation. Someone with a transgender (T) identity may be sexually attracted to males, females, both, or neither. *Questioning* (Q) adolescents are uncertain of their sexual orientation.

What Is Known about Adolescents Who Have an Uncertain Sexual Orientation?

Many LGB adults recall a period of uncertainty and questioning about their sexual orientation during late childhood and early adolescence that gradually gives

The following story by a young woman reveals that uncertainty about one's sexual orientation may continue for some people even into emerging adulthood.

IN THEIR OWN WORDS

At 20 years old, I'm not entirely sure of my sexual identity. If I had been asked to label my sexual identity 2 years ago, I would say heterosexual without a second thought. However, 2 years ago, I also had practically no sexual experience and truthfully had not even considered the possibility that I may be something other than straight. After a few lackluster casual hookups with guys at college and one definitely *not* lackluster relationship with a girl, I now have a little more experience that can be used to determine my sexual identity, but I have yet to come to any definite conclusions.

Following the hookups I'd had with guys in the past, it was like a switch flipped and my feelings for them disappeared. The thought of hanging out with them again would make me anxious and I'd avoid all of their texts and calls. My friends would joke about my "playing hard to get," while I just brushed it off as not having met the right guy yet. I figured the "butterflies" and desire to be in a relationship would come when I found a guy I really liked. However, these feelings of infatuation came immediately after my first hookup with a girl, which led to my first real relationship where I felt truly comfortable and happy.

Now that the relationship with my girlfriend has ended, I'm at a crossroads. I've since had a brief relationship with a guy and had familiar feelings of disinterest, so it seems natural to see what would happen if I were to be with another girl. However, as a stereotypically feminine girl with an entirely straight set of friends at school (though very open-minded and accepting, thankfully!), it's difficult to meet lesbian or bisexual girls. I also think part of me is hoping that I will come across a guy who will give me the feelings I've been looking for, or that my relationship with my girlfriend was a "fluke," so that I can avoid the difficulty of truly exploring the possibility that I could be a lesbian, not just a college girl "experimenting" with her sexuality. In the meantime, I feel most comfortable defining myself as bisexual because I am not willing to write off my past experiences with guys as completely meaningless, but I realize that my sexual identity is definitely subject to change.

way to more certainty and acceptance during late adolescence and emerging adulthood (Igartua, Thombs, Burgos, & Montoro, 2009; Mustanski, Birkett, et al., 2014; Shields et al., 2013).

Data from a health survey of Minnesota youth reveal the clearest picture of sexual orientation as an emergent phenomenon that unfolds during adolescence (Remafedi, Resnick, Blum, & Harris, 1992). The percentage of students who are "unsure" of their sexual orientation steadily declines from a high of about 26% among 12-year-olds to between 5 and 9% among 17- to 18-year-olds. Significantly, the unsure students are especially likely to report sexual experiences with youth of the same sex, suggesting that many unsure students are in the process of developing an LGB orientation. Most heterosexual adolescents are sure of their heterosexual orientation, but many youth who will eventually identify as LGB are unsure of their orientation during early adolescence, and do not reach an achieved sexual identity until late adolescence or even emerging adulthood.

A FOCUS ON RESEARCH

Establishing the true prevalence of homo-sexuality in the United States or in any country is an endeavor plagued by controversy and uncertainty. Estimates range from about two out of 100 based on social science research to 10 out of 100 from Alfred Kinsey and colleagues' (Kinsey, Pomeroy, & Martin, 1948; Kinsey, Pomeroy, Martin, & Gebhard, 1953) clinical research in the 1940s and 1950s. The discrepancy has its roots in three problems inherent in social science survey research: obtaining a representative sample of a population, constructing unambiguous questions, and obtaining valid responses.

Sampling is a problem in social science research where all to often, researchers collect data from convenience samples composed of people who happen to be available. It is not possible to determine a true population figure from data collected from a convenience sample since the sample may not represent the population under study. Most of the research on adolescents is based on data obtained from high school students and most of the research on emerging adults is based on data collected from college students who represent only about 50% of emerging adults. These sampling limitations should be kept in mind when attempting to estimate the percentage of adolescents who are LGB. An additional sampling problem with research on minors is that parents must be fully informed about the purpose of the research and give their permission for their children to participate. The researcher does not know what percentage of LGB adolescents either choose not to participate in the study, or have parents who do not allow their children to take part (Macapagal, Coventry, Arbeit, Fisher, & Mustanski, 2017).

A second problem with survey research emerges from the need to have unambiguous and understandable questions and response alternatives, a problem that may be especially difficult for research on the sexual orientations of adolescents who vary in age from 13 to 19 years. Students who are 13 years old may not have a clear understanding of the terms *heterosexual*, *homosexual*, and *bisexual* in response to a question such as "Which of the following best describes your sexual orientation?" These wordage problems mean that researchers must be certain that their questions and their response alternatives are understandable and have the same meaning for adolescents of all ages.

A third problem concerns response bias. Studies of the prevalence of homo-sexuality may underestimate the true figure because some adolescents with a same-sex orientation are reluctant to admit they are members of a stigmatized group. Some adolescents may be in the closet and want to keep their orientation a secret, even on an anonymous survey. Another type of response bias is that some adolescents may not take sexual surveys seriously and give untrue or misleading answers (Fish & Russell, 2017).

Although there are problems associated with social science survey research, the best studies reflect an attempt to reduce these inherent difficulties. The best research on adolescent sexual orientation is based on data from large representative samples of high school students, with carefully worded and understandable questions and response alternatives, administered to students anonymously. No study is perfect, but results obtained from studies that attempt to minimize survey research problems associated with estimating the prevalence of LGB adolescents provide the most accurate estimates and are more valid than findings from convenience samples or personal experience.

Why the uncertainty? One possibility is that some adolescents are still in the process of forming a sexual identity that is in a state of diffusion in early adolescence. Another possibility is that younger adolescents are unsure of the meaning of the terms *heterosexual, homosexual,* and *bisexual,* an uncertainty that clears up with time and experience. Last, some young adolescents with a same-sex orientation may be reluctant to admit they are members of a stigmatized group, a fear that diminishes for many young people as they become more comfortable with themselves and receive support for their sexual orientation from parents and friends (Saewyc et al., 2004). Uncertainty, misunderstanding, and fear may all be major barriers to labeling oneself and admitting to others that one is LGB.

■ SOME NUMBERS AND STATISTICS

What Percentage of Adolescents Are LGB?

The most recent investigation of the prevalence of sexual orientation among adolescents in the United States is based on data obtained from the Youth Risk Behavior Survey (YRBS), which is a probability sample of almost 13,000 U.S. high school students (Kann, Olsen, et al., 2016). In this study, 88.8% of students labeled themselves heterosexual, 6.0% bisexual, 2.0% gay or lesbian, and 3.2% unsure. A slightly lower percentage of LGB youth was found in a population-based survey of New Zealand secondary school students, in which 5.9% of youth labeled themselves LGB (Lucassen et al., 2015). It appears that between 6 and 8% of high school students label themselves as LGB.

Are There Gender Differences in the Percentage of Adolescents Who Are LGB?

In virtually every study of the prevalence of LGB adolescents, a pattern of gender differences emerges. About the same or slightly more males than females are sexually attracted to same-sex individuals, but more females than males indicate they are bisexual, suggesting that females have a more fluid sexual orientation than males (Mustanski, Birkett, et al., 2014; Priebe & Svedin, 2013; Savin-Williams, Joyner, & Rieger, 2012).

■ SEXUAL ORIENTATION, SEXUAL BEHAVIOR, AND SEXUAL IDENTITY

What Is the Difference between Sexual Orientation, Sexual Behavior, and Sexual Identity?

One useful way of thinking about one's sexuality was developed by Ritch Savin-Williams (2005) at Cornell University, who distinguishes three "primary domains": sexual orientation, sexual behavior, and sexual identity. *Sexual orientation* is based on which gender an individual has a preponderance of erotic feelings, thoughts, and fantasies. One's orientation can be toward the opposite sex, the same sex, both sexes, or neither sex. Sexual orientation may not be a categorical variable, but may exist on a continuum that varies from exclusively heterosexual to exclusively homosexual, making it difficult for some people to define themselves (Savin-Williams, 2014). The second domain is *sexual behavior,* which is broadly defined as engaging in some kind of sexually stimulating behavior with someone of the opposite sex, the same sex, or both sexes. At first glance, an assessment of sexual behavior seems like it would be straightforward, but it is not. Sexual behavior is assessed by a question such as "Have you ever had a sexual experience with someone of the same sex?" Such a general question will corral a broad range of behaviors from vaginal intercourse to anal intercourse, oral sex, erotic fondling, and passionate kissing—a spectrum of behaviors that may be too encompassing for some purposes but appropriate for others. The third domain is *sexual identity,* which is the self-identified sexual label an individual uses to describe him- or herself. It would be assessed with a question such as "Which of the following best describes your sexual identity: heterosexual, gay male, lesbian female, bisexual, transgender, other, or unsure?" For most individuals, these three domains line up and point to one conclusion, but for some people, especially adolescents, there may be inconsistency among the domains, making it difficult for some adolescents to confidently define themselves.

Is a Same-Sex Orientation Enduring and Immutable?

Some gay and lesbian adults report that they were sexually attracted to people of the opposite sex during adolescence or emerging adulthood. Further, some people who eventually identify as gay or lesbian adults engage in sexual behavior, including intercourse, with people of the opposite sex during adolescence and emerging adulthood (Smiler, Frankel, & Savin-Williams, 2011). About half of high school students who label themselves gay or lesbian have had a sexual experience with the opposite sex (Mustanski, Birkett, et al., 2014). These cross-sex attractions and behaviors are difficult to reconcile with the idea that a same-sex orientation is stable and immutable.

Several explanations exist for sexual behavior with the opposite sex among adolescents and emerging adults who will eventually identify themselves as lesbian or gay. One explanation is that these experiences represent experimentation, which is to be expected during the teen and early adult years, since these are periods of exploration and uncertainty (Diamond, 2003).

Another explanation is that some adolescents who will eventually identify as lesbian or gay when they become adults cannot admit to a same-sex orientation when they are young because they cannot accept an orientation that is stigmatized. Thus, these adolescents may view themselves as heterosexual and even engage in sexual behavior with the opposite sex to demonstrate to themselves and to others that they are heterosexual, when they are not.

A third explanation for cross-sex sexual behavior during adolescence and emerging adulthood is that the development of a same-sex orientation is a dynamic process that occurs over a period of years at least through adolescence and emerging adulthood (Li & Hines, 2016; Ott, Corliss, Wypij, Rosario, & Austin, 2011). The idea that one's sexual orientation is established early and permanently is true for the large majority of heterosexuals and most lesbian and gay individuals. But a sizable number of people who will eventually identify themselves as lesbian or gay are sexually attracted to individuals of the opposite sex and have sex with someone of the opposite sex during adolescence and emerging adulthood, all of which suggests that many lesbian and gay individuals do not establish a permanent same-sex orientation until adulthood (Dickson, van Roode, Cameron, & Paul, 2013; Hu et al., 2016).

In the following story, a young, gay male describes his one fulfilling heterosexual experience.

IN THEIR OWN WORDS

When I was about 18 or 19 years old, fresh out of high school, I had a group of friends that I would hang out with three or four times a week. We would always get together and drink and play the guitar and just spend time relaxing and having a good time—this was in large part due to the fact that one of my friends lived on a golf course, and a lot of the time, we would go out to one of the holes and lay out on the green. One of my friends that I hung out with a lot, R., and I were always playfully flirting with one another, but with all my concerns and questions about my homosexuality, I figured nothing would come of the harmless flirting. One night in particular, we were all at R.'s house, drinking more than we probably should have, and she and I ended up alone. I found out that she was a big fan of performing oral sex and the thought of her causing pleasure for someone was a huge turn-on for her.

With this new information, even though I was mainly gay at this point, who was I to pass up an offer like this? We moved to her room and made our way to her bed, where she seductively took off my pants and began performing oral sex. I never returned the favor to her, which now makes me sound like a complete douche bag and makes it seem that I was using her, but she never seemed to be upset by the lack of oral performance on my part. It was a great system for a while, and this went on for a few months and had no effect on our friendship. One night while this was happening, I was getting curious, or my testosterone was high, I'm not really sure why it happened, honestly, but we moved from oral sex to actual intercourse.

While in the middle of her oral act, I stopped her and asked if we could move things further to intercourse, because I was mainly curious as to how it felt and did not want to go my whole life without knowing. She was a great sport about everything and agreed to help me out. Once the act had started, it was only about 20 seconds until I was finished, not really changed at all.

That actually ended up being the last night we ever fooled around with one another. We are still really good friends, and actually ended up working together for 2.5 years. We laugh about our younger years and about how careless we were, but to this day I don't regret a thing. She is still the only woman I've ever done anything sexual with to this day, but that is a story for a different day.

Sexual orientation instability is found even among adults, however, especially among women—findings that are problematic for ideas about sexual orientation permanence (Diamond & Rosky, 2016; Everett, Talley, Hughes, Wilsnack, & Johnson, 2016). Sexual fluidity is somewhat common among females, not only during adolescence but even in adulthood (Ott et al., 2011). As many as 25% of adult lesbians report that they were exclusively heterosexual when they were younger and only became attracted to other females in middle age.

■ THE DEVELOPMENT OF AN LGB IDENTITY

How Does Sexual Identity Develop?

Identifying oneself as LGB is not self-evident to young children, who have yet to experience a true sexual attraction. An LGB sexual identity may be wired into one's DNA, but the knowledge, acceptance, and meaning an individual attaches to that identity is very much a psychological and social process that unfolds over a period of years, typically during the second decade of life.

For most LGB individuals, the formation of a sexual identity is a long-term process that first expresses itself in early childhood with an interest in other-sex toys and activities (Li, Kung, & Hines, 2017). Most models of LGB sexual identity formation propose that individuals progress through a series of stages or phases that begin in childhood with feelings of being different, extend into adolescence, and end years later with the achievement of a sense of one's sexual identity. Two theories lay out the broad outlines of that process, providing roadmaps that describe the sequence of events that eventually lead to the formation of an LGB sexual identity (Eliason, 1996).

In the late 1970s and mid-1980s, Vivienne Cass (1979, 1984), an Australian clinical psychologist, published a groundbreaking theory on homosexual identity formation. According to Cass, the development of an LGB identity progresses through six discrete stages. The first stage is *identity confusion,* which is conscious awareness that homosexuality is relevant to the self. During this stage, young adolescents realize that their thoughts, feelings, or behavior toward same-sex individuals raises the possibility that they are LGB. Stage 2 is *identity comparison,* in which the individual accepts the possibility that he or she may be homosexual. In Stage 3, *identity tolerance,* the individual moves from the idea that "I may be homosexual" to "I probably am homosexual." During this stage, the individual makes contact with other LGB individuals for social support and to counter isolation. Stage 4, *identity acceptance,* includes an increase in contact with other LGB individuals who validate one's LGB identity, which leads to positive feelings that one is normal. The gay subculture becomes an increasingly important part of one's social life in this stage. In the fifth stage, *identity pride,* there is acceptance of one's LGB identity. During this stage, the individual discloses his or her LGB identity to a wider circle of people and becomes far less concerned with the reactions of heterosexuals. In the sixth stage, *identity synthesis,* the individual is able to integrate an LGB identity with other aspects of the self. Instead of viewing oneself as primarily LGB, one's sexual identity is one aspect of the self, and may not even be the most important.

Richard Troiden, a professor of sociology and anthropology at Miami University in Ohio, proposed a four-stage model of the development of a homosexual identity that draws on Cass's (1979, 1984) influential theory (Troiden, 1989). According to Troiden, homosexual identity formation progresses through four stages. Stage 1, *sensitization,* occurs before puberty and is the feeling that one is different in some important way from one's same-sex peers. Usually this feeling of marginality springs from a lack of interest in typical gender activities, such as sports for boys and dolls for girls, and is not based on a same-sex sexual attraction. Stage 2 is *identity confusion.* The next phase of homosexual identity development is to be unsure of one's sexual orientation. Stage 3, *identity assumption,* typically occurs during or after late adolescence, is marked by a definition of oneself as homosexual, and is followed by coming out to significant others.

The following young lesbian describes in detail her feelings about her developing lesbian identity, and her eventual acceptance of who she is.

IN THEIR OWN WORDS

Rainbows, pride, and love were the easiest of things that I welcomed into my life after years of realizing I may be a part of a small subculture of people commonly defined as homosexuals.

A roller coaster is the most accurate analogy I could use to describe this journey, so we will start with the first big hill. Realizing there is a same-sex attraction, sexually acting on this behavior, and personally accepting and identifying with your same-sex orientation make up this first step. For some, it may take years and years to make it all the way through this process. Personally, it took 4 crucial years of my adolescence to sort through what was happening—high school. At a very early age I recall feeling and thinking different in comparison to my female friends, but never understanding what it was or why it was happening. Finally, in high school, these feelings became more fluid and tangible. The experience had evolved from just realizing something new about myself to these thoughts becoming a part of me that was simply apparent, but still I was ignoring, hiding, and afraid of it, and at this

time I had never sexually experimented with any females whatsoever, but I knew what identity I would soon embody. For me, the hardest part was physically acting on this same-sex desire. But in the end, it seemed to be that last step that confirmed everything. When considering behaving as a homosexual, I was fearful for my religious upbringing, my own reaction to the situation, the reaction of anyone that found out, and so many more things.

Eventually, however, those fears were overcome and the feelings I had been attempting to understand became official—I was gay. We have all had the feelings of butterflies, nervousness, and sweaty palms, and for me, certain females happened to set off those triggers. At this point, one would think the fear of that gigantic first hill would be gone, but years and years later I am still left with pulling apart and putting back together the internal dialogue that this is really who I am. It seems silly, because I have been acting on these feelings for almost 8 years now, but the uncertainty that is created within me, by society and religion, is hard to forget.

The following story is from a young woman who had read about Troiden's (1989) theory of homosexual identity formation and explicitly ties her experiences to that theory. Note the distinction she makes between her experience and the last stage of the theory, however.

IN THEIR OWN WORDS

I knew from a very young age that I was different from all of the little girls. I had no interest in playing with Barbie dolls and dressing up; instead I found myself playing touch football with the boys at recess, having way too many Legos, and you couldn't get me into a dress for anything! I also remember having a crush on my substitute teacher in third grade, and was much more drawn to strong female characters in television and film, such as Xena the Warrior Princess. Troiden would call this step "sensitization."

I remember the day that I experienced what Troiden would call "identity confusion," or the day I realized I probably was a lesbian. I was researching on AOL what all these feelings I was beginning to develop for girls in my class could mean and I came across a pamphlet or something similar that didn't cast homosexuality in a negative light. It was a type of moment where everything "clicked," and I realized that I had been having these feelings for the longest time and this was the only thing that made sense.

My "identity acceptance" step followed shortly thereafter, and I remember looking at myself in the mirror and declaring, "You are a lesbian!" I started disclosing my sexuality primarily to online friends in X. and other places, who were also going through the same thing. It took about a year for me to tell my closest real-life friend that I was gay and had a crush on one of our classmates.

Troiden's last step, "identity commitment," involves seeing homosexuality as a way of life, at least in her terms. I have to say that throughout the past decade of my coming-out process, this is not the case for me. I am more of the type to say that I will be with whoever makes me happy, and that in most cases when I think about the future, that person will most likely be a woman. I do not want to limit that based on gender though. It's a way of life in the way that I have accepted that it is a part of me, but not all of me. I identify as many other things before I identify as a lesbian, such as an immigrant or a scholar. I don't like the idea of having one element of my identity define who I am completely.

By the end of this stage, people begin to accept themselves as homosexual. Stage 4, *commitment,* involves adopting homosexuality as a way of life. The main characteristics of this stage are self-acceptance, happiness, and satisfaction with a same-sex sexual identity.

Do Stage Models of LGB Identity Development Fit Every LGB Adolescent?

Empirical examination of stage models of LGB identity development, especially those proposed by Cass (1979, 1984) and Troiden (1989), generally confirm the overall sequence of stages, but research on these models also reveals important variations in sequence and timing (Savin-Williams, 1998b, 2011). One can imagine a boy growing up in a household with homophobic parents, experimenting with a same-sex sexual relationship before labeling himself gay, and, perhaps, never coming out to his parents. Or a girl with very tolerant parents may fall in love with another girl, label herself lesbian, and come out to her parents long before she has a sexual relationship with another girl.

Savin-Williams and Diamond (2000) interviewed over 160 LGB emerging adults about their experience of two *sexual milestones*, which are key events in the formation of an LGB sexual identity. The researchers studied one's first same-sex sexual experience, and labeling oneself LGB. Two groups emerged: a *sex-first* group that included 20% of the females and 51% of the males, who engaged in same-sex sexual contact prior to labeling themselves LGB; and a *label-first* group, comprising 80% of the females and 49% of the males, in which the reverse was true—labeling oneself LGB preceded same-sex sexual behavior. The results suggest that for most females the formation of a lesbian or bisexual identity is not tied to a same-sex sexual experience, while males are evenly split between those who form a gay or bisexual identity before they have a same-sex sexual experience and those who form their identity only after a same-sex sexual experience.

The following story nicely illustrates the progression from same-sex sexual behavior first to a label of bisexual, after, for one young man.

IN THEIR OWN WORDS

I had my first girlfriend midway through my freshman year [in high school]. And I had sex with my girlfriend the beginning of sophomore year. Afterward, sex became a mainstay in my relationships with girls. And I was set. I felt like I knew what I liked, what I didn't, and I was comfortable in my identity. It wasn't until my junior year that I discovered I liked guys and girls. Ha, I never even considered that both could be a choice.

So I bet you're wondering how it happened, right? I was at my friend S.'s birthday party. We were all drinking and having fun and then she had us move into two lines to play the "nervous game." The nervous game was a weird game I had never heard of nor since played. It involved two lines of people and when you got to the front of your line you would face off against the person in the other line to see who could make the other person visibly sexually uncomfortable. I won the first few rounds with little incidence, going up against my girlfriend in the first round and her friend in the second round. I just tweaked both of their nipples; I think girls are easier to embarrass sexually than guys. Anyway, in the last round I came up against my friend D., who also identified as heterosexual. We were both determined not to lose, and the whole two-guys-touching-and-talking-dirty-to-each-other thing had created quite a crowd at the party, so the pressure was on. After some mild groping and whatnot, it had become apparent that neither of us was going to back down. It occurred to me that in order to make D. uncomfortable I would have to make myself uncomfortable. So I kissed him. We were still at a stalemate. Luckily, then we were going to cut the cake so the game was ended.

Later that evening I was like "Wow! I liked kissing a dude." For a brief moment, I wondered if that meant I was gay, but I thought about it and I didn't like girls any less than before I had kissed D. I still watched hetero porn, still liked having sex with my girlfriend, still loved a nice pair of tits. But I definitely liked that kiss and would have been interested in doing more with a guy. So I discovered I was bisexual. I was instantly comfortable with the label. It felt like such a good fit.

Do Ethnicity and Race Influence Sexual Identity Development?

There is a high degree of similarity in sexual identity development across ethnic and racial groups, but with some subtle differences in the process and in the ages of attainment of sexual milestones. No age differences exist in age of first sexual attraction, onset of sexual activity, or in identifying one's sexual identity among LGB white, African American, and Latino youth living in New York City (Rosario, Schrimshaw, & Hunter, 2004). Differences do exist in identity integration, however, and African American LGB youth are less likely to participate in gay-related activities and are more uncomfortable with others knowing about their sexual orientation. African American youth may be more fearful of the stigma attached to homosexuality in the African American community, or, as Rosario et al. suggest, LGB African American youth may experience racism in the largely white LGB community leading to withdrawal from LGB activities. LGB African American youth may be especially vulnerable to social isolation and loneliness because they are not only segregated by sexual orientation but also by race.

■ COMING OUT TO PARENTS AND OTHERS

For LGB youth, coming out is a key developmental milestone. *Coming out* is defined as disclosing one's LGB orientation to others. It is a defining event for most LGB youth and there is not an analogous experience for heterosexual adolescents. Coming out can be a singular event or a gradual process that unfolds over a period of months or even years. It can also be an emotionally challenging event, especially if parents and others do not accept the individual's sexual orientation.

When Do LGB Youth Come Out to Their Parents and to Others?

A recent survey of over 1,000 self-identified LGB adults in the United States reveals that about 86% of respondents say they have told someone about their sexual orientation, and the majority say that all or most of the important people in their lives know. About 66% tell their mothers and about 61% disclose their sexual orientation to their fathers (Pew Research Center, 2013). LGB individuals give several reasons for not disclosing their sexual orientation to parents: it is not important to tell a parent, they assume their parents would not accept them, someone else told the parent, the parent already knows, and the subject never comes up. As one bisexual woman said, "It's just never come up. I rarely discuss details of my love life with anyone since I am a deeply private person. If I were to make a serious commitment to another woman, I would tell my mother about it" (Pew Research Center, 2013, p. 51).

Pew survey researchers found that the median age when gay men tell someone about their sexual orientation is 18 years. It is 21 years for lesbians, and 20 years for bisexuals (Pew Research Center, 2013). Also, it appears that more LGB youth come out, and come out at an earlier age today than they did in the past, perhaps because people today are more accepting of a same-sex orientation than they were in the past (Martos, Nezhad, & Meyer, 2015; Twenge, Sherman, & Wells, 2016).

How Do Parents React When LGB Adolescents Disclose Their Sexual Orientation to Them?

Disclosure to parents is risky business and many LGB adolescents have real concerns about rejection, disapproval, and harmful reactions if they tell their parents about their sexual orientation. After disclosure, youth risk verbal abuse, assault, being thrown out of the house, and loss of the parent–child relationship. On the other hand, not telling is associated with its own problems, such as feeling isolated and alienated from one's family, and a continuing fear of what parents may do if they accidently find out. Keeping one's sexual orientation a secret is especially damaging to lesbians and bisexual females—who are more likely to engage in illicit drug use and experience depression if they do not come out—than lesbian and bisexual females who do come out to a parent (Rothman, Sullivan, Keyes, & Boehmer, 2012).

The majority of LGB individuals say that it is difficult to tell their parents about their sexual orientation, and is especially hard to disclose to their fathers. The good news is that the large majority of LGB individuals report that their relationships with their parents either remain the same or grow stronger after disclosing (Savin-Williams, 1998a).

One common initial response by parents on learning that their child is LGB is to feel somehow responsible. Many parents view homosexuality as a disease in which someone is responsible for what "went wrong," blaming either themselves, a friend, a teacher, the media, or homosexuals who turned the adolescent into one of their own (Savin-Williams, 1998a).

Parental reactions to learning that their adolescent is LGB are not fixed, but may change with the passage of time. In one study of Israeli LGB adolescents, the large majority of parents initially were mostly to fully accepting of their adolescent's sexual orientation. About 25% initially were mostly to fully rejecting, although most of the rejecting parents became more accepting over time (Samarova, Shilo, & Diamond, 2014). Two reasons for the increase in parental acceptance are parents want to remain close to their children, and parents want to maintain a good relationship with their children. The findings show that most parents can overcome what they initially view as a disappointment. Adolescents and parents who are patient with each other and work through feelings of shame and loss may be rewarded in time with a renewed acceptance and understanding of each other.

Is Coming Out to Parents Always a Good Thing?

Disclosing an LGB orientation to one's parents is associated with many positive psychological benefits (Rosario, Hunter, Maguen, Gwadz, & Smith, 2001). Ending concealment of what is a central aspect of the self decreases fear of being inadvertently discovered and lowers stress associated with suppressing and disguising potentially damaging behaviors and emotions. In contrast, some researchers report that coming out to parents has no impact on mental health, while others find that coming out may even precipitate verbal or physical abuse and a variety of other negative responses that worsen psychological and physical health (D'Augelli, Hershberger, & Pilkington, 1998; Kosciw, Palmer, & Kull, 2015). What these mixed findings suggest is that the consequences of coming out depend upon the reactions of parents to the disclosure.

In one study of LGB adults, coming out to parents was associated with less drug use and binge drinking, and a decrease in stress, depression, and emotional problems for females (Legate, Ryan, & Weinstein, 2012). There was no relationship between coming out and mental and physical health for males. For LGB individuals of both sexes, experiencing a lack of emotional support from a parent after coming out is associated with more illicit drug use, depression, and poor health status. Together, these findings suggest that coming out to parents is more beneficial for females than for males, and problematic for adolescents of both sexes when parents reject them after coming out.

LGB adolescents living at home who are financially and physically dependent upon their parents need to be cautious about when and with whom they disclose their sexual orientation. The rewards of honesty can be great, but there are risks. In the following account, one young man describes the dangerous situation he found himself in when his mother found out he was gay.

IN THEIR OWN WORDS

I was about 16 years old the first time I had attempted to "come out" to my mother. I remember hearing my mother scream from the second floor, "J.! Get your ass up here now!" Immediately I knew my mother was angry about something and I became anxious and fearful. My mother and I already didn't have a very good relationship. I peeked into my room where I found her sitting on my bed staring at a collection of porn that she had found from underneath my mattress. She stares at me, and I can immediately sense shame and anger from her eyes. Then all of a sudden my mother jumps up off of the bed and races me down the stairway. All I could feel at the moment was frightened, and thinking what is she going to do to me. I became trapped in the corner of the kitchen where my mother held a knife to my throat. I still hear the yelling fresh in my mind today, "You can't be gay! I raised you better than that!" In order to save my life I responded with, "No mom I was just joking. I'm not actually gay. I just wanted to see how you would react, because I have this friend at school that is gay." There was no friend. Thankfully my grandmother was living with us at the time and she was able to drag my mother off of me. She saved my life that day.

■ RISKY SEXUAL BEHAVIOR AMONG LGB ADOLESCENTS

Do LGB Adolescents Engage in More Risky Sexual Behavior Than Heterosexual Teens?

LGB high school students are more likely to engage in risky sexual behaviors than heterosexual students (Kann, Olsen, et al., 2016; Poteat, Russell, & Dewaele, 2017). LGB students are more likely to have sexual experiences before age 13 years, and this is especially true for gay and bisexual males. Further, the prevalence of having four or more sexual partners is higher among LGB students. In addition, LGB students are less likely to use a condom when they have sexual intercourse. Last, in comparison to heterosexual students, LGB students are more likely to drink alcohol or use drugs before sexual activity (Rosario et al., 2014; Ybarra, Rosario, Saewyc, & Goodenow, 2016).

Researchers have suggested several possibilities for why LGB adolescents engage in more risky sexual behavior than heterosexual teens. One possibility is that LGB adolescents may experience an earlier and stronger sexual drive. LGB adolescents, especially males, may have a more difficult time managing their sexual impulses, which would account for an earlier age of sexual debut, more partners, and impulsive sexual behavior (Ybarra et al., 2016). A second possibility is that some of the higher sexual risk behavior among LGB adolescents may be the result of a history of sexual abuse that is associated with difficulties negotiating safer sexual practices with a partner (Friedman et al., 2011). A third possibility is that some of the risky behavior may be the result of nonconsensual sex, especially among younger LGB adolescents. Last, a lack of sex education for LGB adolescents may lead some teens to unknowingly engage in risky sexual behavior, such as having sex without a condom.

■ BULLYING AND VICTIMIZATION OF LGBTQ ADOLESCENTS

LGBTQ youth are more likely to experience some unique social stressors specifically because of their sexual orientation or gender identity (Kosciw, Greytak, Palmer, & Boesen, 2014). Harassment, victimization, and bullying during the teen years are not problems limited to LGBTQ adolescents, but the extent of the harassment, the motives of the bullies, and the outcome of the victimization has a particularly insidious effect on LGBTQ adolescents (Mueller, James, Abrutyn, & Levin, 2015). Although some LGBTQ youth are not treated badly by their peers and classmates, many are, and those who are experience a variety of mental health and substance use disorders (Saewyc, 2011).

How Many LGBTQ Youth Are Victimized Each Year?

About 85% of LGBTQ students report being verbally harassed at school during the past year (Kosciw et al., 2014). LGBTQ students in the United States and Canada are almost twice as likely to be assaulted as heterosexual students (Friedman et al., 2011). Almost 40% of LGBTQ students report being threatened or attacked. As one male student reported, "I have been so hurt at that school. I have gotten beat up, almost killed, and no one there would do anything about it, except one teacher" (Kosciw et al., 2014, p. 25). In addition, almost 20% of LGBTQ students in comparison to about 7% of heterosexual students report missing school because of fear.

Transgender and gender-nonconforming youth are especially likely to experience victimization (Gordon, Conton, Calzo, Reisner, & Austin, 2016). According to the students, victimization is the result specifically of their transgender identity or lack of conformity to traditional sex role behavior. One young girl reported:

> "This past week has been nothing but 'Is that a boy or a girl?' said loudly behind me or people calling me 'mangirl.' It's making school feel much more unsafe and I hate walking through the halls." (Kosciw et al., 2014, p. 22)

Transgender youth have the highest levels of victimization and psychological distress among LGBTQ youth, revealing the greater visibility and vulnerability of this socially stigmatized group (Ybarra, Mitchell, & Kosciw, 2015). Gender-nonconforming students are also at high risk for harassment, bullying, and name-calling, which is related to poorer relations with peers and depressive symptoms (Martin-Storey & August, 2016; van Beusekom, Baams, Bos, Overbeek, & Sandfort, 2016).

Does Victimization Decrease as LGBTQ Youth Get Older?

Victimization of LGBTQ students decreases between early adolescence and emerging adulthood (Kosciw et al., 2014; Robinson & Espelage, 2011). One longitudinal study of English adolescents reveals that the percentage of lesbian and bisexual girls who were victimized in the past year decreased from about 57% at ages 13–14 to about 6% at ages 19–20, while the comparable percentages for gay and bisexual males declined from about 52 to 9% (Robinson, Espelage, & Rivers, 2013). The greatest decrease in victimization occurs between ages 16 and 19—years corresponding to graduation from secondary/high school. The general decline in victimization between adolescence and emerging adulthood is accompanied by a decrease in psychological distress and depression (Birkett, Newcomb, & Mustanski, 2015). Life does get better for LGBTQ students as they get older, especially after graduating from secondary/high school.

What Effect Does Victimization Have on LGBTQ Adolescents?

Victimization and discrimination at school can undermine students' sense of belonging and feelings that they fit in and are part of their school community. A substantial number of LGBTQ students feel disengaged and detached from their school because of the many negative experiences they have at school. These feelings of isolation and exclusion are related to a variety of academic problems, including low grades and truancy (Birkett, Russell, & Corliss, 2014). In addition, students who experience high levels of victimization are about twice as likely to report that they do not plan to continue their education after high school.

Being harassed or assaulted at school has a negative impact on students' psychological well-being and adjustment (Bontempo & D'Augelli, 2002). LGBTQ students who experience higher levels of victimization, including cyberbullying, have lower self-esteem and higher levels of depression, suicidality, substance use, and sexual risk behaviors than students who do not experience high victimization (Abreu & Kenny, 2018; Birkett et al., 2015).

The pattern of these findings is consistent with *minority stress theory,* which posits that sexual minorities experience stress, including victimization, related to their stigmatized status, and this stigma-related stress produces cognitive, emotional, and social problems that result in an increase in psychopathology (Hatzenbuehler, 2009).

Homophobic name-calling, such as "dyke" and "faggot" can have a detrimental effect on the victims. Homophobic epithets are not benign for youth on the receiving end of this type of harassment. High school students who experience frequent homophobic name-calling show high levels of anxiety, depression, and alcohol use (Tucker et al., 2016). Teachers and school staff should be made aware that such harassment is not harmless teasing, and should make a point of stopping it when they hear it.

■ MENTAL HEALTH ISSUES AMONG LGBTQ ADOLESCENTS

Are LGBTQ Adolescents More Likely to Have Mental Health Problems Than Heterosexual Teens?

Studies of the mental health status of LGBTQ adolescents show that many are psychologically healthy, have friends, and like school (Lucassen et al., 2015). A high percentage of LGBTQ youth have some type of mental health disorder or psychological adjustment problem, however (Mustanski, Garofalo, & Emerson, 2010). Many LGBTQ adolescents report having a mood disorder, especially depression; low self-esteem; an anxiety disorder; using and abusing alcohol and drugs; and thinking about or attempting suicide (Russell & Fish, 2016; Shearer et al., 2016). LGBTQ emerging adults continue to have a high level of psychological distress, including suicidality, binge drinking, and drug use (Kuyper & Bos, 2016). The poorer psychological adjustment of LGBTQ youth is found outside the United States, even among LGBTQ adolescents living in the Netherlands, a country viewed as one of the most tolerant in the world of LGBTQ individuals (Kuyper, de Roos, Iedema, & Stevens, 2016).

One group of LGBTQ adolescents who are at high risk for mental health problems are bisexual adolescents (Shilo & Savaya, 2012). Two related reasons have been proposed to explain the particular vulnerability of bisexuals. One is that bisexuals are stigmatized not only in the straight community but also among lesbian and gay individuals, who are less tolerant of what is perceived to be sexual ambivalence. In addition, this lack of tolerance may discourage many bisexuals from revealing their true identities to other sexual minorities, leading to social isolation and a lack of social support.

In one study of gay and bisexual young men living in the Chicago area, one-third experienced a major depressive episode at some point in their lives, and about the same percentage thought about committing suicide (Burns, Ryan, Garofalo, Newcomb, & Mustanski, 2015). Other common problems include posttraumatic stress disorder, alcohol abuse, and conduct disorder. Over half of these youth had one or more mental health disorder at some point in their lives. Most of these problems first appear between ages 13 and 16 years, demonstrating a heightened vulnerability during early adolescence. The majority of these adolescents never receive any form of treatment, showing the need to find ways to reach sexual-minority youth suffering with psychological problems.

Why Do LGBTQ Adolescents Have a High Rate of Mental Disorder?

The high prevalence of psychological adjustment problems among LGBTQ youth is related to minority stress, especially being stigmatized and bullied by peers (Jones, Robinson, Oginni, Rahman, & Rimes, 2017). In addition, mental health problems are associated with parents who do not accept and even reject their LGBTQ children (Meyer, 2003). Minority stress is thought to be the main cause of the cognitive, emotional, and social problems associated with being an LGBTQ adolescent (Kelleher, 2009; Shilo & Mor, 2014). According to the minority stress model, the heightened psychological problems among LGBTQ adolescents are the direct result of a social environment that is hostile to and unaccepting of LGBTQ individuals. Although sexual minorities are more accepted by mainstream society today than ever before (Twenge et al., 2016), many LGBTQ adolescents continue to experience bias and stigma from parents and peers that leads to rejection, isolation, discrimination, and abuse (Mayer, Garofalo, & Makadon, 2014). The experience of prejudice and rejection, which can be a daily occurrence for some LGBTQ adolescents, may lead to feelings of shame, guilt, and denial that result in internalized homophobia and a negative self-concept that, when coupled with the need to hide and conceal one's true identity, results in stress and poor coping. LGBTQ youth of color are especially vulnerable to minority stress since they must cope with prejudice and discrimination based on their racial/ethnic status in addition to the stresses associated with being a sexual minority (Kuper, Coleman, & Mustanski, 2014).

Another factor related to a high rate of mental disorder among LGBTQ adolescents is social isolation, and low-quality relations with people who matter. In comparison to heterosexual adolescents, LGBTQ teens have poorer relations with parents, peers, and teachers (Bos, Sandfort, de Bruyn, & Hakvoort, 2008; Russell, Seif, & Truong, 2001), which is associated with low social status and social isolation (Hatzenbuehler, McLaughlin, & Xuan, 2012). Adolescents with a same-sex orientation who have friends with a same-sex orientation, or who are in a same-sex romantic relationship, are better adjusted than lesbian and gay youth who are more socially isolated, suggesting that these friendships operate as a buffer against psychological distress (Baams, Bos, & Jonas, 2014; Ueno, 2005).

How Suicidal Are LGBTQ Adolescents?

A high percentage of LGBTQ adolescents report that they have thought about committing suicide or have attempted suicide (Marshal et al., 2008; Stone et al., 2014). There is no reliable way to determine the rate of completed suicides among LGBTQ youth, because death certificates do not routinely include the deceased's sexual orientation. Given the high rates of reports by LGBTQ youth that they have thought about suicide or attempted suicide, experts believe that the suicide rate among LGBTQ youth is higher than among heterosexual youth.

Over the past 20 years, researchers have documented higher rates of *suicidality*—defined as thinking about committing suicide or attempting suicide—among LGBTQ youth (Bostwick et al., 2014). The figures are alarmingly high. LGBTQ youth are at least twice as likely as heterosexual adolescents to contemplate suicide, and two to seven times more likely to attempt suicide (Haas et al., 2011). In one study of LGBTQ youth between 15 and 19 years of age, about one-third reported that they had attempted suicide (D'Augelli et al., 2005). Suicide attempts are especially high among LGBTQ adolescents and emerging adults in comparison to older LGBTQ adults (Russell & Toomey, 2012). Some have speculated that the reason for this age disparity is that suicide attempts are linked to the initial ages at which individuals acknowledge their sexual orientation, and to antigay harassment (Paul et al., 2002).

The high rate of suicidality among U.S. LGBTQ teens does not appear to emerge from unique aspects of U.S. culture. LGBTQ teens living outside the United States also have a high rate of suicidality. In one study of tenth-grade Icelandic students, researchers reported that LGBTQ adolescents were five to six times more likely than non-LGBTQ teens to have thought about committing suicide or to have attempted suicide (Arnarsson, Sveinbjornsdottir, Thorsteinsson, & Bjarnason, 2015).

Two groups with especially high rates of suicidality are transgender adolescents and questioning youth who are unsure of their sexual identity. High rates of suicide attempts among transgender adolescents may be related to the high rates of depression, anxiety, and substance abuse, in addition to problems with parents, including outright parental rejection (Grossman & D'Augelli, 2007). Questioning adolescents are another high-risk group for attempted suicide (Zhao, Montoro, Igartua, & Thombs, 2010). Uncertainty about one's sexual identity coupled with the normal identity crises of adolescence may tax the coping skills of even the most resilient adolescents.

Why Is Suicidality among LGBTQ Youth So High?

A variety of social factors have been implicated in suicidality among LGBTQ adolescents. First, LGBTQ youth experience more frequent discrimination and harassment than heterosexual adolescents, which is often specifically tied to their sexual orientation and to the nonconforming expression of their gender role (Birkett, Espelage, & Koenig, 2009). A negative and unaccepting social environment may be a burden too great for some teens to bear (Almeida, Johnson, Corliss, Molnar, & Azrael, 2009). Second, rejection by peers and the loss of friends because of one's sexual orientation has been implicated in the development of a negative self-concept, and even to internalized homophobia, both of which are associated with suicide attempts (Savin-Williams & Ream, 2003). Third, suicidality is higher among LGBTQ adolescents who feel disconnected from their school, or who feel that school is an unsafe place (Whitaker, Shapiro, & Shields, 2016).

Another factor related to suicidality among LGBTQ adolescents is parental rejection and psychological maltreatment (Puckett et al., 2017). Although the majority of parents accept their LGBTQ children, a substantial minority initially reject them (D'Augelli et al., 1998). The message parental rejection and discomfort sends to LGBTQ adolescents is that something is wrong with the teens, which is an especially destructive message to receive when it comes from the most important people in an adolescent's life. In addition, parents who reject their adolescents because of their sexual orientation or gender identity are not available to console and support their adolescents when they are victimized outside the home. LGBTQ adolescents who feel disconnected from their parents are more likely to think about committing suicide and more likely to attempt suicide than LGBTQ adolescents who feel connected to their parents (Stone, Luo, Lippy, & McIntosh, 2015).

■ LGBTQ ADOLESCENT SUBSTANCE USE AND ABUSE

Are LGBTQ Adolescents More Likely Than Heterosexual Youth to Drink Alcohol and Use Illegal Drugs?

Alcohol use, including binge drinking, is more common among LGBTQ youth than among their heterosexual counterparts (Dermody et al., 2014; Marshal et al., 2008; Ocasio, Feaster, & Prado, 2016). In one recent study of over 37,000 adolescents, more LGBTQ youth report that they drink alcohol and that they began drinking at an earlier age than heterosexual adolescents (Talley, Hughes,

Aranda, Birkett, & Marshal, 2014). LGBTQ adolescents also report drinking more often and participating in more frequent heavy drinking than heterosexual adolescents. Further, LGBTQ youth are more likely to drink alcohol during weekdays than heterosexual youth, primarily as a way of coping with personal worries (Bos, van Beusekom, & Sandfort, 2016).

In addition to alcohol, LGBTQ adolescents are more likely to use marijuana, cocaine, and ecstasy, and to misuse prescription drugs than heterosexual youth (Corliss et al., 2010, 2014). LGBTQ adolescents are also more likely to use multiple substances concurrently (Garofalo, Wolf, Kessel, Palfrey, & DuRant, 1998). Drug use is especially high among gay males and bisexual females (Newcomb, Birkett, Corliss, & Mustanski, 2014).

Why Is Alcohol and Drug Use So High among LGBTQ Youth?

The most common explanation for the high use of alcohol and drugs among LGBTQ adolescents is that alcohol and drug abuse is the result of minority stress

In the following story, a young gay female in college is able to reflect back on her high school years and see the connection between her difficulty accepting her true self and her alcohol use.

IN THEIR OWN WORDS

As I approached the end of my high school career I began to start questioning a lot of things about my life, and inevitably became extremely depressed. I started getting into alcohol my junior year of high school and by my senior year it was a huge problem. I did not know it at the time, but after later reflection I have come to the conclusion that my alcohol use was due to the suppression of my feelings that I could not cognitively tolerate. My cognitive dissonance proved to be too powerful for my rational brain. What the hell do I mean by this? Here is a little bit more into my background: I was raised into an extremely republican, Catholic family. There were definitely set standards for what is acceptable and what was not, and those standards were beat into my head over and over to the point where I knew nothing else to be true. The two major "rules" that I found the hardest to succumb to: no sex before marriage (abstinence is key in Catholicism), and homosexuality is a sin and absolutely unacceptable under any and every circumstance.

So here I am, going through high school, experiencing all of the normal sexual urges that my peers were; yet, I started to find myself becoming attracted to women. This freaked me out more than anything in the world at the time. I knew that having feelings or any sort of attraction toward the same sex was absolutely prohibited. It was mortifying. So what did I do? I lied to myself, told myself that I was not truly experiencing these emotions, and then consciously told myself to stop thinking in that way because it was dirty, unacceptable, and flat out immoral. This is the cognitive dissonance that I was referring to. In my mind, I was experiencing attractions to girls, but I knew that it was not "right," so I constantly was trying to correct my thinking and compensate by forcing myself to have crushes or attractions to boys. This is when the drinking began, which is why I feel like my drinking was to not feel so dirty about my thoughts. More importantly, it allowed me to escape the idea of myself being gay.

(Goldbach, Tanner-Smith, Bagwell, & Dunlap, 2014; Rosario et al., 2014). The stresses associated with being stigmatized include discrimination and bullying, damaging experiences that can lead to isolation and rejection. According to minority stress theory, alcohol and drug use are attempts to cope with these adverse experiences (Burton, Marshal, Chisolm, Sucato, & Friedman, 2013).

A second possible reason for the high rates of alcohol and drug use among LGBTQ youth is that drinking and drug experimentation are part of a gay lifestyle (Green & Feinstein, 2012). The LGBTQ community is heterogeneous, but among many LGBTQ individuals a focus on activities that involve drinking and drug use in bars and at parties is common. Attendance at gay bars and involvement with sex clubs is associated with elevated alcohol and drug problems (Halkitis & Parsons, 2002; Kipke et al., 2007). The easy availability of alcohol and drugs and the presence of many peers who are substance users makes it difficult for LGBTQ youth to avoid peers who are users and to elude triggers for substance use. Further, adolescents who perceive alcohol and drug use as prevalent and acceptable in the LGBTQ community are at risk for substance use and abuse (Mereish, Goldbach, Burgess, & DiBello, 2017).

■ TRANSGENDER ADOLESCENTS

Over the past several years there has been an increase in media attention about *transgender* people, who feel that their psychological gender identity does not match their gender assigned at birth. The very public story of Caitlyn Jenner, plus cover stories in *Time* and *National Geographic* magazines, in addition to the controversy over public bathroom use and transgender individuals in the military, has brought attention to this once invisible minority. In addition, there has been a sharp rise in the number of people who go to gender identity clinics for help with their condition, along with a decrease in the age at which transgender individuals request medical interventions (Wood et al., 2013). In particular, there has been an increase in the number of adolescents who identify themselves as transgender, a rise probably due to more adolescents coming out of the closet than to a bona fide increase in real numbers (Chen, Fuqua, & Eugster, 2016; Zucker, Bradley, Owen-Anderson, Kibblewhite, & Cantor, 2008). The surge in the number of transgender adolescents who seek medical treatment for their condition may reflect a pent-up demand for information and intervention (Spack et al., 2012).

What Percentage of Adolescents Are Transgender?

It is difficult to determine the prevalence of transgender adolescents because a transgender identity is rarely assessed in population-based surveys of adolescent sexuality. In one study of New Zealand high school students, 1.2% of students identified themselves as transgender (Clark et al., 2014). In a survey of high school students in Boston, Massachusetts, only 0.02% indicated they were transgender (Almeida et al., 2009). In other research, a prevalence rate of 0.33% was found for a sample of U.S. emerging adults (Reisner et al., 2014). Most experts believe that the actual number of transgender adolescents is below 1.0% (Connolly, Zervos, Barone, Johnson, & Joseph, 2016).

What Mental Health and Adjustment Problems Do Transgender Adolescents Have?

Many transgender adolescents are harassed, bullied, and physically attacked at school, in their neighborhoods, and online (Mitchell, Ybarra, & Korchmaros, 2014; Reisner, Greytak, Parsons, & Ybarra, 2015). In addition, transgender youth are often rejected by their parents and experience trauma and abuse at home. Given these serious challenges faced by youth with a transgender identity, it is not surprising that many, if not most, transgender adolescents experience significant psychological adjustment and mental health problems (Chen et al., 2016; Veale, Watson, Peter, & Saewyc, 2017). Common mental health problems include depression, anxiety, suicidality, self-harm without lethal intent, poor body image, substance abuse, and posttraumatic stress disorder (Collier, van Beusekom, Bos, & Sandfort, 2013; Connolly et al., 2016; Reisner, Greytak, et al., 2015). There are not differences in the mental health of male-to-female or female-to-male transgender adolescents.

Transgender adolescents have a greater risk for suicidal ideation and suicide attempts than heterosexual peers or LGB youth. In one study, slightly more than 50% of transgender adolescents had attempted suicide (Mustanski & Liu, 2013). Suicide attempts are directly related to feelings of depression and hopelessness, which are themselves associated with peer victimization. Suicide prevention programs are especially important for transgender adolescents, along with programs that help parents cope with the particular issues related to having a transgender adolescent. In addition, school-based programs designed to reduce bullying and victimization in general address a core problem associated with poor psychological adjustment and suicidality specifically among transgender youth.

What Kind of Relations Do Transgender Adolescents Have with Their Parents?

Parents play a key role in the lives of transgender youth. Supportive parents protect and buffer transgender adolescents from negative experiences, and promote positive mental health and psychological well-being, along with greater life satisfaction (Simons, Schrager, Clark, Belzer, & Olson, 2013). In contrast, rejecting and abusive parents have a negative effect on transgender youth and contribute to poor mental health and psychological maladjustment.

Parents of transgender children experience their own adjustment problems. According to one report, parents typically go through the following five stages after they discover they have a transgender child: denial and shock at discovering that their child has a cross-gender identity; anger and frustration;

bargaining, involving threats to disown and disinherit their transgender child; depression and grief; and acceptance of the situation as it is, no longer dwelling on how things could be different (Emerson & Rosenfeld, 1996).

How Do Transgender People Come to Terms with Their Gender Identities?

Transgender adults are not born thinking that they are in the wrong-gendered body. Instead, that perception slowly evolves over a long period of development that starts in early childhood and continues through adolescence into emerging adulthood. One recent attempt to explore how transgender people recognize, acknowledge, and come to terms with their gender identities is based on interviews with a small group of Portuguese adults who made the transition from one gender to the other (Pinto & Moleiro, 2015). The findings may reflect the stages many transgender individuals go through who elect to surgically alter their gender. The results show transgender individuals moving through five developmental stages. Stage 1 is an awareness of being different, accompanied by confusion and distress. During childhood, there is a preference for toys and activities traditionally associated with the opposite sex. In Stage 2, typically during adolescence, individuals discover a label for their experience and realize that there are other people in the same situation. Stage 3 involves exploring options about what to do and when to do it. Searching for information about body modification is common. Stage 4 involves making the transition from one gender to the other. Stage 5 involves living full time as a member of one's new gender. Individual experiences may vary, but the model proposes a general pathway from confusion to understanding, action, and acceptance.

What Is Gender Dysphoria?

The psychiatric diagnosis for a transgender identity is *gender dysphoria* (GD). For there to be a diagnosis of GD in adolescents or adults there must be a persistent feeling lasting at least 6 months that one's biological sex does not match one's experienced gender. GD is manifested in a variety of ways, including a desire to be treated as the other gender, a desire to be rid of one's genitals and other sexual characteristics, and a conviction that one has the feelings typical of the other gender. GD is often experienced as a deeply felt desire to alter one's physical sex to match one's psychological gender.

The majority of prepubertal children who manifest symptoms of GD will become comfortable with their biological sex over time, while a minority will identify as transgender in adulthood (Wallien & Cohen-Kettenis, 2008). It is impossible to make a definitive diagnosis of GD in childhood, and symptoms of GD disappear for 80–90% of children. GD that persists into adolescence is likely to continue into adulthood (Zucker, 2010). It is currently not possible to differentiate children for whom GD will persist from those for whom it will not (Byne et al., 2012).

Given the lack of persistence of GD between childhood and adulthood, drug or surgical intervention in childhood is premature and inappropriate for the large majority of children with symptoms of GD. If one were certain that a child belonged in the persistent group, then it would be possible to treat that child early on with drugs designed to delay the onset of puberty and to suppress the expression of secondary sex characteristics rather than waiting until after the start of puberty, as now typically happens. Clearly, there are serious consequences associated with treating or not treating GD in early adolescence, and adolescents and their parents should be fully aware of the consequences of intervention and of nonintervention (Cohen-Kettenis, Delemarre-van de Waal, & Gooren, 2008).

What about Intervention?

Over the past several years, the ages of youth who seek medical intervention to alter their gender identity has steadily fallen, sometimes including preteens (Milrod, 2014). Some children who strongly identify with the other gender develop psychological problems, such as depression, suicidality, anorexia, or social phobias that are the result of an inability to start treatment for legal or other reasons. The World Professional Association for Transgender Health Standards of Care recommends that irreversible interventions, such as genital surgeries, not be performed until an individual reaches the age of majority in his or her country (Colebunders, De Cuypere, & Monstrey, 2015).

Transgender adolescents in early and mid-puberty are treated with gonadotropin-releasing hormone agonist (GnRHa) to suppress the development of secondary sex characteristics in order to buy time to make an informed decision about gender reassignment surgery. Many adolescents and their parents report that halting puberty brings some immediate relief and an end of suffering.

Puberty suppression by itself does not lead to the amelioration of GD, however, indicating that puberty suppression in conjunction with gender reassignment surgery may be necessary to end GD for some individuals. Puberty suppression and gender reassignment surgery are not risk-free and some researchers and clinicians have expressed concerns about potential risks such as adverse effects on endocrine functioning, interference with brain development, and postsurgical regret (see Cohen-Kettenis, Schagen, Steensma, de Vries, & Delemarre-van de Waal, 2011, for a review). Although biological interventions offer hope to individuals suffering from GD, they are not without risk, and need to be undertaken with great caution.

Why Do Some People Have a Transgender Identity?

The development of a gender identity is a complex developmental process that is the result of the interaction of genetic, hormonal, neurological, and perhaps even psychosocial factors (Kreukels, Steensma, & de Vries, 2014; Sasaki et al.,

2016). GD has no single cause and it is currently unclear what specific biological and environmental factors lead to the development of a transgender identity (Steensma, Kreukels, de Vries, & Cohen-Kettenis, 2013). Researchers have identified a small number of candidate genes that may contribute to the development of GD by influencing the biosynthesis of sex steroids related to the sex differentiation of the brain (Klink & Den Heijer, 2014). Other researchers have found specific brain structures that resemble female brains in male-to-female transgender individuals (Guillamon, Junque, & Gómez-Gil, 2016). Some of these neurological differences are present in adolescence and perhaps earlier (Steensma et al., 2013).

SUMMARY

■ DEFINING SEXUAL ORIENTATION

Three important distinctions used in this chapter include the following: sexual orientation is the gender of the people to whom one is sexually attracted; gender identity is the personal sense that one is a male or a female; and questioning adolescents are teens who are uncertain about their sexual orientation.

Many LGB adults remember a period of uncertainty and questioning about their sexual orientation during adolescence. The percentage of questioning teens steadily declines between early and late adolescence. Several explanations have been offered to explain why some adolescents may be uncertain about their sexual orientation.

■ SOME NUMBERS AND STATISTICS

Between 6 and 8% of U.S. high school students label themselves as LGB, while another 3% are unsure or questioning. These figures may underestimate the true percentages of LGB adolescents for a variety of reasons. More females are attracted to both sexes than are males.

■ SEXUAL ORIENTATION, SEXUAL BEHAVIOR, AND SEXUAL IDENTITY

Three aspects of one's sexuality include sexual orientation, sexual behavior, and sexual identity. Sexual orientation is based on which gender one is sexually attracted to. Sexual behavior focuses on which gender one has had an erotic experience with. Sexual identity is the label one uses to describe one's sexuality. Many lesbian and gay youth have been sexually attracted to and have had a sexual experience with someone of the opposite sex, suggesting that there is some fluidity in sexual orientation and behavior.

■ THE DEVELOPMENT OF AN LGB IDENTITY

For most LGB individuals, the formation of a sexual identity is a long-term process that begins in childhood and extends into adolescence and emerging adulthood. Most LGB individuals go through a sequence of developmental stages that begin with confusion and feeling different in childhood and end in early adulthood with the acceptance and expression of an achieved sexual identity. There is much commonality in the sequence and timing of the stages of sexual identity development, but there is variation as well, depending upon one's gender, race, and ethnicity.

■ COMING OUT TO PARENTS AND OTHERS

Coming out to parents and significant others is a key developmental mile-stone for most LGB youth. The majority of LGB youth eventually come out to their parents, usually in late adolescence or emerging adulthood. LGB youth appear to be coming out at an earlier age than ever before, reflecting a greater acceptance of homosexuality by heterosexuals. Most parents accept their child's sexual orientation, but a minority do not. Disclosing one's sexual orientation is associated with many positive outcomes, but there are risks that include verbal and physical abuse, rejection, and even being thrown out of the house. Coming out to parents initiates a process that can take a long time to complete.

■ RISKY SEXUAL BEHAVIOR
AMONG LGB ADOLESCENTS

LGB teens and emerging adults engage in more risky sexual behavior than heterosexual youth. LGB adolescents are more likely to have a sexual experience before age 13 years, have more sexual partners, are more likely to drink alcohol and use drugs before sex, and are less likely to use a condom before sexual intercourse. Several explanations focusing on strength of sex drive and early sexual experiences have been proposed to explain these differences.

■ BULLYING AND VICTIMIZATION
OF LGBTQ ADOLESCENTS

A large majority of LGBTQ students report that they have been verbally harassed, and a substantial minority have been threatened or injured at school. Victimization rates and psychological distress decrease between early adolescence and emerging adulthood, especially after students graduate from high school.

■ MENTAL HEALTH ISSUES
AMONG LGBTQ ADOLESCENTS

Most LGBTQ adolescents are emotionally healthy, but a substantial minority have a variety of psychological problems, with depression being the most common. Minority stress, coupled with poor relations with parents and peers, is the primary explanation for LGBTQ psychological problems.

A substantial minority of LGBTQ adolescents have thought about or attempted suicide. Several explanations have been proposed for the high suicidality rate among LGBTQ adolescents, such as discrimination and victimization, poor relations with peers leading to internalized homophobia, and parental rejection. LGBTQ adolescents who express their gender roles in nontraditional ways are more likely to think about suicide and attempt suicide than heterosexual youth who express their gender roles in traditional ways.

■ LGBTQ ADOLESCENT SUBSTANCE USE AND ABUSE

Use and abuse of alcohol and drugs is more common among LGBTQ youth, a pattern usually attributed to minority stigmatization. High substance use can also be an attempt to cope with depression and discrimination. Last, alcohol and drug use is a central part of some gay communities composed of individuals who encourage and support alcohol and drug use.

■ TRANSGENDER ADOLESCENTS

Less than 1% of adolescents have a transgender identity. Many transgender adolescents are harassed, bullied, and physically attacked at school, in their neighborhoods, and online. Mental health problems, including depression, suicidality, and substance abuse, are common among transgender adolescents. Supportive parents can protect and buffer youth from some of these negative experiences and promote positive mental health.

GD is a persistent feeling that one's biological sex does not match one's experienced gender. The majority of children who express symptoms of GD will become comfortable with their biological sex over time. This inability to distinguish persistent from nonpersistent GD makes treatment difficult. Some adolescents are treated with hormones that delay the onset of puberty, giving the adolescent more time to decide on the advisability of surgical intervention.

Intervention involves a combination of psychotherapy; hormonal treatment; and, in some cases, sex reassignment surgery. There is risk to medical interventions that involve the suppression of puberty and surgery, but there is also risk to doing nothing. GD has no single cause but is the result of an interaction of genetic, hormonal, neurological, and perhaps even psychosocial factors.

SUGGESTIONS FOR FURTHER READING

Goldbach, J. T., Tanner-Smith, E. E., Bagwell, M., & Dunlap, S. (2014). Minority stress and substance use in sexual minority adolescents: A meta-analysis. *Prevention Science, 15,* 350–363.

Hu, Y., Xu, Y., & Tornello, S. L. (2016). Stability of self-reported same-sex and both-sex attraction from adolescence to young adulthood. *Archives of Sexual Behavior, 45,* 651–659.

Mayer, K. H., Garofalo, R., & Makadon, H. J. (2014). Promoting the successful development of sexual and gender minority youths. *American Journal of Public Health, 104,* 976–981.

Russell, S. T., & Fish, J. N. (2016). Mental health in lesbian, gay, bisexual, and transgender (LGBT) youth. *Annual Review of Clinical Psychology, 12,* 465–487.

Savin-Williams, R. C. (2005). *The new gay teenager.* Cambridge, MA: Harvard University Press.

Steensma, T. D., Kreukels, B. P. C., de Vries, A. L. C., & Cohen-Kettenis, P. T. (2013). Gender identity development in adolescence. *Hormones and Behavior, 64,* 288–297.

CHAPTER 9

Teen Mothers, Their Children, and the Fathers

In 2013, New York City launched a $400,000 media campaign designed to educate teens about the negative effects of teen pregnancy in order to aid in the prevention of pregnancies among adolescents. A series of posters portraying the dire consequences of teenage pregnancy and parenthood were posted in subways and bus shelters in neighborhoods with high rates of teen pregnancy. One poster features a picture of a curly-haired infant with sad eyes and tears streaming down his cheeks with the caption "I'm twice as likely not to graduate high school because you had me as a teen." Another poster shows a young girl with the caption "Honestly mom . . . chances are he won't stay with you. What happens to me?" The campaign has drawn much criticism and little praise from organizations dedicated to reducing the incidence of teen pregnancy and to helping young mothers and their children. For example, Planned Parenthood of New York City denounced the campaign, claiming that the posters will have little effect on the true causes of teen pregnancy and will further shame teen mothers, who are already one of the most stigmatized groups in America.

The campaign is built on two underlying assumptions about teenage pregnancy. First, teen pregnancy is the result of irresponsible sexual behavior. Second, a teen pregnancy has enduring negative consequences to all involved, including the children, the mothers, and the fathers. In this chapter, these two assumptions are examined by focusing on two questions: What are the causes of teen pregnancy? and What are the consequences of teen pregnancy and parenthood for the mothers, their children, and the fathers?

■ SOME NUMBERS AND STATISTICS

What Is the Teen Pregnancy Rate in the United States and in Other Countries?

In 2013, the pregnancy rate among U.S. 15- to 19-year-olds was 43.4 per 1,000 females, a rate only exceeded by Azerbaijan, Georgia, and Romania in countries outside of Africa (Kost, Maddow-Zimet, & Arpala, 2017; Sedgh, Finer, Bankole, Eilers, & Singh, 2015). By way of comparison, Switzerland has a teen pregnancy rate of about eight per 1,000 females. Teen pregnancy rates are especially high in sub-Saharan Africa, where many pregnancies are to young girls who marry and become pregnant early in their lives.

What accounts for cross-cultural differences in teen pregnancy rates? There are two proximal determinants of adolescent pregnancy rates: first, the percentage of adolescents who are sexually active; and second, the percentage of adolescents who consistently use an effective contraceptive. Cross-cultural differences in pregnancy rates may be the result of both factors, but the differences are mainly due to the percentage of adolescents who use reliable birth control (Santelli, Sandfort, & Orr, 2008).

Social, economic, and cultural factors also influence teen pregnancy rates. A lack of economic opportunity plays an important role in global differences in teen pregnancy rates, which generally are higher in poor countries and in countries with high income inequality (Santelli, Sharma, & Viner, 2013).

How Are Teen Pregnancy, Birth, and Abortion Rates in the United States Changing?

As can be seen in Figure 9.1, beginning in the early 1990s, teen pregnancy rates and birth rates in the United States began to drop sharply and continuously after yearly rises during the 1970s and 1980s. Teen abortion rates began to decline in the late 1980s after several years of stability. All of these rates have fallen for every racial and ethnic group. Teen pregnancy rates, birth rates, and abortion rates have reached historic lows in the United States and continue to fall (Kost et al., 2017; Romero et al., 2016).

These relatively low rates translate into large numbers of teens, however. In the United States in 2013, 448,440 teens became pregnant, which resulted in 273,105 births, 109,740 abortions, and 65,590 miscarriages (Kost et al., 2017). We should not forget that each of these numbers is a story that represents a life-changing event for all involved.

In most Western nations, teen pregnancy rates peaked in the mid-1970s, after which they declined precipitously. The decline in these rates is similar across developed nations, which suggests that whatever is responsible for the decrease in teen pregnancy rates is not unique to the United States but is shared by the community of developed nations.

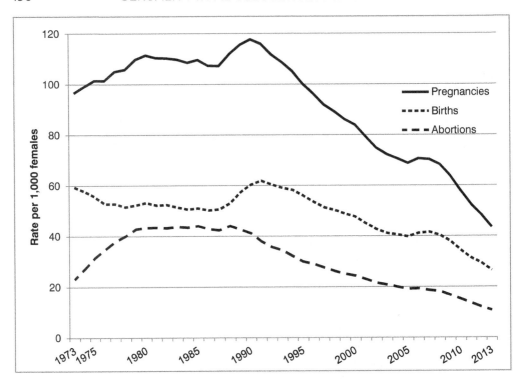

FIGURE 9.1. Trends in U.S. pregnancy, birth, and abortion rates per 1,000 females 15–19 years of age, 1973–2013. Adapted from Kost, Maddow-Zimet, and Arpala (2017).

Why Are Teen Pregnancy Rates Declining?

One reason for the decline in teen pregnancy rates is that over the past 25 years there has been a decrease in the percentage of U.S. high school students who have ever had sexual intercourse, falling from about 54% in 1991 to about 41% in 2015 (Kann, McManus, et al., 2016). This decline has not been constant during this period, however. The decrease mainly occurred between 1991 and 2001, and has not significantly changed since 2001. Pregnancy rates continue to fall even after 2001, however, suggesting that the more recent decline in pregnancy rates is mainly due to an increase in contraceptive use and not to a decrease in sexual activity (Boonstra, 2014; Lindberg, Santelli, & Desai, 2016).

Several changes in teenage contraceptive use have occurred over the past few years, each of which could lead to a decrease in pregnancy rates, and taken together indicate that teens today are more sexually responsible than they were in the past. More teens today report that they used some form of contraception the first time they had intercourse, used contraception the last time they had intercourse, and used multiple kinds of contraception (Finer & Philbin, 2013; Kann, Olsen, et al., 2016; Santelli, Lindberg, Finer, & Singh, 2007).

There are several possible explanations for the increase in contraceptive use among adolescents over the past few years. First, there has been a spread of school-based comprehensive sex education programs with an emphasis on safer sex. Second, there is greater awareness of AIDS and an increase in AIDS education programs, which have emphasized the importance of using condoms during sexual intercourse. Third, there has been more media attention paid to the problems associated with a teen pregnancy, in shows on TV such as *16 and Pregnant* and *Teen Mom*. And fourth, condoms are more available and easier to purchase than before, when they had to be bought from a pharmacist.

The policy implications of these findings are clear. Emphasizing the importance of waiting to have sex is a worthwhile goal of any sex education program, but it is also critical to convince sexually active teens to use contraception consistently and to make effective, inexpensive forms of contraception easily available to adolescents.

Is Every Teen Pregnancy an Unintended Pregnancy?

The phrase *teen pregnancy* is often preceded by the word *unintended,* the implication being that pregnancies to unmarried teens are accidental and unplanned (e.g., Hall, Kusunoki, Gatny, & Barber, 2015). Further, the use of the word *unintended* implies that there are two types of pregnancies, unintended and intended, with no room for degree of intendedness, including ambivalence. Research suggests that intendedness is not easily divided into two categories, but is better thought of as a continuum ranging from 100% intended to ambivalence to 100% unintended.

Not all teens think that a pregnancy is something to be avoided at all costs. In one study, Jaccard, Dodge, and Dittus (2003) found that 16% of females between the ages of 15 and 19 years either do not think that being pregnant is a terrible situation to be in, or they have an ambivalent attitude about becoming pregnant. Attitudes about pregnancy matter, and results from other studies indicate that adolescents with more favorable attitudes about pregnancy are considerably more likely to intend to get pregnant or get pregnant than adolescents with less favorable attitudes (Atienzo, Campero, Herrera, & Lozada, 2015; Farrell, Clyde, Katta, & Bolland, 2017; Rocca, Doherty, Padian, Hubbard, & Minnis, 2010). Some of the adolescents who become pregnant expect the relationship they are in to last, and they view their pregnancy as unplanned but not unwanted (McMichael, 2013). The mechanism that accounts for the connection between ambivalent attitudes about a pregnancy and a pregnancy is consistency of contraceptive use (Sipsma, Ickovics, Lewis, Ethier, & Kershaw, 2011).

These findings have implications for interventions, virtually all of which are based on the assumption that teen pregnancies are unwanted. Counseling adolescents about the demanding reality of taking care of an infant may help some adolescents make a more responsible decision about whether they truly want a child at their stage of life.

What Is the Teen Birth Rate and How Has It Changed over the Past Several Years?

There is good news and bad news about the number births to teenage mothers in the United States in the past few years. The good news is that the number is way down and continues to fall. The bad news is that an awful lot of children continue to be born to teens, 90% of whom are unmarried. In 2016, there were 209,480 children born to females in the United States between 15 and 19 years of age, a rate of 20.3 births for every 1,000 females in this age group, the lowest rate ever recorded in U.S. history (Hamilton, Martin, Osterman, Driscoll, & Rossen, 2017). The teen birth rate has declined 67% since 1991 when it was at its peak. Further, the birth rate has declined across the board, for younger and older teens, and for teens who are white, Hispanic, and African American.

Births to teens are not just a problem in the United States, but are a worldwide problem. Since the mid-2000s about 16 million teen girls worldwide give birth each year (Chandra-Mouli, Camacho, & Michaud, 2013). Approximately two million of these births are to girls 14 years old and younger, many of whom suffer grave long-term health and social consequences, including 70,000 teens who die each year from complications due to pregnancy and childbirth (United Nations Population Fund, 2013).

Why Are There More Births to African American and Hispanic Teens Than to White and Asian American Teens?

There are substantial racial and ethnic differences in teen birth rates. In 2013, Hispanic girls were more likely to give birth than any other group of teens, with a rate of 41.7 per 1,000 girls between 15 and 19 years of age, closely followed by African American girls with a birth rate of 39.0. The birth rate drops to 18.6 among white girls, reaching its lowest rate of 8.7 among Asian American girls (Martin, Hamilton, Osterman, Curtin, & Mathews, 2015). These large racial and ethnic differences in teen birth rates are troubling for many reasons, one of the most important being that the burden of teenage pregnancy is particularly great in Hispanic and African American communities. Why do these group differences exist?

William Julius Wilson's (2012) book *The Truly Disadvantaged* provides one compelling explanation for high pregnancy and birth rates among African American teens, an analysis that also applies to Hispanic teens. Wilson argues that racial differences in teen birth rates are highly related to differences in socioeconomic status. Poverty creates the conditions that lead to social disorganization, unstable relationships, and out-of-wedlock pregnancies, including teen pregnancies and births. According to Wilson, when traditional pathways to success are impeded or perceived to be blocked, people will seek other ways to find meaning and purpose in their lives. When a college education and a good job seem unattainable, many African American and Hispanic young women turn to motherhood as a meaningful alternative route to purpose and fulfillment. As a result of this way of thinking, many African American and Hispanic sexually active teens develop a casual attitude about birth control, the outcome of which for all too many sexually active girls is an early pregnancy and a birth.

Among many African Americans, especially those who are poor, a girl's social status is enhanced when she becomes a mother because of the high value put on having children in the African American community (Jacobs & Mollborn, 2012). Indeed, among many low-income minority young women, motherhood is viewed as a necessity for personal happiness and fulfillment (Edin & Kefalas, 2005). In addition, motherhood conveys on many low-income minority girls a sense of purpose and accomplishment, signifying passage into adulthood when other achievements of adulthood, such as graduation from college, landing a good job, and marriage, seem unattainable (Merrick, 1995).

Consistent with these ideas are findings that pregnancy and early parenthood are more acceptable among African American and Hispanic adolescents than among white adolescents. African American and Hispanic youth, especially those in economically disadvantaged communities, report that they would be less embarrassed and upset if they became pregnant or got someone pregnant than white youth from more advantaged communities (Mollborn, 2010; Myers & Geist, 2015). These findings suggest that race, ethnicity, and economic conditions shape attitudes about adolescent parenthood, which have an impact on the contraceptive use of sexually active teens, and on the probability of early parenthood.

If this analysis is correct, then reducing the pregnancy and birth rates of African American and Hispanic teens not only depends on effective sex education programs and access to contraception but also on improving educational success, decreasing poverty, reducing income inequality, and enhancing job prospects for disadvantaged teens.

Does Teen Parenthood Lead to Poverty?

Teen parents complete fewer years of school, are more likely to be unemployed, and more likely to live in poverty than teens who do not become teen parents (Furstenberg, 2003; Kearney & Levine, 2012). These impoverished socioeconomic circumstances are typically thought of as *consequences* of teenage parenthood, and there is evidence that they are, but they also are *predictors* of teen parenthood (Kearney & Levine, 2012). Luker (1996) makes the point that poverty precedes parenthood for many teens. According to Luker, "Teenage parents are not middle-class people who have become poor simply because they have had a baby; rather, they have become teenage parents because they were poor to begin with" (1996, p. 108). It is true that dropping out of school, unemployment, and poverty increase the risk of teen parenthood, but teen parenthood is also a risk factor for dropping out of school, unemployment, and poverty. Thus, poverty is both a cause and a consequence of teen parenthood.

■ TEEN MOTHERS

What Are Some of the Characteristics of Teen Girls Who Become Pregnant?

There is no one type of girl who is at risk for becoming pregnant during her adolescence. Teenage pregnancy is found in every social strata, race/ethnicity, family type, and psychosocial makeup, but some factors do increase the risk that a girl will experience a teen pregnancy. African American and Hispanic adolescents, especially if they are poor, are much more likely to experience a pregnancy than white adolescents (Woodward, Fergusson, & Horwood, 2001). Being minority, poor, and living in circumstances in which few people ever escape their poverty leads some girls to engage in risky sex, accepting an early pregnancy and young motherhood as a route to a meaningful life (Kearney & Levine, 2012).

Teen pregnancy is not just about race/ethnicity and economics, however. Family factors play an important role in increasing the risk of an early pregnancy. Specifically, teen girls are more likely to become pregnant if they are raised by a single mother, especially one who was never married (Maness, Buhi, Daley, Baldwin, & Kromrey, 2016; Woodward et al., 2001). Never-married mothers, particularly those who were mothers when they were teens, model premarital childbearing for their daughters, increasing the odds that the daughters will follow in their mothers' footsteps. Genes also matter, and daughters of never-married single mothers may inherit characteristics such as high risk-taking and low impulse control from their mothers that might lead to inconsistent contraceptive use and an early pregnancy (Harden et al., 2007).

Girls with stepparents, most of whom are stepfathers, are also more likely to become pregnant during adolescence than girls with two biological parents (Gaudie et al., 2010). Both the breakup of the original family and the arrival of the stepparent are transitions that can have a disruptive effect on family relations. These multiple family transitions create unstable environments that lead to poor parent monitoring, an increase in parent–teen conflict, and a decrease in parent–adolescent contact and closeness, which are all related to risky teen sex that can lead to an early pregnancy.

Another family factor related to teen pregnancy is maltreatment. Girls who are maltreated by family members are more likely to become pregnant during adolescence than girls who are not maltreated (Noll & Shenk, 2013; Young, Deardorff, Ozer, & Lahiff, 2011). Sexual abuse is especially predictive of teen pregnancy. Some have suggested that sexual abuse leads to a live-for-the-moment attitude, leading to impulsive sex and inconsistent contraceptive use (Herrman, 2014).

Another route to an early pregnancy is associating with deviant peers who use alcohol and drugs, and engage in delinquency, which exposes adolescents to other risky behaviors, such as casual sex (Hoskins & Simons, 2015). Members of deviant peer groups are themselves likely to be sexually active, and some may even be young mothers, providing models of risky sex and early motherhood.

Two behavioral characteristics related to teen pregnancy are antisocial behavior and low self-control. Girls who become pregnant during adolescence often engage in antisocial behavior, such as bullying, arguing, fighting, and delinquency (Gaudie et al., 2010). Other research has shown that conduct problems in childhood predict teen pregnancy (Woodward & Fergusson, 1999). Underlying many of these antisocial behaviors is low self-control, which is related to impulsive sex and inconsistent contraceptive use (Moffitt et al., 2010; Moffitt, Poulton, & Caspi, 2013).

One group of teen girls at risk for an early pregnancy are bisexual young women, a group not often thought of as a teen pregnancy risk group. Bisexual females have a higher pregnancy rate than either heterosexual or lesbian females (Goldberg, Reese, & Halpern, 2016). The main reason for the high pregnancy rate is that bisexual females engage in high-risk sexual behaviors that include an early age of sexual debut, more sexual partners, and inconsistent contraceptive use. One implication of these findings is that pregnancy prevention efforts should include some material specifically targeted at young bisexual females, most of whom are ignored in traditional sex education courses.

There is no simple explanation for teen pregnancy. A teen pregnancy is the result of a complex set of characteristics that include race/ethnicity, socioeconomic status, family type, parenting, peers, biology, and individual behavioral characteristics that put girls at risk for an early pregnancy. Teen pregnancy is more than just irresponsible sexual behavior. It is the result of life circumstances that narrow choices and lead to poor judgment (Leadbeater, 2014).

Are Daughters Like Their Mothers When It Comes to Teen Pregnancy?

The daughters of mothers who were mothers when they were teens are more likely to become mothers themselves when they become teens, perpetuating what is referred to as the *intergenerational cycle of teenage motherhood*. This intergenerational cycle is not unique to the United States but also exists in other countries where it has been studied, such as Britain (Manlove, 1997) and New Zealand (Jaffee, Caspi, Moffitt, Belsky, & Silva, 2001). The effect of having a mother who was a mother when she was a teen is substantial, ranging from a 66% increase in the probability of teen motherhood among U.S. teens (Meade et al., 2008), while in New Zealand, daughters of teen mothers are almost three times more likely to become teen mothers themselves (Jaffee, Caspi, Moffitt, Belsky, et al., 2001), all in comparison to girls born to mothers who were not teen mothers.

Researchers have uncovered four factors that increase the risk of the intergenerational cycle: poverty, being African American or Hispanic, lower parental monitoring, and deviant peer group membership (Meade et al., 2008). The authors suggest that when life opportunities are limited, daughters are more likely to follow in the footsteps of their own mothers, especially daughters who are African American or Hispanic, two groups that emphasize the importance

A FOCUS ON RESEARCH

Studying the consequences of teen motherhood is a complex task for at least two reasons. First, it is difficult to determine the direction of causality between teen motherhood and the many factors associated with teen motherhood. For example, poverty is an antecedent to teen motherhood, but poverty is also an outcome of teen motherhood, the result of the inability of teen mothers to financially support themselves and their children. Substance use is another example of a problem that can be both a cause and a consequence of teen motherhood. Adolescents who use and abuse alcohol and other drugs are at risk for inconsistent contraceptive use and an unplanned pregnancy, but becoming a teen mother is itself a risk factor for further use and abuse of alcohol and drugs. Thus, many of the characteristics associated with teen pregnancy and motherhood can be both causes and consequences.

A second problem facing researchers studying teen pregnancy is differentiating between the specific impact of pregnancy on teens from outcomes that might occur even if the teens do not become pregnant. For example, some girls doing poorly in school become pregnant and drop out before they graduate, suggesting that teen pregnancy causes early school leaving, which it does, but doing poorly in school is itself a risk factor for dropping out, even for girls who do not become pregnant. What is difficult to ascertain is the probability that a pregnant girl doing poorly in school would have dropped out even if she had not become pregnant.

Establishing the causes and consequences of teen pregnancy is a complex affair because it is often difficult to determine which events precede the pregnancy and which follow from the pregnancy. Further, what appears to be a consequence of teen pregnancy may have occurred even if a girl had not become pregnant. Researchers attempt to untangle these complexities through the use of longitudinal research designs and sophisticated data analyses that make it possible to construct a plausible model of the sequence of events that best fits the data.

of motherhood as a road to a life with purpose. Going down that road may lead to an early pregnancy and motherhood for girls who are not monitored very well and who associate with friends who engage in deviant behavior, including early sex.

Genetic influences are another explanation for the intergenerational cycle of teenage motherhood. One possible connection is through daughters' inheritance of maternal traits, such as sensation-seeking and impulsivity, both of which have a genetic basis and are implicated in risky sexual behavior (Donohew, Zimmerman, Cupp, Novak, Colon, et al., 2000). Mothers who possess these traits may pass them on to their daughters, increasing the daughter's risk for an early pregnancy and teen motherhood.

Are There Certain Behavioral Profiles of Young Girls Who Become Mothers?

Several profiles exist for teen mothers (Kneale, Fletcher, Wiggins, & Bonell, 2013). For some adolescents, teen motherhood occurs at the end of a long developmental sequence that begins in early childhood and continues throughout adolescence. Many future teen mothers have conduct problems in early

> The young woman in the following story comes across as a good student disconnected from her parents and from the father of her son, a young man she never mentions. She has some, but not all, of the characteristics of young women who become pregnant, illustrating the complex nature of teen pregnancy.

IN THEIR OWN WORDS

Less than 2 months after turning 17 years old, I found out that I was pregnant. From that moment I was a mother. I spent time trying to come to terms with the idea and coming up with a plan for my immediate future. I knew my father was going to kick me out of the house so I had made arrangements to move in with my best friend's family.

As for my personal experience. . . . I was born into an upper-middle SES [socioeconomic status], had never had an STI, used contraception regularly, no drug/alcohol use, and I was a good student with a 3.7 GPA [grade point average]. My teen years were definitely lacking in family connectedness. I spent most of my teens alone in my room not interacting with my father and stepmother. There was limited contact with just my father, but when all three of us were in a room, I was mostly invisible. They never even noticed that I was having morning sickness and had developed a baby bump.

childhood, leading to high parent–child conflict that extends into adolescence (Lehti et al., 2011). Some of these children possess poor cognitive abilities that result in academic difficulties and disengagement from school (Hardy, Astone, Brooks-Gunn, Shapiro, & Miller, 1998). Many students who do poorly in school form friendships with other students doing poorly in school, friendships that are associated with deviant activities, including risky sexual behavior (De Genna, Larkby, & Cornelius, 2011). For adolescents with this background, early sex and inconsistent contraceptive use are common, increasing the risk of an early pregnancy (Xie, Cairns, & Cairns, 2001).

Another teen mother profile is one that includes low emotional support at home, leading to low self-esteem and depression (Hammen, Brennan, & Le Brocque, 2011). Some of these girls attempt to find a meaningful relationship with a boyfriend to substitute for the lack of connection with parents. Many of these girls expect their current romantic relationship to last and perhaps even include a future pregnancy, an expectation that can lead to inconsistent contraceptive use, increasing the risk of an early pregnancy.

What Problems Are Common among Teen Mothers?

On average, teen mothers complete fewer years of school and are more likely to drop out of school than girls who are not mothers (Mollborn, 2007). There is a real educational penalty for becoming a teen mother, and the reason is that many teen mothers do not have adequate housing, access to child care, and financial support, which interferes with their ability to continue their schooling. Most teen mothers have to work and take care of their children, while living in substandard housing, conditions that make it difficult for the young mothers to finish school. Programs that provide child care to teen mothers so they can stay in school are good investments that help the mothers reduce their reliance on public assistance, which helps us all.

Teen mothers are also beset with a variety of psychological and adjustment problems. For example, adolescent mothers experience significantly higher rates of depression than either teens who are not mothers or in comparison to adult mothers (Hodgkinson, Beers, Southammakosane, & Lewin, 2014). Further, teen depression lasts, often persisting for many years after the birth of the child (Boden, Fergusson, & Horwood, 2008). Although completed suicides are rare among teen mothers, feelings of hopelessness and despair are not, leading to suicidal ideation among many adolescent mothers (Bayatpour, Wells, & Holford, 1992). Some of these adjustment problems may be present before the birth of the child, but they are made worse by the demands of parenthood during adolescence, which exacerbates any preexisting problems and difficulties.

Some girls abuse alcohol and drugs before they become pregnant (De Genna & Cornelius, 2015), and many of these girls use alcohol and drugs during their pregnancy, habits that continue after the birth of the baby (Ebrahim

---

Not all teen pregnancies end badly, as the following story told by a college student about a friend illustrates. As we try to understand why the following situation seems to have turned out well, note that the couple were in college, the father was involved with his daughter, and the couple had the help of a supportive therapist.

IN THEIR OWN WORDS

During my freshman year of college, one of my best friends became pregnant. M. and C. met during our senior year and began to date. During this time, C. was not a very good boyfriend and he would cheat on her constantly. They would fight all the time and even break up for a couple days, but it would never last. Finally, M. decided she wasn't going to put up with it anymore and tried to end things for good. However, 2 months later she found out she was pregnant with his child. She went a little over a month not realizing that she was pregnant. During that time, she was very irresponsible. She would drink a lot, take Adderall every day, and eat unhealthy. Naturally, she was devastated when she found out she was pregnant because she was no longer with the father, and she was worried that her actions during the first month of her pregnancy would affect her baby's health. M. and C. decided to work through their issues and get back together for the sake of their child. They moved in together and started planning their futures together.

M. hated being pregnant. She was emotional, and hated her body. She would cry to me almost every day because she wanted her old life back. Even though C. had completely changed his ways, it was really hard for her to forgive him for all he had done in the past. She did not have an easy pregnancy, to say the least, and she was terrified for her future. It has been over 2 years now since M. gave birth. C. and M. are still together and have a beautiful and healthy baby girl. They go to a therapist together twice a month to help them work through their issues. C. is graduating this year and going to law school next year. While M. would never trade A. for anything, she wishes she would have done things differently. Young motherhood is really hard, but she has done the best she could do. They have made a terrible situation into something happy and good.

& Gfroerer, 2003). Substance use for some teen mothers may be an attempt at self-medication in the face of difficult life circumstances.

The lives of teen mothers are considerably more stressful and violent than the lives of girls who are not mothers. One study found that a typical teenage mother experiences more than five stressful and violent events after the birth of her baby, including physical attacks by her partner, neglect, abuse by a parent, and criminal behavior (Coyne, Fontaine, Långström, Lichtenstein, & D'Onofrio, 2013). Girls who experience these adverse events pay a psychological price for the traumas they undergo. Almost 50% of the teen mothers in one study met the full criteria for posttraumatic stress disorder (Leplatte, Rosenblum, Stanton, Miller, & Muzik, 2012).

Although problems with depression, substance use, stress, and violence are common among teen mothers, many young mothers do not fit this profile, and there is considerable variability in the adjustment of teen moms. Many young mothers do as well as their peers who do not have children, especially when the teen mothers receive emotional, social, and financial support from their own parents, the father of the baby, and from friends (Hodgkinson, Beers, Southammakosane, & Lewin, 2014).

What about Repeat Pregnancies?

One circumstance that can have a major negative effect on the life of a young mother is the arrival of another child. Repeat pregnancies, defined as a pregnancy within 24 months of a previous pregnancy, are all too common among teen mothers. In 2013, one in six births to 15- to 19-year-olds were to females who already had a child (Martin et al., 2015). Researchers in another study of urban, mainly African American adolescent mothers found that over 40% of the mothers had a repeat pregnancy (Crittenden, Boris, Rice, Taylor, & Olds, 2009). The immediate cause of the second pregnancy is that many of the repeat pregnancy mothers are inconsistent contraceptive users who did not use any type of contraception the last time they had intercourse. Many of the repeat pregnancy mothers have positive attitudes about being a mother, and are not strongly motivated to avoid a second birth, attitudes associated with careless contraceptive use and a repeat pregnancy (Barr, Simons, Simons, Gibbons, & Gerrard, 2013).

■ THE CHILDREN

What Are Some of the Medical and Health-Related Risks to Infants Born to Teen Mothers?

Infants born to teen mothers are at higher risk for premature birth, low birthweight, and birth defects than infants born to adult mothers (Khashan, Baker, & Kenny, 2010; Yasmin, Kumar, & Parihar, 2014). Low-birthweight infants have a higher risk of brain damage and cognitive impairment. Many adolescents drink alcohol while they are pregnant, increasing the risk to the newborn of fetal alcohol syndrome, which is characterized by growth retardation and central nervous system disorders (Allard-Hendren, 2000). In addition, infants born to teen mothers, especially those under the age of 15 years, are more likely to be stillbirths or to die in the first year of life from all causes, including sudden infant death syndrome, than infants born to adult mothers (Malabarey, Balayla, Klam, Shrim, & Abenhaim, 2012).

Why Are Children Born to Teen Mothers at Risk?

Two explanations have been proposed to account for the high rate of birth problems and neonatal difficulties (neonatal refers to the first month of life) of children born to teen mothers. One explanation focuses on the mother's immature reproductive system, and on the nutritional needs of the growing mother (Chen et al., 2009; Scholl, Hediger, & Ances, 1990). Pregnancy-related problems are attributed to the fact that the fetus is developing in a reproductive environment that is itself continuing to grow and mature. The young girl's reproductive system simply is not yet ready to provide a healthy environment for a developing fetus. In addition, there is competition for nutrients between the still-growing adolescent mother and her fetus. As a result, fetal development suffers, deliveries are difficult, and the baby is more likely to be born in an unhealthy state.

A second explanation focuses on the behavior of the teen mom before and after the birth of the baby (Raatikainen, Heiskanen, Verkasalo, & Heinonen, 2006). Pregnant teens are less likely to seek prenatal care, and more likely than adult pregnant women to smoke cigarettes, drink alcohol, use drugs, and have a poor diet. Any one of these factors can have an adverse effect on pregnancy, birth, and neonatal health. In combination, these behaviors can have a devastating effect on the developing fetus that continues long after birth.

In the following story, one young woman discusses her negative experiences being a teen mother that included an early birth and being treated badly by the medical staff at her hospital, perhaps because she was a teen mother.

IN THEIR OWN WORDS

My freshman year of college I found out that I was pregnant. I was 19 and scared of what the future would hold. I was in disbelief as I was then on the pill and taking it regularly. I thought I was safe.

I delivered my daughter at [hospital]. She was born at 35 weeks and was small at 5 pounds 8 ounces. I had no complication during pregnancy so I didn't understand why she came early. She was in the special care nursery for 8 hours. My experience at the hospital was not the best either—my doctor was awesome, the other staff in postpartum was not. I was treated like I was a single teen mom—a stigma I was not happy to fall into. The nursing staff was not helpful—they pushed me to bottle feed even when I repeatedly asked for help breast-feeding.

One integration of these two explanations suggests that the problems experienced by infants born to young teens are due to the immature reproductive system of the young teen and to her unhealthy lifestyle (Gibbs, Wendt, Peters, & Hogue, 2012). The reproductive system of younger adolescents is still developing, which can have an adverse effect on the developing fetus, especially in combination with unhealthy maternal behaviors. The problems experienced by infants born to older teens whose reproductive system is more fully developed are more highly related to the mother's negligent lifestyle and irresponsible behavior.

What Are the Long-Term Risks of Being Born to a Teen Mother?

Given the many short-term problems infants have who are born to teen mothers, it is not surprising that the long-term prognosis of many of these children is poor. Teen motherhood puts infants and young children at risk for injury through abuse or neglect (Barczyk, Duzinski, Brown, & Lawson, 2015). Many risk factors for childhood injuries are present in the lives of teen mothers, including low socioeconomic status, social isolation, lack of social support, family disorganization, and household crowding. The presence of these social forces are conducive to child abuse no matter how old the mother is, but they are especially powerful when they are part of the family life of a young teen who lacks the personal and social resources to cope with the incessant demands of an infant.

Even if the infants of teen mothers are not physically injured, the infants are at risk for low-quality mother–infant relationships that include many negative interactions and little positive play time (Crugnola, Ierardi, Gazzotti, & Albizzati, 2014). It is common for the infants of adolescent mothers to have an insecure attachment style characterized by a weak emotional bond with a mother who is insensitive to her infant's needs. Infants with insecure attachments often grow into adults who have difficulty understanding their own emotions and the feelings of others, and tend to form unsuccessful, superficial relations with others.

Children born to teen mothers have a difficult and disturbed adolescence that includes having sex at an early age (Pogarsky, Thornberry, & Lizotte, 2006), which is associated with contracting an STI, and an early pregnancy. Children born to teen mothers are more likely to drink alcohol and use marijuana during adolescence than youth born to adult mothers (De Genna & Cornelius, 2015; De Genna, Goldschmidt, & Cornelius, 2015). Many children born to teen mothers have externalizing behavior problems, which develop into antisocial and delinquent behavior during adolescence. The findings suggest that many young mothers do a poor job of raising and supervising their children, who then become involved in sex, drugs, and delinquency when they become adolescents.

Children born to teen mothers are at risk for a variety of poor life outcomes that extend into adolescence and emerging adulthood. Boys born to teen mothers, in comparison to boys born to adult mothers, are more likely to join a gang, and become teen fathers during adolescence, while girls are more likely to become teen mothers themselves (Pogarsky et al., 2006). Offspring of teen mothers in comparison to offspring of adult mothers are more likely to do poorly in school and to be convicted of a criminal offense (Coyne, Långström, Lichtenstein, & D'Onofrio, 2013). As adults, offspring of teen mothers have lower life satisfaction, are more likely to be unemployed, and make less money than offspring of adult mothers (Lipman, Georgiades, & Boyle, 2011). The larger point is that children born to teen mothers typically do not grow out of their early childhood deprivation, but become adolescents and emerging adults who have a variety of adjustment problems.

Why Are Children Born to Teen Mothers at Risk for Negative Outcomes?

Researchers have developed two frameworks to explain why children born to teen mothers are at risk for adverse outcomes. The first is called *social influence effects,* which is that teens are ill equipped to raise their children well because of their young age and immature psychological development. As a result of their immaturity, teens do a poor job socializing their children, who suffer the negative consequences of their upbringing throughout their lives. According to the social influence idea, if only the young mothers had waited to have children until the mothers were older, their children would have turned out better. The second framework is called *social selection effects,* which is the idea that some mothers possess certain characteristics that are detrimental to the healthy growth and development of their children. Some of these characteristics include maternal impulsivity, irritability, and depression that interfere with a mother's ability to successfully socialize her children no matter how old the mother is. Mothers who lack the skills to properly care for their children will have children who are at risk for problem behavior because of how the children are raised, whether the mothers are teens or adults. Thus, the problem for the child is not having a teen mother—it is having a mother who lacks the qualities necessary to be a good mother.

Results from one 20-year longitudinal study of children born to teen mothers demonstrates both social influence and social selection effects (Jaffee, Caspi, Moffitt, Belsky, et al., 2001). Teen mothers are more likely to respond to child misbehavior with inconsistent discipline, and have more negative interactions with their children than do adult mothers. According to the social influence idea, the negative interactions teen mothers have with their offspring are mainly the result of a mother's immaturity and poorly developed parenting skills. If only the girls had waited to have children until they were older, the quality of their interactions with their children would have been better, improving the life chances of the offspring. However, social selection effects also matter. Teen mothers who do poorly in school have children who do poorly in school, but adult mothers who do poorly in school also have children who do poorly in school. In other words, poor school performance has little to do with having a teen mother and more to do with having a mother of any age who does poorly in school. The poor school performance of a child is tied to characteristics of the mother more than to the age of the mother.

These findings have important implications for intervention programs designed to improve the lives of children born to teen mothers. The social influence idea suggests that interventions should be designed to delay the onset of a pregnancy until after girls grow out of their teen years. Merely delaying a first pregnancy is not enough, however. The social selection idea suggests that some young women have cognitive and personality traits that will make it difficult for them to be effective mothers, whenever they become mothers. From this perspective, successful programs to improve the life chances of children are those that attempt to help girls develop the characteristics they need to be successful mothers, such as learning to control their impulses, avoiding alcohol and drugs, and improving their interpersonal skills, all of which will enhance their parenting, whenever it occurs (Harden, Brunton, Fletcher, & Oakley, 2009).

Do All Children Born to Teen Mothers Turn Out Badly?

The bleak prognosis for the offspring of adolescent mothers, while true, ignores the heterogeneity and resilience of some children who manage to more than survive their perilous life circumstances, who thrive, and do quite well. Findings from one 10-year longitudinal study of children born to teen mothers reveals that 20% of the third graders display few behavioral problems, have good social relations, and are doing well in school, while the large majority of the children are adjusted in at least one area of their lives (Rhule, McMahon, Spieker, & Munson, 2006). Children of teen mothers who are thriving have good language skills, are securely attached to their mothers, and have mothers who are effective parents, all of which improves the life chances of the offspring.

Other research on a small group of Navajo adolescents born to teen mothers uncovered three groups of teens (Dalla & Kennedy, 2015). A *well-adapted* group, which includes 42% of the total sample, is composed of adolescents who do well in school, participate in extracurricular activities, and have high aspirations for themselves. These adolescents respect their parents, have parents who provide material and emotional support to the adolescents, and live in a nurturing family environment. An *overcoming* group, which is 29% of the sample, includes youth who are getting average grades and have vocational/technical career plans. These adolescents have an emotionally close and supportive relationship with at least one family member, but also experience significant family adversity, sometimes including physical abuse. Many of the parents in this group abuse drugs and alcohol and are chronically unemployed. A third group, *struggling,* which includes 29% of the sample, do poorly in school, are teen parents themselves, and are unemployed. These youth live in single-parent homes with depressed mothers who are out of work and who receive public assistance.

These findings demonstrate that children born to teen mothers do not inevitably become problem children and adolescents. In the right family environment, many children of teen mothers do well psychologically, socially, and academically on their way to successful, productive lives.

■ THE FATHERS

Teen fathers are the largely forgotten member of the teen pregnancy triad that includes the mother, the child, and the father, a situation that leads to the impression of teen fathers as uninterested and uninvolved with their children. While it is true that some young fathers are disengaged from their children and from the mothers of their children, others are involved with the mothers and take an active role in raising their children, while still others would like to participate in family life, but do not for a variety of reasons.

We know less about teen fathers than teen mothers for several reasons. First, many young men who father children with teen girls are not teens themselves, but may be well into their 20s and even beyond. Second, it is more difficult to determine paternity than maternity, since birth certificates contain limited information about the birth father, which makes it difficult to locate the fathers. Third, teen mothers are more accessible for research through their visits to clinics and hospitals than teen fathers, some of whom do not make themselves available for research. Despite these limitations, some characteristics of teen fathers are known, which are examined in this section.

Who Are Teen Fathers?

Most young men who father children with teen mothers are older teens between 18 and 19 years of age (Scott, Steward-Streng, Manlove, & Moore, 2012), but some are even older. In one Texas study, about 30% of births to teen mothers were fathered by males over the age of 19 years (Castrucci, Clark, Lewis, Samsel, & Mirchandani, 2010).

Less than 10% of teen fathers are married to the mother at the time of the birth of the child. About 25% of teen fathers are cohabiting with the mother when the child is born, a fragile relationship associated with problems for the children when they become adolescents, such as delinquency, substance use, and early sexual behavior (Waldfogel, Craigie, & Brooks-Gunn, 2010).

What Are Some Characteristics That Predict Teen Fatherhood?

Teen fathers come from every socioeconomic strata, but they are likely to be impoverished. Having an impoverished socioeconomic background is also true for teen fathers in other countries, such as Sweden, which suggests that poverty is a general risk factor for teen fatherhood (Ekéus & Christensson, 2003).

Socioeconomic status matters, but individual, psychological, and behavioral characteristics are also associated with adolescent fatherhood. Boys who become teen fathers, in comparison to boys who do not, are more likely to have emotional problems in childhood, including conduct disorders, and during adolescence, are more likely to engage in delinquent behavior, use alcohol and drugs, have sex at an early age, and be inconsistent contraceptive users (Jaffee, Caspi, Moffitt, Taylor, & Dickson, 2001; Pears, Pierce, Kim, Capaldi, & Owen, 2005; Wei, Loeber, & Stouthamer-Loeber, 2002). Many teen fathers receive poor grades in school, are suspended from school, or convicted of a criminal offense. The pattern of these characteristics suggests that many teen fathers are impulsive adolescents who engage in reckless, risk-taking activities, and who flout authority (Garfield et al., 2016).

Two sexual characteristics related to teen fatherhood are a high number of lifetime sexual partners and negative reactions to condom use (Lau, Lin, & Flores, 2015). Having many sexual partners, coupled with negative attitudes about condoms, can lead to inconsistent condom use, which is a recipe for an unplanned pregnancy. These results suggest a pattern of risky sexual behavior that increases the probability of teen fatherhood.

The attitudes of adolescents about becoming a teen father play a role in whether a teen becomes a father. In one study, almost 41% of Latino adolescent males and 33% of African American adolescent males reported that they would be pleased by a pregnancy, in contrast to only 16% of white adolescent males (Lau, Lin, & Flores, 2016). Some marginal young men involved in deviant activities may have ambivalent or even positive attitudes about a teen pregnancy, perhaps because fathering a child may lead to an increase in social status, or to an enhancement of the father's sense of manhood (Augustine, Nelson, & Edin, 2009).

One in-depth study of 26 teen fathers reveals the thinking of these young fathers and provides an inside look at how these young men explain the pregnancy (Weber, 2012). One common explanation is based on the idea that the woman is in charge of preventing pregnancy and she is responsible if a pregnancy occurs. One young man admitted that he does not like to wear a condom because "it didn't feel good," and went on to say:

> "I was always, like, let's go get you on birth control. And she was always, like, 'No, I just got off because it messes up my body.' And I was like, well, there's different things. And she was always just like, yeah. . . . But she never did. And then we got pregnant." (Weber, 2012, p. 910)

Another theme is that the pregnancy was an accident that occurred in "the heat of the moment." As one teen said:

> "It's just one of those things where you just wanna have sex. You're not thinking of anything else . . . I mean . . . I'm a guy, you know . . . I'm like, I just wanna have sex. And, when you're a man and your hormones are raging, and it's like you

In the following story, one young man who had a brush with a teen pregnancy describes the freedom he had to do as he pleased, since neither he nor his girlfriend were well monitored, a situation that led to a pregnancy scare.

IN THEIR OWN WORDS

My [girlfriend's parents] did not pay much attention to their kids while they were in high school. My [girlfriend's mother] had a boyfriend who she frequently saw on the weekends out of town. [My girlfriend's father] pretended everything was always great and that his kids could not ever be deviant.

My parents never cared where I stayed on the weekends. I spent those weekends staying with my [girlfriend] in high school, her mother was out of town and sometimes she did not care if I stayed as long as she was home much earlier than curfew. Of course we spent all those times having sex on the weekend or whenever I would stay there. My [girlfriend] in high school was getting off birth control because it hurt her stomach too much, we were still having sex and began to use condoms again because she was not taking birth control any longer. In the process of quitting birth control, her hormones took a major change, causing her menstrual cycle to skip a month. I felt like my life was over. When I say I felt like my life was over I meant that there will be no more fun, no college, and that was it. I even remember going to lunch with my school counselor and telling him, asking him what should I do. The thought crossed my mind that I was going to be buying his minivan from him. I was completely lost and unsure for what was going to happen. We were fortunate that did not happen.

can't think about anything else besides having sex . . . so you just do it." (Weber, 2012, p. 912)

A third theme is based on the idea that the two teens are in love, and although the pregnancy is unplanned, it is not unwanted. As one young man said:

"I mean, I was using [protection] at first, but I thought she was the one. I mean, it wasn't like I was just sleeping with all these girls . . . I loved her. We was talkin' about gettin' married and all this stuff. And then I wanted to have kids with her. And then we did. But, like it just didn't work out." (Weber, 2012, p. 916)

Is Teen Fatherhood Passed from Father to Son?

An intergenerational cycle of parenthood not only exists between mothers and daughters but also between fathers and sons. In one study, sons of fathers who had a child when they were teens are more than three times as likely to have a child when they are teens than sons with fathers who did not have a child during their adolescence (Sipsma et al., 2010). One explanation for a father–son intergenerational cycle is that fathers communicate their values and expectations about sex to their sons by the way they raise their sons, which shapes the sexual attitudes and behaviors of sons. Sons with fathers who were teen fathers may develop positive attitudes about casual sex that are associated with early fatherhood. Many of the sons who become adolescent fathers do not live with their fathers, however, which suggests that fathers can have a powerful influence on their sons, even when the father is not present. Perhaps fathers pass on their genetic makeup to their sons for characteristics such as risk-taking and low impulse control, which would result in a father–son intergenerational cycle.

What Consequences Are Associated with Becoming a Teen Father?

Teen fatherhood is associated with several negative socioeconomic consequences that persist into adulthood. For example, teen fathers are more likely to earn a general equivalency diploma (GED) than a high school diploma, and will spend more time unemployed than youth who do not become teen fathers (Assini-Meytin & Green, 2015; Fletcher & Wolfe, 2012). Teen fathers often drop out of school before they graduate, which means that they rarely have the financial resources to provide much support for their children, perpetuating a cycle of poverty for the teen parents and their children (Bunting & McAuley, 2004). In addition, teen fathers are more likely to be incarcerated than teens who do not father a child (Dariotis, Pleck, Astone, & Sonenstein, 2011).

Low educational achievement is both a cause and a consequence of teen fatherhood. For example, academic difficulties predate teen fatherhood by as much as a decade, which suggests that many of these young men are on the verge of dropping out of school before they become teen fathers (Dearden, Hale, & Woolley, 1995).

Almost half of teen fathers have a second and even a third child by the time they are 24 years old. The large majority of these second and third births are to the same mother of the first child. The negative educational and economic consequences to the fathers of having more than one child in adolescence and emerging adulthood are substantial (Manlove, Logan, Ikramullah, & Holcombe, 2008).

Why Are Some Teen Fathers Involved with Their Children, While Others Are Not?

Positive father involvement with their children includes contact with the children, providing financial support, participating in activities with the children, being emotionally supportive, and taking on parenting tasks such as supervision and discipline. How involved are teen fathers with their children? One study of mainly African American teen fathers found that approximately 50% of fathers are involved to some degree with their children when the children are infants, a figure that drops to about 33% when the children are 1 year old, where it remains into the child's second year of life (Lewin, Mitchell, Burrell, Beers, & Duggan, 2011). High father involvement is related to having only one child, high maternal self-esteem, low maternal depression, few conflicts with the mother, and respect for the mother. Fathers are more likely to be involved with their children if they have a romantic relationship with a well-functioning mother. Results from this study suggest that interventions designed to enhance fathers' involvement with their children need to address the romantic relationship between the father and the mother of the child, which plays a large part in how involved fathers are with their children.

Other researchers report that father involvement significantly decreases during the first year of a child's life, but remains high if the father has a good relationship with the maternal grandmother of the child (Kalil, Ziol-Guest, & Coley, 2005). Fathers who are not involved with their children tend to have a poor relationship with the child's mother and with the maternal grandmother. The authors suggest that maternal grandmothers matter, both for relations between teen mothers and the fathers of their children, and between young fathers and their children.

Many parents of teen mothers, as well as social programs designed to improve the lives of children born to teen mothers, may discourage romantic and coparenting relationships between teen parents (Mollborn & Jacobs, 2015). Many teen fathers want to be involved in the lives of their children, but feel excluded or pushed out by the mother's parents and even by social service agencies that want to focus on the mothers and their infants. Although some young mothers and their children are better off without the involvement of an unemployed, substance-abusing father, other mothers and children could receive much needed help and support from a responsible, involved young father.

What Effects Do Teen Fathers Have on Their Children?

In one study of teen parents and their infants, researchers reported that infants are less distressed in families where the father is present, especially when the father provides some financial support (Lewin et al., 2015). Financial assistance helps the mother, who is less stressed, and who then has more quality time to spend with her infant. Another avenue by which teen father involvement decreases infant distress is by buffering infants from the negative effects of maternal depression, which is high among teen mothers. A young father involved with his child may help the young mother cope with her postpartum depression, in addition to providing the infant with a nondepressed parent.

Other research on teen mothers and fathers reveals that children with residential fathers for the first 3 years of the child's life have fewer problems, and are more securely attached to their mothers than children with nonresidential fathers (Martin, Brazil, & Brooks-Gunn, 2012). The positive effects of co-residence are not explained by higher household income, which is only slightly higher in two-parent households than in households with a nonresident father. It is what fathers do with their children that matters, not just how much they earn. The findings reveal that many responsible young men who choose to live with their child and with the mother of the child can have a positive effect on the life of the child. It is important to remember that not every teen father adds to the health of his child, however. Some teen mothers and their children are better off without the presence of a young father who is unemployed and delinquent, characteristics in young fathers associated with negative outcomes for the children (Bunting & McAuley, 2004).

In general, children who reside with their teen mothers and fathers fare better than children of teen mothers with nonresidential fathers (Mollborn & Lovegrove, 2011). These are generalizations, however, and there is much variability among fathers. At the very least, we can say that not all teen fathers are a detriment to their children. Some are responsible young men who contribute to the healthy development of their children. Identifying these young men and encouraging them to be involved with their children should be a goal of every social service program designed to help teen mothers and their children.

■ INTERVENTIONS TO IMPROVE THE LIVES OF TEEN PARENTS AND THEIR CHILDREN

Teen pregnancy and parenthood not only affect the lives of the teens and their children but also have steep social and economic costs that have an impact on us all. Teen pregnancies come with an expensive price tag, costing U.S. taxpayers approximately $9.4 billion annually (National Campaign to Prevent Teen and Unplanned Pregnancy, 2013). Successful interventions that decrease the rate of teen pregnancy not only improve the lives of teens and their children but benefit us all.

The problems of teen parents and their children are not inexorable, and several intervention programs have shown varying degrees of success, increasing the odds that the teen parents and their children will thrive.

A substantial number of teen mothers have a repeat pregnancy within 2 years of their first pregnancy, a situation related to further adjustment problems for the mothers and their children and continuing public assistance. Several in-home teen pregnancy prevention programs have as one of their primary goals the prevention of rapid repeat pregnancies. The programs typically include weekly home and clinic visits that focus on a broad range of services for teen families, one component of which is to provide the parents with effective contraceptives (Hayter, Jones, Owen, & Harrison, 2016). In general, programs designed to prevent adolescent repeat pregnancies and births have a positive effect on adolescent outcomes (Maravilla, Betts, Abajobir, Cruz, & Alati, 2016). One evaluation of these programs found an average 50% reduction in the odds of another pregnancy 19 months after the start of the intervention, although the impact of the interventions disappeared by 31 months (Corcoran & Pillai, 2007). Another program led to an increase in contraceptive use and a lower rate of repeat pregnancies 24 months after the start of the program (Patchen, Letourneau, & Berggren, 2013). Even a relatively short-term effect can have long-term advantages for the child, since during the time the young mother has only one child she can devote more of her time and resources to raising that child during the critical first few years of life, increasing the odds that the child will be well cared for and flourish.

Many in-home interventions for teen mothers are designed to enhance the developmental outcomes of the children by improving the child-rearing skills of the mothers. As a group, teen mothers tend to be relatively insensitive and unresponsive mothers, so improvement in their parenting styles can go a long way toward ameliorating some of the disadvantages of being born to a teen mother (Beers & Hollo, 2009). Some of these in-home programs have shown modest short-term improvements in the involvement of mothers with their children, in parenting knowledge, and in decreasing parenting stress (Ruedinger & Cox, 2012).

Most school-based programs are grounded on the theory that children of teen mothers are benefited if the mother can continue her education after the birth of her baby. Not surprisingly, school-based child care facilities for teen moms increase school attendance and reduce school dropout rates. Keeping mothers in school is also related to higher-quality mother–child interactions and a more supportive home environment, demonstrating that improvements in mothering are a by-product of educational attainment (Sullivan et al., 2011).

School health clinics are another means of reaching teens who are pregnant or parenting. These clinics offer contraceptive services, prenatal exams, counseling, and classes in child care. There is some evidence that these clinics are successful in reducing repeat pregnancies, enhancing parenting skills, and improving infant development (Strunk, 2008). Unfortunately, many adolescents do not have access to a school clinic, either because the school does not have a clinic or because the teen mom drops out of school after she becomes pregnant.

Another venue for programs for pregnant teens and teen mothers is a medical clinic, often affiliated with a hospital. These clinics typically focus on the entire family and offer services that go beyond medical care, such as support groups, counseling, and parenting classes. Some of these programs show modest successes, reducing repeat pregnancies and increasing child immunization rates (Akinbami, Cheng, & Kornfeld, 2001).

Although rates of teen pregnancies and births have been declining in the past several years, teen parents and their children continue to be a large and vulnerable group in need of support services. Goals include less reliance on public financial assistance; continued schooling; gainful employment; a reduction in repeat pregnancies; improvement in parenting skills; and, ultimately, healthy and happy children on their way to successful lives. These are lofty goals that may not be reachable by many intervention programs, but they are the standards by which these programs should be evaluated. Recent reviews of intervention programs indicate that some of these goals are attainable for some teens enrolled in these programs. Getting teens into these programs and keeping them in remains the elusive goals of just about every pregnancy prevention and teen parenting program.

SUMMARY

■ SOME NUMBERS AND STATISTICS

Teen pregnancy is a worldwide problem. Teen pregnancy rates have been declining in the United States and around the world, mainly because teens use some form of contraception more consistently than ever before. Although teen pregnancy is found in every socioeconomic strata, it is more common among adolescents who are poor, minority, and from single-parent homes. Girls who become pregnant tend to have antisocial tendencies, low impulse control, and are likely to become members of deviant peer groups.

■ TEEN MOTHERS

Although births to teens are down, 209,480 children were born to U.S. teens in 2016. This high number includes many unintended pregnancies, but some teens have ambivalent and even positive attitudes about becoming pregnant— attitudes that are associated with an early pregnancy. Many young African American and Hispanic females find meaning and purpose in becoming a mother when other avenues to success are blocked. Many teen mothers have mothers who were themselves teen mothers, a phenomenon referred to as the intergenerational cycle of teenage motherhood. Many teen mothers are impoverished before they become teen mothers, and having a child contributes to further poverty. In addition to an impoverished background, several individual factors are related to becoming a teen mother, which include below-average school performance, conduct disorder, low self-esteem, having deviant friends, and inconsistent contraceptive use. Becoming a teen mother furthers many of these problems in addition to creating new difficulties for the young mother. This negative picture of teen motherhood is not true of every teen mother, however. Some resilient young mothers manage to beat the odds and do well in spite of being a teen mother.

■ THE CHILDREN

Children born to teen mothers are at risk for a variety of health problems, including premature birth and low birthweight. Two explanations have been offered to account for the greater risks to neonates born to teen mothers: the biological development of very young mothers is not complete, which puts a strain on the developing fetus; and many teens, even older teens, do not properly care for themselves during their pregnancy, not eating well, smoking cigarettes, drinking alcohol, and using drugs, all of which adversely affects fetal development.

Children born to teen mothers are at risk for a variety of adjustment problems and poor outcomes that extend beyond childhood into adolescence and emerging adulthood. Two frameworks have been proposed to explain the difficulties children of teen mothers have: the social influence framework, which suggests that teen mothers do a poor job raising their children, because of their young age and immature psychological development; and the social selection framework, which refers to the idea that some mothers possess characteristics that make it difficult for the mother to be a good parent, whether the mother is a teen or an adult. Not all children born to teen mothers do poorly. Some resilient children manage to thrive and do quite well. These children typically have good cognitive skills, allowing them to do well in school, and have good relations with their mothers, who are effective parents.

■ THE FATHERS

Less is known about teen fathers in comparison to teen mothers, which contributes to the impression many people have that teen fathers are uninvolved and irresponsible, a characterization true for some, but not all, teen fathers. Only a minority of teen fathers are married to or living with the mother of the child at the time of the child's birth. Teen father involvement with his child decreases as the child gets older, especially when the father does not live with the mother. Teen fathers tend to be involved with their children if they are living with the mother at the time of the birth of the child, are romantically involved with the mother, and have a good relationship with the maternal grandmother of the child. Many teen fathers will become a teen father for the second time before the father is in his mid-20s. Teen fathers frequently have fathers who were teen fathers themselves. Although teen fathers often have emotional problems and behavioral difficulties in childhood and adolescence, they can have a positive effect on their children if they can financially contribute to their family and develop a positive relationship with their children.

■ INTERVENTIONS TO IMPROVE THE LIVES OF TEEN PARENTS AND THEIR CHILDREN

Several interventions aimed at teen parents, especially the mothers, have shown positive effects on the lives of teen families. One of the most basic requirements of any successful intervention is to prevent a second pregnancy through an improvement in contraceptive use, and several programs have had a positive effect on this problem. Other interventions are designed to enrich the lives of the children by upgrading the parenting skills of the mothers. Some school-based programs focus on keeping the mothers in school in order to improve the chances of the mothers for a productive job after graduation from high school, or for additional schooling. School health clinics reach teen mothers at school and provide help in a variety of ways, including prenatal exams, contraceptive services, counseling, and parenting classes. Some medical clinics in and out of hospitals offer services specifically addressed to the problems of teen families.

Getting teens into these programs and keeping them in remains a high priority, but an elusive goal, of most teen parent intervention programs.

SUGGESTIONS FOR FURTHER READING

Beers, L. A. S., & Hollo, R. E. (2009). Approaching the adolescent-headed family: A review of teen parenting. *Current Problems in Pediatric and Adolescent Health Care, 39,* 216–233.

Boonstra, H. D. (2014, Summer). What is behind the declines in teen pregnancy rates? *Guttmacher Policy Review, 17*(3). Retrieved July 24, 2016, from *www.guttmacher.org/sites/default/files/article_files/gpr170315.pdf.*

Bunting, L., & McAuley, C. (2004). Teenage pregnancy and parenthood: The role of fathers. *Child and Family Social Work, 9*(3), 295–303.

Gibbs, C. M., Wendt, A., Peters, S., & Hogue, C. J. (2012). The impact of early age at first childbirth on maternal and infant health. *Paediatric and Perinatal Epidemiology, 26,* 259–284.

Ruedinger, E., & Cox, J. E. (2012). Adolescent childbearing: Consequences and interventions. *Current Opinion in Pediatrics, 24,* 446–452.

Sedgh, G., Finer, L. B., Bankole, A., Eilers, M. A., & Singh, S. (2015). Adolescent pregnancy, birth, and abortion rates across countries: Levels and recent trends. *Journal of Adolescent Health, 56,* 223–230.

CHAPTER 10

STIs, Condom Use, and Risky Sex

Almost 40% of sexually active female teens in the United States have an STI; Forhan et al., 2009). A comparable figure for adolescent males is not available, but there is every reason to think that the percentage of teen males with an STI is as high. These figures may be surprising to some people, especially adolescents, many of whom are not well-informed about STIs and do not realize how prevalent STIs are in their age group (Cherie & Berhane, 2012; King, Vidourek, & Singh, 2014; Samkange-Zeeb, Spallek, & Zeeb, 2011).

The young woman in the following story describes her reaction to learning that she had human papillomavirus (HPV). She also discusses her frustration about the poor quality of the sex education she received, which did not include material on STIs or contraception.

IN THEIR OWN WORDS

I lost my virginity about 5 months after I began taking birth control, and because most of my sex education had been based on pregnancy, I did not take extra precautions to avoid getting an STD. I was fortunate to not get an STD from the person I first had sexual intercourse with, but I was still very lenient with forms of contraception, other than the pill. After I became sexually active with my current boyfriend (my third partner), I became scared that he had given me an STD because he had had sex with five people before me and we almost never use condoms.

I found out about a year later that I do, in fact, have a form of HPV and I was devastated. Luckily, it is the least harmful form of HPV, but it still rocked my world. The only people who knew (until now) were my boyfriend and my mom. I am telling you this because I feel that if I had had a sex education that did not try to scare me with a pregnancy video and focused more on the likelihood of contracting an STD, I would have been better informed and might have made better decisions. I was ill informed and have suffered the consequences.

Sexually transmitted infection is a term that is replacing the term *sexually transmitted disease* (STD; Handsfield, 2015). One reason for the change is that STD suggests a medical problem with obvious symptoms, while several of the most common STIs have no signs or only mild or occasional symptoms, even though the individual is infected. Individuals with an STI without symptoms may think of themselves as disease-free, even though they have an infection that can be passed on to someone else. Similarly, a potential sexual partner may have an STI but not have any obvious symptoms.

■ SEXUALLY TRANSMITTED INFECTIONS

STIs are mainly transmitted from one individual to another through sexual contact, including vaginal, anal, or oral sex. Some people have the mistaken belief that an STI cannot be transmitted or acquired through oral sex, but it is possible. There are at least 25 different STIs, but there are eight that are significant problems among adolescents. Some are bacterial, such as chlamydia, syphilis, and gonorrhea. Others are viral, such as herpes simplex virus, type 1 (HSV-1, sometimes referred to as oral herpes); herpes simplex virus, type 2 (HSV-2, referred to as genital herpes); human papillomavirus (HPV); and HIV/AIDS. Trichomoniasis is parasitic; bacterial and parasitic STIs are curable, while viral STIs can be treated but are incurable.

Although some STIs only cause minor discomfort, others can have lasting health consequences, including complications leading to death. Trichomoniasis symptoms include itching or irritation in the genital area and burning after urination. HSV-1 and HSV-2 symptoms include intermittent sores around the genitals, rectum, or mouth. Chlamydia, syphilis, and gonorrhea can cause

---

In addition to the physical consequences of contracting an STI, there are the emotional reactions of embarrassment, shame, and guilt that accompany an infection, as the following story by a young woman illustrates.

IN THEIR OWN WORDS

That night [after having intercourse accompanied by bleeding] I went home crying because all I could think about was that I must have an STD. I was so puzzled because I was so consistent with condom use. I did not know who I got it from, considering I had sex with two other people in two other isolated incidents in that time frame. I was so ashamed. I did not call any of my friends or tell my parents. I told myself that I was not going to tell D. or J. or any other sex partners that I was worried unless I really had an STD. I felt like they would never have sex with me again and I would lose both of them. I also feared that they would tell everyone and then everyone would know they got an STD from me. I knew I had to go see a doctor for my first vaginal exam in the morning.

The results came back and all I had was a yeast infection and a UTI [urinary tract infection]. I was so relieved. It was then when I asked for birth control and began taking it regularly. Today I still use condoms and I will never forget that experience.

infertility, pelvic inflammatory disease, and increased risk of HIV infection. HPV is linked to cervical cancer. HIV/AIDS does not have one set of symptoms, but is linked to opportunistic infections that can lead to serious illness and death among infected individuals with a compromised immune system.

STIs not only cause pain and suffering for the infected individuals but are expensive for society as a whole. The 2010 estimate of the direct medical costs, including visits to doctors and medications associated with STIs, was close to $17 billion for the United States (Chesson et al., 2011), a yearly amount probably higher today.

The most common STI among individuals in the United States between the ages of 15 and 24 is HPV, with a prevalence of about 18 million infections (Satterwhite et al., 2013). About 30% of young women 15–19 years old are infected with HPV, while slightly over 50% of women 20–24 years old are infected. Two other common STIs among young people are HSV-2, with a prevalence of about 2.5 million infections, followed by chlamydia, with about one million infections. In 2014, there were about 20 million new STI infections in the United States, with nearly 50% of them acquired by individuals 15–24 years of age, a disproportionately high incidence for that age group (Centers for Disease Control and Prevention, 2015).

The World Health Organization estimates that over 300 million STIs occur each year worldwide, most in the developing world (Dehne & Riedner, 2005). The highest number of new infections are to people under the age of 25 years, with the highest incidence among emerging adults 20–24 years old, followed by teens 15–19 years old. STIs are more common among youth in Africa and the Caribbean than in other regions, primarily because more young people in those parts of the world are sexually active, and are less likely to use condoms consistently (Hokororo et al., 2015; Hughes et al., 2001).

This chapter examines the determinants of STI risk among adolescents. The focus is on risky sexual behaviors, such as having sexual intercourse at an early age; engaging in sex without a condom, especially with a casual partner; and having multiple sex partners. The chapter does not focus on the biochemistry or symptoms of STIs, or on any particular STI. This is a chapter about the behavior of adolescents related to the acquisition of an STI, and of the antecedent conditions associated with that behavior. The chapter focuses on heterosexual adolescents, although much of the research on risky sex also applies to LGBTQ youth. Research on risky LGBTQ sex is examined more fully in Chapter 8.

■ CONDOM USAGE

How Can Adolescents Prevent Contracting an STI?

Sexual abstinence and the correct and consistent use of a condom are two methods of decreasing the probability of acquiring an STI. Having a long-term sexually monogamous relationship with someone who does not have an STI is

The following story reveals what happened to one young woman who trusted her boy-friend and thought he was in a monogamous relationship with her, which turned out not to be true. The story begins after she went to see a doctor about her symptoms.

IN THEIR OWN WORDS

When my gynecologist came back to my examination room, she told me that I had been diagnosed with chlamydia. She told me this as if it was a normal occurrence and something to be taken lightly. As she wrote my prescription, I was thinking about the multiple ways in which my world was about to fall apart. My mom would find out since I was a minor at the time. She did not even know I was sexually active at this point. Also, since I had been completely faithful to A., this confirmed the fact that he was being unfaithful. I was emotionally disturbed and more embarrassed than I had ever been. I did not even know how to go about telling A. When I did, I ended our relationship right there. He said that I was being unreasonable and he had just slept with the other girl once. I told him that it only took once for him to contract an STI, give it to me, and lose all my trust in the process. (What a loser/idiot!)

another method of decreasing the probability of contracting an STI. Two problems associated with this last method are that it is impossible to know whether a person has an STI, and during adolescence, stable, long-term relationships are uncommon. Abstinence is the only method that is 100% effective in preventing STIs. Condoms are highly effectively in preventing STIs, but failures do occur (Crosby, Charnigo, Weathers, Caliendo, & Shrier, 2012). Typical condom failures are due to breakage, leakage, slipping off, reuse, late application, or early removal.

How Common Is It for Adolescents to Use Condoms When They Have Sexual Intercourse?

Adolescents are more likely to use condoms than adults, with the highest condom use rate among teens 14–17 years of age (Reece et al., 2010). Recent public health efforts to encourage the use of condoms, coupled with comprehensive sex education programs, suggest that the message about using condoms is getting through to many adolescents.

The good news is that the percentage of U.S. high school students who report they used a condom the last time they had sexual intercourse increased from about 46% in 1991 to a high of about 63% in 2003. The bad news is that between 2003 and 2015, condom use declined slightly to about 57% in 2015 (Kann, Olsen, et al., 2016). The birth control pill is the second most frequently used form of contraception among high school students, with about 21% of sexually active females reporting that they use birth control pills. About 14% of high school students indicate that they did not use any form of birth control the last time they had sexual intercourse.

A FOCUS ON RESEARCH

Rates of actual condom use may be lower than reported because of the uncertain validity of self-reports of condom use. Adolescents may report what they consider to be the "correct" answer—that they used a condom the last time they had sex when they did not. This bias is revealed in one study in which 100% of a group of African American girls ages 15–21 years old attending a health clinic reported that they used a condom the last time they had sexual intercourse, although 34% showed biological evidence of sperm in their vagina (Rose et al., 2009). It is possible that condoms were used incorrectly, but another explanation for the discrepancy is that these youth may have given socially desirable answers rather than truthful answers.

Social desirability bias is thought to be a problem in research on sexuality, although the extent of the problem is unknown. Social desirability bias is the tendency for people to give responses on questionnaires or in interviews that reflect positively on the self, instead of giving truthful answers that may reflect negatively on the self. The bias may be due to self-deception, based on a desire to validate an idealized conception of the self, or it may be due to other deception, which is an attempt to create a positive image of oneself in the minds of others. The bias takes the form of overreporting "good" behavior and underreporting "bad" behavior. Social desirability bias is a problem in many areas of research where there is an acceptable or socially correct answer, and research on sexuality is considered one of those areas, since some people may be reluctant to admit that they engage in behavior that many might consider inappropriate, wrong, or undesirable. The most common method of managing social desirability bias is to administer a social desirability scale in order to determine the extent to which a person is responding in a socially desirable manner. Unfortunately, social desirability scales are rarely used in research on adolescent sexuality, where answers are assumed to be valid.

Why Don't Adolescents Use Condoms Consistently?

The *theory of planned behavior* (TPB) provides a framework for understanding condom use (Ajzen, 2012). According to TPB, an outcome is the result of attitudes about a behavior followed by a belief that one can achieve the outcome by behaving in a certain way. This belief leads to intentions to act in a certain way, followed by a behavior that affects the outcome. According to TPB, people who have positive attitudes about condoms and believe that by using condoms they can prevent STIs are likely to intend to use a condom the next time they have sexual intercourse, leading to condom use (Albarracin, Johnson, Fishbein, & Muellerleile, 2001; Shilo & Mor, 2015). Negative attitudes about condoms are associated with weak intentions to use condoms, leading to nonuse or inconsistent use.

Two cognitions that increase condom use include worry about contracting an STI, and the belief that a condom offers protection against an STI. Adolescents who believe that the threat of infection is high, and also believe a condom will protect them, are more likely to use a condom when they have sexual intercourse than adolescents who believe that the threat is low, or that condoms are ineffective (Bermudez, Castro, & Buela-Casal, 2011).

Negative attitudes about condoms related to nonuse include beliefs that condoms are difficult to use, decrease sexual pleasure, and too expensive to buy on a regular basis (Novak & Karlsson, 2005). Other attitudes associated with the nonuse of condoms include the belief that they feel unnatural, and interfere with one's ability to have an orgasm (Brown et al., 2008). These negative attitudes are not without foundation, and they should not be ignored or devalued. Condoms do come between skin on skin, which is the price one has to pay to be safe.

One cognitive process associated with the nonuse of a condom is *delay discounting,* which is the preference for an immediate reward over waiting for a later reward (Rachlin, Raineri, & Cross, 1991). A variation of delay discounting is *sexual discounting,* which is a preference for immediate sex, even if it is risky sex, over waiting to have safer sex with a condom at some later time. The longer the delay, the less likely it is the individual will wait to use a condom, and the more likely it is the individual will have sex without a condom. Results from one study reveal that a delay as short as 1 hour to obtain a condom reduces the likelihood of waiting to have safer sex, while delays longer than an hour lead to a drastic reduction in a willingness to wait to have safer sex. This impatience is especially strong when individuals are sexually aroused (Dariotis & Johnson, 2015), or when the sexual partner is viewed as especially desirable (Collado, Johnson, Loya, Johnson, & Yi, 2017). The implication of sexual discounting is that having a condom available in one's wallet or purse might tip the scale toward using a condom, while the need to delay sex, even for a few hours, in order to obtain a condom, may lead to unprotected sex.

An additional cognitive distortion related to the nonuse of condoms is called the *optimistic bias,* which is a self-serving belief that the risk of a negative outcome to oneself is less than the risk to others. Research on Dutch adolescents and emerging adults found that the majority of inconsistent condom users thought that the risk of contracting an STI was greater for others than for themselves, primarily because they indicated they knew their partners well and were certain their partners did not have an STI, attitudes related to acquiring an STI, since it is not possible to know with certainty that another individual is STI-free (Wolfers, de Zwart, & Kok, 2011).

Are There Gender Differences in Attitudes about Condom Use?

One stereotype about condoms is that men have more negative attitudes about condom use than women, but one study of young men and women found that many women also have negative attitudes about condoms (Crosby et al., 2013). Many women, and men, report that they feel closer to their partner when they have sexual intercourse without a condom.

In the following story, one young woman describes her negative feelings about condoms and indicates that she is on the pill but does not use condoms when she has sex.

IN THEIR OWN WORDS

I hate condoms. They are sticky, annoying, expensive. . . . [I read in a book] that only half of young adults feel comfortable buying condoms. I am not in that half. To this day, I have never gone to the store to purchase any. Only half also reported being able to talk with a partner about condom use. I made my partner get tested before we started having sex and I take my birth control religiously so I have mainly avoided that discussion. Less than half of teens said they felt comfortable carrying a condom "just in case." I've never had a random encounter and I rely on my pill.

Is Condom Use Related to Communication between Sexual Partners?

One factor strongly associated with condom use among adolescents is communication between partners about condoms (Noar, Carlyle, & Cole, 2006; Widman, Noar, Choukas-Bradley, & Francis, 2014). In particular, teens who clearly indicate their desire to use a condom, or insist their partner use a condom, are more likely to actually use a condom than adolescents who do not talk to their partners about this issue or do not stand up for their rights (Schmid, Leonard, Ritchie, & Gwadz, 2015).

Conversations about sex are sensitive and can be difficult, not only for adolescents but even for adults. In one study of young adults, only 41% indicated that they had ever talked to their sexual partner about condoms, conversations that often focused on the importance of avoiding an STI or an unwanted pregnancy (Horan & Cafferty, 2017). Adolescents may have an especially difficult time talking about sexual topics with their partners, because they lack the conversational skills and the language to do so and are negotiating sexual

The following story by a college female reveals the strong position she took about using condoms, which she communicated to her boyfriend, who reluctantly went along with it.

IN THEIR OWN WORDS

After I felt ready to have sex, I made sure my boyfriend knew that he would be using a condom. I did NOT want to become pregnant, and I was also (somewhat) afraid of catching some type of disease. He was OK with this; he felt the same way.

As time went on, my boyfriend began to ask for sex without a condom more and more. He claimed it would feel better, he could pull out, and many other typical excuses for not using a condom. Every time, I said, no way. I knew that unprotected sex was a BAD idea; my boyfriend never became upset, but I think he'd just hoped to create the same experiences his buddies had (even though the same buddies had gotten their girlfriends pregnant).

issues for the first time. Whatever the reasons for the difficulty of talking about contraception, many adolescents do not discuss condoms or safe sex with their sexual partners, a silence related to a lower condom use rate (Ryan, Franzetta, Manlove, & Holcombe, 2007).

Are Relations between Parents and Adolescents Associated with Condom Use?

Adolescents who usually use a condom when they have sexual intercourse report that they have a good relationship with their parents and do not want to let their parents down by contracting an STI or experiencing a pregnancy. In contrast, adolescents who are less likely to use a condom are less satisfied with the overall quality of their relations with their parents (Deptula, Henry, & Schoeny, 2010; Dittus & Jaccard, 2000). The association between parent–adolescent relationship quality and condom use decreases as adolescents get older and peers begin to exert a stronger influence on sexual behavior. Parents do not become irrelevant, however, and even emerging adults are more likely to use a condom if they have good relations with their parents (Gillmore et al., 2011; Pingel et al., 2012).

Are Condoms More Likely to Be Used in a Short-Term or a Long-Term Relationship?

Condoms are more likely to be used with casual sexual partners than with long-term sexual partners (Ewing & Bryan, 2015; Kerr, Washburn, Morris, Lewis, & Tiberio, 2015). Once individuals enter into a monogamous relationship they may feel safer and more comfortable using other forms of contraception, even though these other forms of birth control are not as effective against STIs (Ashenhurst, Wilhite, Harden, & Fromme, 2017).

In one qualitative study, most young men endorsed the idea that a condom should be used the first time one has sexual intercourse with a new partner, or in a hookup (Raine et al., 2010). The longer a relationship continues, the less likely these young men felt a condom needed to be used as the primary form of contraception, since many men believe that the risk of contracting an STI decreases the longer a relationship lasts (Vaughan, Trussell, Kost, Singh, & Jones, 2008). In addition, according to these young men, a woman might get mad if a man insisted on using a condom in a long-term relationship, because insisting on a condom implies that the woman might have an STI or could not be trusted to remain monogamous.

One study of French adolescents and emerging adults revealed that a switch from condom use to another form of birth control frequently occurs in the early stages of a sexual relationship, often as soon as the second time the couple has intercourse (Lantos, Bajos, & Moreau, 2016). This alteration in contraceptive use indicates a shift from a concern about STI prevention to a worry about an unwanted pregnancy, even though most other forms of contraception, such as the birth control pill or the female diaphragm, do not prevent contracting an STI.

■ INDIVIDUAL INFLUENCES ON RISKY SEXUAL BEHAVIOR

In the following sections, the various factors that influence risky sexual behavior among adolescents are examined using a modification of a scheme developed by DiClemente, Salazar, Crosby, and Rosenthal (2005) at Emory University, a scheme that itself was adapted from Bronfenbrenner's (1979) ecological systems theory of social behavior. A *social-ecological perspective* on adolescent sexual behavior involves examining sexual risk-taking from various levels of influence. The first level is the individual level, which includes individual adolescent factors such as knowledge and attitudes about STIs, sexual self-concept, and psychological characteristics. The second level includes interpersonal influences, especially partners, peers, and parents. The third level is the community level, which encompasses one's neighborhood. From a social-ecological perspective, sexual behavior is embedded in an ever-widening circle of influences that begin with the individual, expand to include interpersonal relations, and extend out to neighborhood characteristics.

What Is the Relationship between Age of Sexual Debut and Contracting an STI during Adolescence?

Having sex at a young age is one of the most robust predictors of contracting an STI among adolescents (Epstein et al., 2014; Palmer et al., 2017). The odds of contracting an STI during one's lifetime are significantly greater for adolescents who first have sex before age 16 years for two reasons: they are less likely to use condoms consistently; and they have more lifetime sexual partners than late starters (Finer & Philbin, 2013; Michael, 2016; Vasilenko, Kugler, & Rice, 2016). Early starters are often poorly informed about contraceptive use and have less access to contraceptives than older teens, factors related to the nonuse, and inconsistent use, of condoms (Lee, Lee, Kim, Lee, & Park, 2015).

What Is the Relationship between Age and Sexual Risk-Taking?

Sexual risk-taking increases between early and late adolescence, peaks in late adolescence, and declines during emerging adulthood when individuals form serious romantic relationships, especially when they cohabit or marry (Moilanen, 2015; Moilanen, Crockett, Raffaelli, & Jones, 2010). Early substance use is a strong predictor of early sexual risk-taking, while continued substance use is associated with an increase in sexual risk across adolescence (Bryan, Schmiege, & Magnan, 2012).

How Informed Are Adolescents about STIs?

The United States and other industrialized countries spend the bulk of their sexuality education resources teaching adolescents about HIV/AIDS, which is rare among teens, and put fewer resources into teaching about other more common STIs, about which adolescents know little. The typical high school student in the United States is poorly informed about STIs other than HIV/AIDS (Clark, Jackson, & Allen-Taylor, 2002; Nsuami, Sanders, & Taylor, 2010). Ignorance about STIs is not confined to U.S. teens, and adolescents in many countries, such as Africa, Italy, and Iran, are also poorly informed about the characteristics of many STIs other than HIV/AIDS (Amu & Adegun, 2015; Pelucchi et al., 2010; Rahimi-Naghani et al., 2016).

One study of African American girls in Atlanta, Georgia, revealed the extent of ignorance about STIs (Voisin, Tan, Salazar, Crosby, & DiClemente, 2012). Slightly more than one-third of the girls did not know that females are more susceptible to sexually transmitted infections than males, or that having an STI increases the risk of contracting HIV. Almost half of the girls did not know that most men with an STI do not have any observable symptoms. Knowing about the characteristics of STIs and how they are transmitted does not automatically lead to a reduction in risky sexual behavior, but knowledge is the first step in changing behavior and preventing disease.

Knowledge about STIs varies by gender and personal experience. Females and older adolescents know more about STIs than males and younger adolescents. Adolescents learn about STIs and contraception mainly in school, followed by parents and friends (Jones, Biddlecom, Hebert, & Mellor, 2011). Personal experience with an STI is another route by which adolescents learn about STIs. Results from one U.S. survey of sexually active 14- to 18-year-old girls found that most of these teens acquired what knowledge they had about chlamydia, gonorrhea, and syphilis only after they were infected (Downs, Bruine de Bruin, Murray, & Fischhoff, 2006).

What Are Some Attitudes and Beliefs That Lead Adolescents to Engage in Risky Sexual Behavior?

Many adolescents have the mistaken belief that they are not at risk for an STI when, in fact, they are. The majority of girls in one study perceived themselves to be at little or no risk for an STI despite their reckless background that included sex at a young age, sex with multiple partners, and unprotected sex (Ethier, Kershaw, Niccolai, Lewis, & Ickovics, 2003). Clearly, there is a mismatch between perception and reality, a cognitive distortion that can easily lead to risky sex and an infection. There are several possible explanations for this distortion. Many adolescents believe that their sexual partners are not likely to have an STI, which leads to unprotected intercourse (Wolfers et al., 2011). In addition, some adolescents feel invulnerable, believing they are immune from the negative consequences of risky sexual behavior that affects others but not themselves.

In the following story, one young woman describes her feeling of invulnerability, which led her to engage in risky sex without a condom.

IN THEIR OWN WORDS

In my less educated days (bogus excuse, I know) I was more likely to not use a condom. I was in one relationship where we rarely used condoms after we had been together a while. I am and was on birth control, which was obviously being used as a preventative measure to pregnancy. However, I was not worried about STIs since I thought *It can't happen to me.*

The invulnerability illusion is the cloud I was under when considering using a condom and deciding against it. I have never had an STI, but I now realize that I am very lucky, considering my thoughtless experiences. You could trust someone with all that you have, but they may not have told you about an STI that they have had.

Whatever the explanation, many adolescents think they are safe when they are not, a cognitive distortion that can have dire consequences on their health.

Another explanation for the high rate of adolescent risky sex, and risky behavior in general, is that adolescents tend to focus on the possible positive results of their behavior and de-emphasize potential negative consequences—a way of thinking rooted in the functioning of the teen brain (Defoe, Dubas, Figner, & van Aken, 2015). Data from functional magnetic resonance imaging (fMRI) brain scans reveal that adolescent risk-taking has a biological basis to it. Adolescents who engage in risky behavior show more activity in brain systems associated with rewards, including the ventral striatum, than in areas of the brain implicated in cognitive control, especially the prefrontal cortex (Chein, Albert, O'Brien, Uckert, & Steinberg, 2011). Thus, adolescents who engage in risky sex focus on the rewards of sex, which they expect to receive, and minimize the probability they will experience any potential costs, which they do not expect to experience.

What Is the Relationship between Adolescent Self-Concept and Risky Sexual Behavior?

Self-concept includes the attitudes, beliefs, and cognitions a person has about him- or herself. One's self-concept has an influence on one's sexual behavior. For example, if being in a relationship with a boy is an important component of a girl's self-concept, she will engage in riskier sexual behaviors, including having unprotected sex, anal sex, and sex when her partner is high on alcohol or drugs, than a girl who is less invested in the need to be in a relationship (Raiford, Seth, & DiClemente, 2013). In one study of African American girls, refusing unprotected sex was related to having a positive self-concept, which includes high self-esteem, strong ethnic identity, and a good body image (Salazar et al., 2004). A girl with these qualities is more likely to demand that her partner use a condom, and refuse to have sex if he does not.

Sexual self-concept is defined as how an individual perceives his or her own sexual qualities (Hensel, Fortenberry, O'Sullivan, & Orr, 2011). Sexual self-concept is a domain-specific aspect of the self that includes factors such as sexual interest, sexual desire, and sexual self-efficacy, which is the ability to assert your sexual needs.

One aspect of a sexual self-concept especially important for effective contraceptive use is accepting oneself as someone with sexual interests and desires. In one longitudinal study, it was found that adolescent females who accept their own sexual desires communicate more often with their sexual partners about sex and consistently use effective forms of contraception (Tschann & Adler, 1997). In contrast, young women who do not accept their own interest in sex are inconsistent contraceptive users, and are hesitant to bring up the topic of contraception with their partner, perhaps because they fear they would appear to be promiscuous or sexually assertive if they talk about sex and contraception.

Another way one's sexual self-concept is related to engaging in risky sex is by defining oneself as a person unlikely to contract an STI. There is a stigma attached to people who have an STI that is not attached to individuals with other types of infections, such as the flu (Newton & McCabe, 2008). Because STIs are transmitted through sexual contact, people who have an STI, especially infected females, are often perceived as sexually reckless and promiscuous (Nack, 2000). Most women do not perceive themselves as possessing these undesirable characteristics—a perception of the self leading to the belief that they are not at risk for contracting an STI. In one study, young women who did not view themselves as the type of woman who could contract an STI were more likely to engage in unsafe sex than women who thought they could contract an STI (East, Jackson, Peters, & O'Brien, 2010).

What Is the Relationship between Sensation-Seeking and Risky Sexual Behavior?

Sensation-seeking is a personality trait with a biological basis defined by a desire for experiences and emotions that are novel, exciting, and intense (Zuckerman, 1994). Sensation seekers are people willing to take risks in order to have thrilling experiences. High sensation seekers are willing to engage in risky sexual behavior, such as having unprotected sex, having sex with many partners, and having sex under the influence of alcohol or drugs (Charnigo, Garnett, Crosby, Palmgreen, & Zimmerman, 2013).

Not only is sensation-seeking related to risky sex, but more specifically, *sexual sensation-seeking* (SSS) is related to risky sexual behavior. SSS is a desire for sexually novel and exciting experiences. Girls who are high in SSS are likely to engage in risky sexual behavior, such as having casual sex with someone the girl does not know very well (Spitalnick et al., 2007; Voisin, Tan, & DiClemente, 2013).

The findings on SSS suggest a troubling possibility that risky sex is exciting to some adolescents precisely because it is somewhat dangerous. For adolescents high in SSS, making an impulsive decision to hook up with someone adds to the excitement of the sexual experience and gives it a charge that safer sex lacks. If this is true, then it should not be surprising that admonitions to practice safer sex fall on deaf ears of some adolescents, who do not want to eliminate sexual risk but who relish it.

What Is the Relationship between Depression and Risky Sexual Behavior?

Symptoms of depression, such as feeling hopeless and sad, are predictors of risky sex (Elkington, Bauermeister, & Zimmerman, 2010; Seth et al., 2011; Seth, Raiji, DiClemente, Wingood, & Rose, 2009). Negative thoughts and cognitive distortions associated with depression can interfere with rational decision making, leading to poor decisions and risky behavior, including unsafe sexual behavior.

The connection between symptoms of depression and risky sex is especially strong among adolescent females (Brawner, Gomes, Jemmott, Deatrick, & Coleman, 2012). Depression can be an outcome of risky sex, but it can also lead to a sexual situation in which a female who is coping with feelings of sadness and hopelessness may acquiesce to noncondom use and undesired sexual activity because the girl is worried that she may lose a romantic partner if she insists that he use a condom. A quest for emotional comfort and self-validation may lead to a risky sexual encounter that goes against a girl's better judgment but which feels right at the time. As one adolescent girl reported, " . . . it's like you wanna give your feelings up to somebody, you just don't know who to give 'em to so you'll just do anything that'll make your feeling more better . . . you'll try anything" (Brawner et al., 2012, p. 623).

Depressed adolescent females are not alone in their willingness to engage in risky sex, as illustrated by the findings from one study of Spanish secondary school students (Ramiro, Teva, Bermúdez, & Buela-Casal, 2013). Depressed boys more than nondepressed boys are also likely to engage in risky sex as a means of validating their self-worth through casual sex and sexual conquest.

Other research indicates that risky sexual behavior in adolescence is associated with adolescent depression brought on by physical abuse in childhood for boys, and sexual abuse for girls (Braje, Eddy, & Hall, 2016). The authors suggest that some adolescents who are victims of childhood abuse may develop a live-for-the-moment outlook and engage in risky sex to temporarily relieve feelings of sadness and isolation.

What Is the Relationship between Substance Use and Risky Sexual Behavior?

Substance use—including using cigarettes, alcohol, marijuana, and cocaine—is linked to having multiple sexual partners and inconsistent condom use, increasing the risk for an STI among adolescents (Merianos, Rosen, King, Vidourek, & Fehr, 2015; Ritchwood, Ford, DeCoster, Sutton, & Lochman, 2015; Rossi,

The following story illustrates the dangerous effect alcohol intoxication can have on sexual behavior. Note that getting drunk and having sex with a casual acquaintance is a theme in this girl's life.

IN THEIR OWN WORDS

Another factor in my unsafe sex decisions has been alcohol. Every time I have failed to use a condom I have been highly intoxicated. Some instances I was even blacked out and barely remembered having sex. It's pretty embarrassing to admit that I could be that dumb, but it still happened. And I'm not on the pill, so not only were STIs a huge concern but pregnancy could have happened as well. Compounding this already incredibly risky situation is the fact that most of the guys I was with were complete strangers. I knew absolutely nothing about them or their sexual histories. My one saving grace is that I have made sure to get tested after every risky encounter and thankfully have contracted no STIs.

The most recent incident happened a few months ago. I met a guy at a bar, got very drunk, and went home with him. We had sex and I remember telling him he couldn't come in me. After, I remember his saying something about he didn't want to have babies and I agreed but didn't think much about why be brought that up. I was actually so drunk I ended up puking before I left his house and actually didn't even remember where his house was. When I woke up the next morning, I had flashbacks from the night before and finally put together that he had came in me. I panicked and took some of my friend's birth control pills instead of buying Plan B and immediately made a doctor's appointment. My friends have made the same mistake and we end up laughing about it later and sharing our stories, but at the same time I realize how serious the situation could have been.

Poulin, & Boislard, 2017). Occasionally drinking alcohol and experimental marijuana use are not associated with risky sexual behavior, but heavy episodic drinking and frequent marijuana use are (Vasilenko, Kugler, Butera, & Lanza, 2015).

Substance use predicts risky sex and is not just correlated with it (Scott-Sheldon, Carey, Cunningham, Johnson, & Carey, 2016). Alcohol and drug use can have an influence on STI risk during adolescence and emerging adulthood in several ways (Khan, Berger, Wells, & Cleland, 2012). Substance use impairs good judgment, which can lead to risky sexual behavior. Further, substance use is related to higher levels of sexual arousal, which may make people less cautious about their sexual behavior. Last, substance use may lead to membership in a deviant peer group in which unprotected sexual behavior is normative.

■ INTERPERSONAL INFLUENCES ON RISKY SEXUAL BEHAVIOR

Do Sexual Partners Have an Effect on Adolescent Risky Sexual Behavior?

A long-term sexual partnership between adolescents who are monogamous and not infected with an STI protects against the acquisition of an STI, but such partnerships are rare among adolescents. Adolescents who have many short-term sexual relationships are at risk for contracting an STI or spreading an STI if they are already infected (Ott, Katschke, Tu, & Fortenberry, 2011). Further, among late teens and emerging adults, overlapping sexual partners is common, especially at the end of one relationship and the start of another, a pattern associated with an increased risk of contracting or spreading an STI (Foxman, Newman, Percha, Holmes, & Aral, 2006; Kelley, Borawski, Flocke, & Keen, 2003).

One relationship factor related to risky sex is the age difference between the two partners. Males who are 2 or more years older than their female adolescent partners are less likely to use a condom when they have intercourse than males who are less than 2 years older than their partners (Chirinda & Peltzer, 2014; DiClemente et al., 2002). One possible explanation for this association is that males who are much older than their female partners have more relationship power than younger females who fear that their older male partners may react negatively if they bring up the topic of condom use (Morrison-Beedy et al., 2013). This social power imbalance may result in a lack of condom use among males who do not want to use a condom, and who have partners who do not insist they must. Interventions designed to increase condom use among adolescents should address the interpersonal power difference between males and females, and help females learn how they can negotiate this difference and demand that their partner use a condom.

Another explanation for the riskier sexual behavior of romantically involved adolescents with a large gap in their ages is that adolescents who date older partners engage in an overall riskier lifestyle, and this is especially true for younger girls who date older boys (Oudekerk, Guarnera, et al., 2014). The larger the gap in ages between the two individuals who are sexually involved, the more likely it is that the youth engage in substance use and delinquency. One possibility is that younger females might date deviant older males because the risky lifestyle of the older males makes them seem "cool" to some younger females who are then drawn into a deviant lifestyle that includes early sex and unprotected intercourse (Morrison-Beedy et al., 2013).

What Effect Do Peers Have on Adolescent Risky Sexual Behavior?

Peer norms are strongly related to adolescent sexual behavior, including condom use and risky sex (Ajilore, 2015; Buhi & Goodson, 2007). Both peer selection and peer socialization often operate in a reciprocal manner; adolescents select friends who hold sexual values and norms similar to their own, and those friends in turn have an influence on adolescent sexual behavior.

Both peer selection and peer socialization were found in one longitudinal study of the relation between the risky sexual behavior of peers and adolescent risky sex. Adolescents who engage in risky sex choose friends who also participate in these risky behaviors, demonstrating peer selection. In turn, the risky sexual behavior of friends predicts the further involvement of adolescents in risky sex, including inconsistent condom use, demonstrating peer socialization (Voisin, Hotton, Tan, & DiClemente, 2013).

Another study illustrates the operation of both negative and positive peer selection and peer socialization (Henry et al., 2007). Adolescents in this study selected friends who shared attitudes about sex similar to their own, confirming the idea of peer selection. When those attitudes supported risky sex, there was an increase in the probability of an unintended pregnancy or an STI diagnosis during emerging adulthood, confirming peer socialization (Henry, Deptula, & Schoeny, 2012). When those attitudes supported sexual caution, adolescents were more likely to use some form of contraception and had lower rates of unintended pregnancies and STI diagnoses in emerging adulthood. One implication for intervention that follows from all these studies is that adolescents need to understand that the sexual attitudes and behavior of friends can have an effect on their own sexual behavior, so it is important to have sexually responsible friends and to avoid sexually irresponsible peers.

Results from one study examined one mechanism by which peer socialization might operate—talk. Latino adolescents who used condoms talked to their friends about contraception and STIs, and had friends who used condoms (Kapadia et al., 2012). Condom-supporting talk gets translated into condom use, and adolescents who believe in the importance of practicing safer sex actively encourage and support one another to be sexually responsible.

Sexting is another peer behavior associated with risky sexual activity. Adolescents who sext are more likely to engage in risky sex, including having sex without a condom, than adolescents who do not sext (Rice et al., 2012). LGBTQ adolescents who sext are especially likely to engage in unsafe sex. Sexting itself does not pose a risk for the transmission of STIs, but sexting may be a warning sign of other risky sexual behaviors.

Do Parents Matter?

Parents and Peers

Given the strong relationship between what peers think and do and what adolescents think and do, can parents have any influence on adolescent risky sex? The short answer is Yes, they can. One way parents matter is that relationships with parents set the stage for peer influence, leading to a greater or lesser effect of peers on adolescent sexuality. Poor relationships with parents are associated with greater susceptibility to the pressures and norms of peers. More specifically, the more parents use *psychological control* with their adolescents, the more likely it is that the teens will associate with peers who have sex at an early age and will, themselves, have sex at an early age (Oudekerk, Allen, et al., 2014). Psychological control is when parents use guilt, anxiety, shame, and love withdrawal to obtain compliance to parental wishes. When parents are low in psychological control, adolescents are not as likely to engage in risky sex, even when their peers have risky sex.

Parents may also buffer the effect of negative peer influences on risky adolescent sex by providing a supportive home environment that can reinforce positive sexual attitudes and behavior, counteracting undesirable peer influence.

Consistent condom use is highest when adolescents have positive relations with parents and are friends with responsible peers, and lowest when teens have poor relations with parents and have friends who engage in risky sex (Elkington, Bauermeister, & Zimmerman, 2011; Saftner, Martyn, & Lori, 2011).

Parent Monitoring

One aspect of parenting that discourages adolescent risky sex is effective *parent monitoring*. When adolescents think their parents are not well-informed about where they are, who they are with, and what they are doing, teens are more likely to engage in risky sex, such as having sex at an early age, and having multiple sex partners (DiClemente et al., 2001). These results have been replicated in studies of parents and teens around the world, including Indonesia (Suwarni, Ismail, Prabandari, & Adiyanti, 2015), the Bahamas (Wang, Stanton, Deveaux, Li, & Lunn, 2015), the Netherlands (de Graaf et al., 2010), and Scotland (Wight, Williamson, & Henderson, 2006), revealing a robust, cross-cultural consistency between monitoring and adolescent sexual behavior. Further, effective monitoring in early adolescence is a predictor of safer sex in later adolescence, demonstrating a possible causal relationship between monitoring and adolescent sexual behavior (Crosby, DiClemente, Wingood, Lang, & Harrington, 2003). Monitoring consistently emerges as one of the most important parenting techniques parents can employ to deter adolescent dangerous and unhealthy behavior, including risky sex (de Graaf, Vanwesenbeeck et al., 2011).

Monitoring is a deterrent to risky sex even for adolescents who live in dangerous environments with a high level of community violence (Voisin, Tan, Tack, Wade, & DiClemente, 2012). The pathway from community violence to risky sex often passes through gang membership and participation in peer groups with deviant peer norms. To the extent that parents can influence friendship choice and adolescent time use, which are difficult but not impossible tasks for parents living in dangerous environments, parents can inhibit the emergence of risky sexual behavior by steering adolescents away from negative influences.

■ NEIGHBORHOOD EFFECTS ON RISKY SEXUAL BEHAVIOR

Microinfluences are the effects individual and interpersonal factors have on adolescents. There are other larger, background influences on adolescent behavior that also have a powerful effect on adolescent sexuality. These background influences are referred to as *macroinfluences,* which are influences exogenous to individuals and include the physical, social, and economic features of the environment in which adolescents live. One of the most important macroinfluences on adolescent risky sexual behavior is the neighborhood in which an adolescent resides.

What Effect Do Neighborhoods Have on Adolescent Sexual Behavior?

Adolescents and emerging adults living in disadvantaged neighborhoods have a higher rate of risky sexual behavior than youth in more advantaged neighborhoods (Warner, 2018). Youth living in impoverished neighborhoods are more likely to be sexually active, have an earlier sexual debut, and have many more sexual partners than youth in neighborhoods with less poverty (Browning, Burrington, Leventhal, & Brooks-Gunn, 2008; Cubbin, Brindis, Jain, Santelli, & Braveman, 2010; Warner, Giordano, Manning, & Longmore, 2011). Several studies of adolescents and emerging adults in the United States and South Africa find that neighborhood disadvantage is also associated with inconsistent condom use (Burgard & Lee-Rife, 2009; Oman et al., 2013) and with contracting an STI (Wickrama, Merten, & Wickrama, 2012). Although the relationship between neighborhood disadvantage and risky adolescent sexual behavior is not always present (e.g., Bauermeister, Zimmerman, & Caldwell, 2011), the results from most studies show that risky sexual behavior is high among adolescents living in disadvantaged neighborhoods. These descriptive findings leave unanswered an important explanatory question: Why are youth from impoverished neighborhoods more likely to engage in risky sexual behavior than adolescents who do not live in socioeconomically disadvantaged neighborhoods?

Social disorganization theory is an attempt to account for the association between disadvantaged neighborhoods and poor health, including risky sexual behavior (Kawachi & Berkman, 2003). According to social disorganization theory, neighborhood structural features such as poverty, unemployment, a high crime rate, many single-parent households, and residential instability often cluster together and lead to neighborhood social disorganization. These disadvantages have a negative effect on adolescent health because they produce weak social ties among neighbors who are not highly involved with one another; limit exposure to positive role models; increase exposure to negative role models; increase contact with deviant peers; and undercut conventional social norms, including norms regarding sexual behavior and childbearing. As a result of social disorganization and isolation from mainstream values, adolescents living in disadvantaged neighborhoods are more likely to manifest higher rates of problem behaviors, including risky sexual behavior, than youth in more advantaged neighborhoods.

How Do Disadvantaged Neighborhoods Influence Teen Sexual Behavior?

What precisely is the disadvantage of being disadvantaged? One answer to this question focuses on the problems associated with single-parent families. Risky sexual behavior is high among adolescents who live in neighborhoods with a high proportion of single-parent families, and risky sexual behavior is even higher if the adolescent also lives in a single-parent family (Cleveland & Gilson,

2004). There are at least three ways in which a high proportion of single-parent families in a neighborhood could lead to risky sexual behavior, especially among boys. First, a high proportion of single-parent families reduces the number of adults in the neighborhood who can monitor the behavior of adolescents and deter deviant behavior of every kind. Nothing discourages adolescent unacceptable behavior so much as the presence of watchful, responsible adults, so in neighborhoods where there are few adults present, adolescent deviant behavior is high. Second, because of the high demands of work and family life, single parents have less time to contribute to the general social welfare of their neighborhood. Single parents are not well integrated into their neighborhood, so they are not likely to talk to neighbors about the behavior of their own adolescents or attempt to deter the deviant behavior of their neighbors' adolescents. Third, a high proportion of single-parent families reduces the number of mainstream adult role models, especially male role models, available to adolescents, since most single-parent households are female headed. With few positive male role models in the neighborhood, boys are more likely to develop a macho, hypermasculinity that includes risky sexual behavior.

Another problem associated with disadvantaged neighborhoods is that adolescents are at risk for being drawn into the exciting world of deviant peer groups. In these groups, peer norms associated with risky behavior exert a powerful influence on the behavior of adolescents. In disadvantaged neighborhoods, peers can become a second family to adolescents, even more influential than the adolescent's biological family, which leads to the unfortunate situation of adolescents raising one another, with other adolescents as the primary models of how to behave (Upchurch et al., 1999).

In addition, youth living in neighborhoods with a high concentration of impoverished families do not have many opportunities for future achievement. Poverty encourages grabbing immediate pleasure over waiting for a better future that may never appear (Crandall, Magnusson, Novilla, Novilla, & Dyer, 2017). Disadvantaged neighborhoods do not provide adolescents with reasons for responsible sexual behavior in the form of the promise of future opportunities, the motivation to delay gratification, or a normative system to guide responsible sexual behavior (Billy, Brewster, & Grady, 1994).

Another effect on adolescent sexuality that can be attributed to living in a disadvantaged neighborhood is the high risk of having sex with someone who already has an STI. STIs are found in every neighborhood, but they tend to cluster in certain neighborhoods (Jennings et al., 2010). Adolescents are more likely to have a sexual relationship with someone from the same neighborhood where they live than with someone from another neighborhood. If a neighborhood has a high number of individuals who have an STI, then adolescents from that neighborhood have a high risk of having a sexual relationship with someone who is already infected.

Last, disadvantaged neighborhoods have high rates of incarceration, which leads to the removal of many young males from the community, producing a low male-to-female sex ratio (Thomas & Sampson, 2005). Under these conditions

The following story is not about living in a disadvantaged neighborhood, but life in a small town has some of the same characteristics as life in a disadvantaged neighborhood. When one of the adolescents is diagnosed with an STI, the results reverberate throughout the entire group of teens.

IN THEIR OWN WORDS

Living in a small town, there were a limited amount of "eligible boys" to choose from. This issue resulted in a lot of partner swapping and at very high rates. I became part of a large delinquent peer group that actually spanned the county I lived in. Members of this group hung out on the weekends at various house parties. In addition to drinking and drug use, a lot of sex went on at these gatherings. Among the group, there was a lot of male infidelity within these romantic relationships. Instead of teaching us we were choosing bad partners, the behavior fueled a major competition among the girls to see who could "win" their man back. Unsurprisingly, the guys took advantage of this and basically slept with whoever would let them, knowing that their girlfriend(s) would take them back in order to get even.

There was obviously a high amount of emotion involved in these behaviors and a lot of people were psychologically harmed. In addition to the mental pain it caused all of us, one of the males informed us all that he had been diagnosed with chlamydia.

The news was a shock to all of us. Not only was this news a shock, but seeking treatment was a whole other bag of worms. Fortunately, the city we lived in had a Planned Parenthood that was open once a week for a very limited number of hours. Obviously, we didn't want our parents to know about the predicament we had gotten ourselves into so we all opted to go this free/secretive route. But remember, all of the parties involved basically hated each other! Let me just say that sitting knee-to-knee in a waiting room with 20 of my worst enemies was not a comfortable situation, especially when we were all there for the same reason. After most people checked in, the office workers made the connection and decided to give us all an antibiotic rather than individually testing all of us. Even though I'll never know if I actually contracted chlamydia, the lengthy process and embarrassment I had to go through was enough of a wake-up call for me. We were all very lucky that it was a curable infection and not something that would follow us for the rest of our lives.

of male scarcity, many urban adolescent females living in disadvantaged neighborhoods report that there are few ideal sex partners in their neighborhood, which leads to a reluctant acceptance of male infidelity (Matson, Chung, & Ellen, 2014). Females in these neighborhoods often find themselves sexually involved with nonmonogamous males, a situation related to the acquisition of and spread of STIs, especially in neighborhoods with a high prevalence of STIs.

Can Parents Counteract the Effects of Disadvantaged Neighborhoods?

Parents are not powerless to influence their adolescents in a positive direction, even in the face of seemingly insurmountable obstacles found in impoverished crime-ridden neighborhoods. The idea that parents can counteract the negative effect of disadvantaged neighborhoods is called the *family compensatory effects model*. Researchers in one study examined the association between parenting and adolescent risky sexual behavior among black adolescents living in disadvantaged neighborhoods in South Africa (Goodrum, Armistead, Tully, Cook, & Skinner, 2017). Results indicate that even in unsafe, dangerous neighborhoods, risky sexual behavior is low when parents engage in positive parenting, consisting of emotional support and high monitoring. A positive parent–adolescent relationship combined with effective monitoring can offset the negative effects of high-risk neighborhoods.

Another study based on the family compensatory effects model investigated adolescent sexual behavior and its relationship to parent monitoring and family routines, which included eating together, doing homework, and going to bed at a certain time. The adolescents resided in neighborhoods with problems such as drugs, gangs, burglaries, abandoned houses, and unsupervised children (Roche & Leventhal, 2009). Results are consistent with the family compensatory effects model. Adolescents who live in disadvantaged neighborhoods are less likely to become sexually active if they think their parents know where they are when they are away from home, and when the teens participate in many family routines. High parent monitoring deters youth from associating with peers who are engaged in deviant activities, such as early sexual activity, drug and alcohol use, and delinquent behavior. In addition, family routines provide adolescents with predictable schedules in contrast to the unpredictable environments of adolescents living in chaotic families. Parents may not be able to completely shield their adolescents from the dangers present in disadvantaged and disordered neighborhoods, but they can act as a buffer between exposure to unhealthy behaviors and participation in those behaviors.

SUMMARY

■ SEXUALLY TRANSMITTED INFECTIONS

STIs are mainly passed from one individual to another through sexual contact, including vaginal, anal, and oral sex. The most common STIs among U.S. adolescents are HPV, HSV-2, and chlamydia. Worldwide, the highest number of new infections each year are to emerging adults and teens. In addition to the pain and suffering associated with an STI, sexually transmitted infections come with a high price tag of over $17 billion dollars a year in the United States.

■ CONDOM USAGE

About three out of five adolescents report that they consistently use a condom when they engage in sexual intercourse. According to the theory of planned behavior, condom use is the outcome of having positive attitudes about condoms, believing that condoms can prevent STIs and pregnancy, and intending to use a condom. Two cognitive processes associated with the nonuse of a condom are delay discounting and the optimistic bias. Several beliefs are related to not using a condom, such as that they decrease sexual pleasure, are too expensive to buy, and interfere with one's ability to enjoy the sexual experience. Adolescents who have a positive relationship with their parents are more likely to use a condom when they have intercourse than teens who have a negative relationship with their parents.

■ INDIVIDUAL INFLUENCES ON RISKY SEXUAL BEHAVIOR

An early sexual debut is one of the best predictors of contracting an STI. Having sex at an early age is a risky sexual behavior associated with other risky sexual behaviors such as inconsistent condom use and having multiple partners.

Many adolescents are uninformed about STIs, a situation related to the attitude that they are not at risk for an STI, when in fact they are, because of their risky sexual activity. There are several aspects of one's psychological makeup that are associated with risky sexual behavior, including focusing on possible positive outcomes and de-emphasizing potential negative outcomes. Further, risky sexual behavior is associated with one's self-concept, sexual self-concept, the trait of sensation-seeking, especially sexual sensation-seeking, depression, and substance use.

■ INTERPERSONAL INFLUENCES ON RISKY SEXUAL BEHAVIOR

Sexual partners, peers, and parents have an influence on the risky sexual behavior of adolescents. Adolescents are less likely to use a condom if there is a large age difference between the two individuals in a sexual relationship.

Both peer selection and peer socialization are associated with adolescent risky sexual behavior. Adolescents choose friends who have attitudes about risky sex and condom use that are similar to their own, and those friends have an influence on later sexual behavior. Membership in a deviant peer group is related to the acquisition of an STI.

What parents do can have a powerful influence on risky adolescent sexual behavior. Parents who use psychological control are more likely to have adolescents who have sex at an early age than parents who do not use psychological control. In contrast, parental monitoring curbs risky adolescent sexual behavior.

■ NEIGHBORHOOD EFFECTS ON RISKY SEXUAL BEHAVIOR

The neighborhood in which an adolescent lives has an influence on adolescent risky sexual behavior. According to social disorganization theory, negative neighborhood characteristics can lead to risky adolescent sexual behavior. One problem associated with disadvantaged neighborhoods is the presence of many single-parent households. In addition, teens in disadvantaged neighborhoods are exposed to deviant peer groups, which encourage risky sexual behavior. Further, neighborhood disadvantage may shape norms about sexual activity that lead to valuing immediate pleasure over restraint. Another problem associated with living in a disadvantaged neighborhood is that disadvantaged neighborhoods have a high concentration of individuals with an STI, increasing the odds of acquiring an STI. It is difficult to be an effective parent in a dangerous neighborhood, but parents are not powerless to compensate for some of the disadvantages, especially by being good monitors.

SUGGESTIONS FOR FURTHER READING

Albarracin, D., Johnson, B. T., Fishbein, M., & Muellerleile, P. A. (2001). Theories of reasoned action and planned behavior as models of condom use: A meta-analysis. *Psychological Bulletin, 127,* 142–161.

de Graaf, H., Vanwesenbeeck, I., Woertman, L., & Meeus, W. (2011). Parenting and adolescents' sexual development in Western societies: A literature review. *European Psychologist, 16,* 21–31.

Deptula, D. P., Henry, D. B., & Schoeny, M. E. (2010). How can parents make a difference?: Longitudinal associations with adolescent sexual behavior. *Journal of Family Psychology, 24,* 731–739.

Noar, S. M., Carlyle, K., & Cole, C. (2006). Why communication is crucial: Meta-analysis of the relationship between safer sexual communication and condom use. *Journal of Health Communication, 11,* 365–390.

Roche, K. M., & Leventhal, T. (2009). Beyond neighborhood poverty: Family management, neighborhood disorder, and adolescents' early sexual onset. *Journal of Family Psychology, 23,* 819–827.

CHAPTER 11

Teaching Sex
in and out of School

Are schools an appropriate place to teach children and adolescents about sex? If they are, what should be taught? Are there some topics that should not be covered? Does sex education work? These are some of the questions examined in this chapter.

In the United States and in most of the developed world, school-based sex education is the most common intervention employed to instruct children and adolescents about the mysteries of sex (Ponzetti, 2016). School-based sex education remains rare in some parts of the world, such as in the Middle East, where Muslim traditions regard sexual information as dangerous knowledge that can lead to sexual experimentation (Tabatabaie, 2015). Even in the United States, a large percentage of adolescents do not receive any school-based instruction in sex education.

There has been a significant decrease in the percentage of U.S. adolescents who receive formal school-based sex education over the past few years (Lindberg, Maddow-Zimet, & Boonstra, 2016). The decline is especially great for adolescents living in rural areas. The overall decrease in sex education instruction is part of a long-term trend that extends back to at least 1995, when 81% of adolescent males and 87% of adolescent females reported receiving some sex education in school, percentages that have fallen to 55% of males and 60% of females by 2011–2013.

It is not clear what impact, if any, this decrease in sex education may have on teen pregnancy rates in the United States, which have been falling at the same time access to sex education has been declining. One British study found no evidence that cuts in government spending for teen pregnancy prevention programs are associated with an increase in teen pregnancies (Paton & Wright, 2017). These findings need to be interpreted cautiously, however—the authors suggest ineffective programs may be the first programs cut, but the findings do indicate that the relationship between access to sex education programs and pregnancy rates is not straightforward.

Although school-based sex education is the typical intervention designed to have an impact on adolescent sexual behavior, it is not the only attempt to influence adolescent sexuality. Virginity pledges, parent education programs, peer-led sex education classes, media interventions, and school-based health clinics (SBHCs) are other attempts designed to have an impact on adolescent sexuality. This chapter examines those interventions, mainly focusing on school-based sex education. The basic question is What works? The chapter begins with a brief history of sex education in the United States in an attempt to better understand contemporary approaches to sex education and the controversies surrounding those approaches.

■ THE HISTORY OF SEX EDUCATION IN THE UNITED STATES

The movement for sex education in U.S. public schools began in the second decade of the 20th century in response to the double-edged social problems of prostitution and venereal disease (Luker, 2007). Prostitution was viewed as a public nuisance, a failure of personal morality, and the main conduit for the spread of venereal disease. Most importantly, prostitution and sex outside marriage were seen as threats to the sanctity of marriage and the family. Social reformers argued that something needed to be done on a national scale to combat these assaults on public health and private morality. As a consequence of what was perceived as a national crisis, a group of social activists met in New York City in the early 1900s to mount a response to these problems out of which emerged the social hygiene movement, with school-based sex education as its central component.

Sex education was viewed optimistically as a cure for sexual ignorance, thought to be the root cause of public and private problems related to sexuality. Social reformers believed that an antidote to the problems of prostitution and venereal disease was accurate sexual knowledge delivered to young people by trusted experts (Carter, 2001). Those who opposed sex education at the time feared that sex education would open the door to sexual behavior and encourage sexual experimentation. This belief in the transformative power of sexual knowledge to influence sexual behavior continues to be the cornerstone of contemporary sex education, and remains a concern for many who worry that knowledge about sex will lead to sexual activity among the young.

An emphasis on the acquisition of sexual knowledge was coupled with the main message of most sex education courses, which was to "Just say no" to premarital sex. The primary aim of much of sex education in the United States was, and continues to be, to deter young people from having sex until they marry (Moran, 2000). Early sex educators viewed sex as primarily procreative and the foundation of the family. Sex was seen as healthy and wholesome when it occurs in marriage, and debased outside of marriage.

The history of sex education is the story of the various attempts by sex educators to dissuade adolescents from having sex outside of marriage, initially by emphasizing the importance of preventing disease, later by stressing the need to avoid an unintended pregnancy, and more recently by schooling students on the dangers of STIs, especially HIV/AIDS. More recent still is the ascension of the abstinence movement with its emphasis on sex within marriage as the only circumstance in which sex is appropriate, an approach that returns sex education to its early roots.

Sex education has been controversial for as long as it has existed, initially between those who believed that school was an appropriate place to educate students about sex and those who thought sex education belonged in the home. Today the controversy is between those who believe that the purpose of sex education is to reduce the potential harm to adolescents of risky, irresponsible sexual behavior versus those who believe that the purpose of sex education is to preserve the sanctity of marriage by teaching sexual abstinence before marriage.

From its early beginnings, sex education set for itself the formidable goal of imparting knowledge about sexuality to students in order to influence their out-of-school behavior. Having an effect on adolescent sexual activity is an especially ambitious goal, given the limited amount of school time that can be devoted to sex education and the multiple influences on adolescent sexual behavior. The rest of this chapter is an assessment of the degree to which sexuality education has achieved the lofty goal set for itself and had a positive effect on adolescent sexual behavior.

■ COMPREHENSIVE SEX EDUCATION

What Is Comprehensive Sex Education?

There is no single definition of comprehensive sex education. Several organizations provide an outline of what comprehensive sex education should be, with the one by the Sexuality Information and Education Council of the United States (SIECUS) typical. According to SIECUS (2009, October), a comprehensive sex education program should:

1. Provide young people with the tools to make informed decisions and build healthy relationships.
2. Stress the value of abstinence while also preparing young people for when they become sexually active.
3. Provide medically accurate information about the health benefits and side effects of all contraceptives, including condoms, as a means to

prevent pregnancy and reduce the risk of contracting STIs, including HIV/AIDS.

4. Encourage communication about sexuality between parent and child.

5. Teach young people the skills to make responsible decisions about sexuality, including how to avoid unwanted verbal, physical, and sexual advances.

6. Teach young people how alcohol and drug use can affect responsible decision making.

Points 2 and 3 above, which are that a comprehensive sex education program should teach both the value of sexual abstinence and provide information about contraceptives, including their correct use, are viewed by some as especially problematic. Some wonder whether such a combination is feasible, or if an attempt to include material on both approaches sends a confusing double message to adolescents, perhaps inadvertently encouraging teen sexuality (Weed & Lickona, 2014).

Comprehensive sex education is more than just a narrow focus on contraception. It also includes material on personal decision making, life-skills training, parent–child relations, and drug and alcohol use. Few courses cover all these topics, but this list provides a blueprint for what an ideal comprehensive sex education program might look like.

Comprehensive sex education programs are designed to prevent or reduce the risk of an unintended pregnancy and of contracting an STI. Some programs promote abstinence and sexual risk reduction, mainly condom use (abstinence-plus education), while others focus on sexual risk reduction (safer-sex education).

The following account of a comprehensive high school sex education course is brief, but the student describes a program that contains many of the basic elements of a good sex education program.

IN THEIR OWN WORDS

My high school had a comprehensive sex education program as part of a required health class that all sophomores had to take. It is likely that many of the teens [in the class] already had sexual experiences before sex education was taught. The portion of the course that talked about sexual development and contraception lasted about 3 or 4 weeks. It included us being tested on diagrams of both male and female sexual organs, learning about different kinds of hormonal and nonhormonal forms of contraception, transmission and symptoms of STIs, and had one of those infamous jars where students could anonymously submit questions for the teacher to answer. The instructors for these health classes were always physical education teachers, but we got extremely lucky with the instructor for our class. She knew what she was talking about and talked about it easily. A student club came in to do a presentation about sexual abstinence, but it also had another student club do a presentation on abstinence from alcohol. The course seemed to be balanced quite well.

Some programs even include condom distribution to students. Most programs are taught in school, but some are based in a community setting. Most programs are taught by adults, but some also employ trained adolescent instructors.

What Is Contained in Comprehensive Sex Education Programs?

One review of the content of 10 comprehensive sex education programs reveals that the majority of programs provide information about abstinence, contraceptive use, STIs, and unplanned pregnancies (Schmidt, Wandersman, & Hills, 2015). Few programs contain information about romantic relations, dating violence, or gender roles, and even fewer programs have material on LGBTQ issues, which are largely ignored in most sex education programs.

Does Comprehensive Sex Education Work?

Several evaluations of comprehensive sex education report generally positive effects on adolescent sexual behavior that include reductions in the following: percentage of adolescents who become sexually active, age of sexual debut, frequency of sexual activity, number of sexual partners, and occurrence of pregnancies (Chin et al., 2012; Glassman, Potter, Baumier, & Coyle, 2015; Goesling, Colman, Trenholm, Terzian, & Moore, 2014). These are impressive results that reveal an overall pattern of success in influencing the sexual behavior of adolescents. Some effects may be short-lived, not always significant for all measures, or significant only for a particular subgroup such as young adolescents or girls, however (Picot et al., 2012). In addition, there is heterogeneity in program effectiveness, and about one-third of programs fail to demonstrate an effect on any aspect of sexual behavior (Haberland & Rogow, 2015).

These positive findings are mirrored in other reviews of comprehensive sex education, which report that some interventions designed to reduce risky sexual behavior are associated with a small increase in condom use, and some decrease in unprotected sexual intercourse (Johnson, Scott-Sheldon, Huedo-Medina, & Carey, 2011; Kirby & Laris, 2009; Scott-Sheldon, Huedo-Medina, Warren, Johnson, & Carey, 2011; von Sadovszky, Draudt, & Boch, 2014).

Comprehensive sex education is associated with a reduction of many sexual risk-taking behaviors, but one outcome has been particularly intractable. On the whole, there is little evidence that school-based sex education programs effectively prevent contracting HIV or another STI (Mirzazadeh et al., 2017), despite the puzzling finding that several programs lead to an increase in knowledge about HIV and STI prevention, and a small increase in condom use. Apparently, knowing what to do does not automatically lead to actually doing something when the situation arises for large numbers of adolescents. The authors suggest that the reason sex education programs have only a minor effect on condom use is due to the difficulty of influencing a complex behavior such as condom use, especially for a long period of time.

Although many comprehensive sex education programs have a positive effect on teen sexual behavior, one review of abstinence-plus sex education programs reveals that the effects are limited (Bennett & Assefi, 2005). The authors conclude that some abstinence-plus programs have a positive effect on some teen sexual behaviors, but " . . . the effects are relatively modest and may last only short term" (Bennett & Assefi, 2005, p. 78), a conclusion echoed in other more recent reviews (Haberland & Rogow, 2015; Johnson et al., 2011).

A FOCUS ON RESEARCH

Does sex education work? The basic technique for answering that question is to compare the sexual behavior of students who complete one sex education course with the sexual behavior of students who take another sex education course, or no course at all. This deceptively simple approach in reality is difficult to implement, and many assessments of sex educations courses are limited for several reasons. Some evaluations are based on small samples. Sample size matters, and researchers are more confident of results from studies with large sample sizes. The dependent variables in many assessments of sex education are sexual knowledge or sexual intentions. Sex education courses are meant to have an impact on adolescent sexual behavior, so assessments of behavior are more persuasive than measurement of sexual attitudes. Further, many evaluations assess the dependent variables immediately after the intervention, or a short time later. Demonstrating that an intervention has a long-term effect months or even years after completion of the program is more compelling than finding an effect immediately after the intervention. Unfortunately, small samples are common in the evaluation of sex education programs, as is the assessment of sexual knowledge and intentions measured a short time after completion of a program, limitations that compromise the validity and generalizability of the assessment.

A fundamental requirement for a valid evaluation of a sex education program is random assignment of students to a treatment group or to a nontreatment control group. Random assignment, especially when the sample size is large, is an attempt to ensure that no differences exist between the treatment group and the control group at the beginning of the study. For example, with random assignment, about the same number of students who are liberal, or religious, or risk takers should be in each group. If a difference in sexual behavior emerges after the intervention, then that difference must be due to the treatment since the treatment is the only difference between the groups.

For practical and ethical reasons it can be difficult to randomly assign students to a treatment group or a control group. Practically, it may be difficult if not impossible for researchers to randomly assign students to one of two courses, or to a no-treatment control course, because of the needs of students to take a particular course, the willingness of parents to allow researchers to randomly assign their children to one course or another, and the requirements of schools. Further, many might consider it unethical to place students in an untested program or withhold a sex education course from students who want the course and could benefit from it.

Despite these hurdles, several impressive assessments exist of sex education programs with random assignment of students. In addition, some of these studies are based on large samples, and include self-reports of behavior over a relatively long time frame. Any evaluation of a sex education program in a naturalistic setting includes some compromises, but the best of these assessments are credible and persuasive.

In the following description of a comprehensive sex education program, the student reports that learning about contraception did not encourage her to have sex, but had the opposite effect, and may have delayed the age when she first became sexually active.

IN THEIR OWN WORDS

In fifth grade, the teachers separated us by gender and took us into different rooms, where we watched videos about puberty, sex, etc. From then on, the NY education system had us in a health class, or some variation of health class, from sixth grade all the way until senior year of high school. In these classes, we learned the ins and outs of puberty, pregnancy, delivery, STDs, prophylactics, birth control, abstinence, etc. The most memorable thing I can recall from these classes occurred in ninth grade "Parenting" class, where my teacher (who happened to have nine and a half fingers), chose to use my desk as her demonstration table. On the desk in front of me were plastic gadgets, foams, creams, condoms, and ointments. Over the next 80 minutes of class, my teacher demonstrated and explained (vividly) how to insert and use all of these materials in order to prevent pregnancy and STDs. This was enough to scare me out of sex until I had graduated from high school. As traumatizing as this experience was, I'm thankful for the information that was given to me within the NY education system; I feel very confident in my knowledge regarding sex, pregnancy prevention, and STD prevention. I'm also sure my parents are thankful for this education, considering they didn't have to confront the inevitable awkward sex talk with their first teenage daughter.

No comprehensive sex education program is associated with an increase in adolescent sexual behavior, dispelling the myth that teaching students about sex and contraception leads to an increase in sexual activity (Bennett & Assefi, 2005; Chin et al., 2012).

Two Comprehensive Sex Education Programs with Positive Results

One example of a comprehensive sex education program with positive results is It's Your Game: Keep It Real, a program for eighth- and ninth-grade students. Some of the specific topics covered in the course include setting limits, developing refusal skills, defining a healthy dating relationship, and condom use. In one evaluation, schools were randomly assigned to either the intervention condition or a control condition in which students received their regular health classes. Evaluation of the program reveals that students in the intervention group are somewhat less likely to engage in vaginal, oral, and anal sex in the ninth grade in comparison to students in the control group (Tortolero et al., 2010). The study is a demonstration of the effectiveness of an intervention program to delay the onset of risky sexual behavior among young teens in the eighth and ninth grades.

Reducing the Risk (RTR; Langley et al., 2015) is a comprehensive sex education program that focuses on delaying the initiation of sexual intercourse in conjunction with teaching students about contraceptive use for those students who become sexually active. RTR+ is a variation of RTR that emphasizes learning general information about STIs and condom usage. In one study, teens were randomly assigned to an RTR+ group, an RTR group, or a control group. Results reveal that RTR+ delays the onset of sexual intercourse, and reduces the number of sexual partners of teens who become sexually active in comparison to the other two groups (Reyna & Mills, 2014). Students in the RTR+ group who become sexually active are not more likely to use condoms, however. Overall, the results show that the RTR+ program has a positive impact on some, but not all, aspects of sexual risk-taking in adolescence.

What Are Some of the Characteristics of Successful Comprehensive Sex Education Programs?

Some comprehensive sex education programs reduce sexual risk-taking and some do not. What accounts for this variation in effectiveness? This is an important question to answer in the continuing attempt to develop more and better intervention programs. Some common themes of successful programs have emerged.

In general, successful programs teach students about the transmission of STIs, including HIV/AIDS; stress the importance of using condoms to avoid those infections (Escribano, Espada, Morales, & Orgilés, 2015); provide information on how to practice safer sex, such as the need to consistently and properly use a condom; and focus on increasing the motivation of students to use condoms as a highly effective way to avoid STIs and unwanted pregnancies (Johnson et al., 2011); In addition, successful programs teach students how to refuse unprotected sex and how to communicate with a partner about sexual matters, especially about the importance of discussing contraceptive use, a necessary but difficult discussion for many adolescents (Protogerou & Johnson, 2014).

The positive impact of a comprehensive sex education program is increased when classroom instruction is combined with other sexual health interventions into a multicomponent intervention. For example, combining in-school sex education instruction with a program designed to increase parent–adolescent communication about sexuality is more effective in reducing risky sexual behavior and teen pregnancies than either program is by itself (Shackleton et al., 2016). Multicomponent interventions that tie school-based sex education with face-to-face counseling and the provision of contraceptives are more effective in lowering the incidence of STIs and reducing pregnancy rates among adolescents than stand-alone sex education programs (Salam et al., 2016).

■ ABSTINENCE SEX EDUCATION

Since its inception, sex education in the United States has mainly been abstinence education, an approach that was advanced in 1981 by the passage of the Adolescent Family Life Act (AFLA), which authorized funding sex education demonstration projects that emphasize the importance of abstaining from sexual activity until marriage, an approach expected to lead to a decrease in the rates of STIs and unintended pregnancies among adolescents (Perrin & DeJoy, 2003). The next step in the promotion of abstinence sex education occurred in 1996, with an increase in federal funds specifically earmarked for sex education programs that met the criteria for abstinence sex education.

What Is Abstinence Sex Education?

The U.S. Department of Health and Human Services (Social Security Act, 2018) precisely defined abstinence sex education as an educational or motivational program that adheres to the following eight points:

(a) Has as its exclusive purpose, teaching the social, psychological, and health gains to be realized by abstaining from sexual activity.

(b) Teaches abstinence from sexual activity outside marriage as the expected standard for all school-age children.

(c) Teaches that abstinence from sexual activity is the only certain way to avoid out-of-wedlock pregnancy, sexually transmitted diseases, and other associated health problems.

(d) Teaches that a mutually faithful monogamous relationship in the context of marriage is the expected standard of human sexual activity.

(e) Teaches that sexual activity outside of the context of marriage is likely to have harmful psychological and physical effects.

(f) Teaches that bearing children out of wedlock is likely to have harmful consequences for the child, the child's parents, and society.

(g) Teaches young people how to reject sexual advances and how alcohol and drug use increases vulnerability to sexual advances.

(h) Teaches the importance of attaining self-sufficiency before engaging in sexual activity.

There are several noteworthy omissions in this approach to sex education. Most notably, there is no mention of contraception, since abstinence education exclusively focuses on self-restraint. Also, the points assume a heterosexual orientation, and there is no accommodation for adolescents or adults who are LGB. Further, there is no provision made for single adults who are expected to remain celibate unless they marry. Sex and marriage are intimately tied together for individuals of all ages.

Abstinence sex education is based on the deeply held belief of abstinence sex educators that unmarried adolescents should not engage in sexual activity, even if it could be made safe. It is a philosophy that challenges the foundation of comprehensive sex education, which is based on the principle that sex between unmarried adolescents is not inherently wrong or immoral, and that the purpose of sex education is to reduce the potential harm that may arise from sexual activity, mainly by teaching adolescents how to correctly use contraceptives, especially condoms. Arguments for and against abstinence sex education are rarely dispassionate, but are usually heated disagreements, driven not only by scientific data but also by political and religious ideologies.

Does Abstinence Sex Education Work?

The Mathematica Study

The largest, most ambitious, and best-known evaluation of abstinence sex education is a study by Mathematica Policy Research Inc., which received approximately $5 million of federal funds to conduct an independent assessment of abstinence sex education programs (Trenholm et al., 2007). Four abstinence programs in four cities were evaluated. Two of the programs included students in the fourth and fifth grades, and two served youth in the seventh and eighth grades. Approximately 2,500 students participated in the study. One strength of the study is that students were randomly assigned to one of four abstinence sex education programs or to a control group, which included courses in health education normally taught in each school. The control groups were fairly heterogeneous, but most included some material on the importance of sexual abstinence. The sexual behavior of students was assessed 4–6 years after the students completed the program in which they were enrolled. The findings indicate that there are no differences between the abstinence groups and the control groups in the percentage of students who have sex, in the age of sexual onset, number of sexual partners, occurrence of pregnancies, incidence of STIs, or percentage of students who engage in unprotected sex. The results show that sex education programs focused on sexual abstinence have no more long-term impact on teen sexual behavior than standard health education courses.

The Mathematica study is an impressive evaluation, and the finding of no-treatment effect is a blow to abstinence sex education, but the study has shortcomings, which limit validity and generalizability. First, the study is not proof that abstinence sex education in general is ineffective, since it is an evaluation of only four programs. We cannot generalize the findings from this small sample of programs to the many abstinence sex education programs that were not evaluated. Second, there is not perfect separation between the treatment groups and the control groups, some of which included information about abstinence. In addition, since the two groups are in the same school, some of the students in the treatment group may have talked to students in the control group about what they were learning, contaminating the treatment and control groups. Third, looking for an effect 4–6 years after the end of an intervention is a high standard for any sex education program, one that even comprehensive sex education programs might not meet had they been evaluated. In order to gain a better perspective on the effectiveness of abstinence sex education programs, we need to examine other evaluations.

Other Evaluations of Abstinence Sex Education

A more recent evaluation of 23 abstinence sex education programs leads to a mixed conclusion about the efficacy of abstinence sex education (Chin et al., 2012). According to this review, a few abstinence sex education programs lead to some reduction in the percentage of adolescents who become sexually active, a delay in the onset of sexual activity, and a decrease in the frequency of sexual activity among those adolescents who are sexually active.

Adolescents who take an abstinence sex education course and then become sexually active are no less likely to use condoms when they have sex than adolescents who take a comprehensive sex education course (Chin et al., 2012). This finding is especially important because some critics of abstinence sex education argue that adolescents who take an abstinence sex education course and become sexually active are unlikely to use contraceptives correctly, or unlikely to use them at all, since abstinence sex education either does not include lessons on correct contraceptive use, or sometimes provides incorrect information about condom use (Lin & Santelli, 2008). One study did find an increase in unprotected sex at a 3-month assessment for African American adolescents who took an abstinence sex education course, but the effect disappeared at 9 months (Shepherd, Sly, & Girard, 2017). In general, abstinence sex education is not associated with an increase in unprotected sexual activity.

Other evaluations of abstinence sex education indicate that most programs have no effect on adolescent sexual behavior, although a small number of programs have a positive effect on some aspects of sexual activity (Bennett & Assefi, 2005). Kirby (2008) evaluated nine abstinence sex education programs and finds no overall effect of abstinence sex education on sexual behavior, although two programs do delay the initiation of sexual intercourse, and one also decreases the frequency of sexual activity.

A third review examined the effectiveness of 13 abstinence sex education programs and found that abstinence sex education has no effect on any aspect of teen sexual behavior (Underhill, Montgomery, & Operario, 2007). Results from this review suggest that in general, abstinence sex education programs have little effect on adolescent sexual behavior, but the authors did not look for possible differences among programs.

Based on these reviews and other studies (Johnson et al., 2011; Kohler, Manhart, & Lafferty, 2008; Silva, 2002), it appears that in general, abstinence sex education has no effect on adolescent sexual behavior. It would be a mistake to conclude that no program works, however, since there is evidence that some programs delay the onset of adolescent sexuality. It seems time to move beyond the tired debate of whether abstinence sex education works to the next phase of this issue, which is for abstinence sex educators to identify those specific

In the following story, one young woman describes her experience with an abstinence sex education program and wonders whether the program did have an effect on her sexual behavior.

IN THEIR OWN WORDS

I remember once, my freshman year in high school, they brought in special guest speakers to talk about abstinence. These two women told us how we definitely should wait to have sex in marriage. Their big convincing point—that I do remember 8 years later (with lots of memory triggering), is that I should wait to have sex because I wouldn't want my future spouse being intimate with other women before me. Therefore, if I want my husband to wait for me, then I should for him. This made logical sense, so I decided to follow it, for as long as I could. Before the program I was not having sex, and after the program I was not having sex. It was my freshman year and it wouldn't be until senior year in high school when I lost my virginity. The talk originally made an impression on me, but by my senior year I didn't remember why I should wait, just that it seemed good. But when deciding between engaging in the awesome experience of sex, you have to have good reasons to wait. And I didn't. Overall, the sex education didn't have the effect my educators may have wanted. But who knows, maybe without it I would've had sex sooner.

features of programs that delay the onset of sexual activity and to develop and evaluate programs that contain those components.

One Abstinence Demonstration Program with Positive Results

Jemmott, Jemmott, and Fong (2010), at the University of Pennsylvania, developed an abstinence sex education program and evaluated the program over a period of several years. The course they developed and evaluated did not meet federal criteria for abstinence sex education programs, and is not designed to teach students to abstain from sexual relations until marriage. Instead, the course is designed to delay sexual behavior until the adolescents are older and more prepared to cope with the psychological and emotional issues related to sexual activity. Over 660 low-income African American students in grades 6 and 7 participated in the study, which took place on Saturdays in the schools. Students were randomly assigned to either an abstinence program, a comprehensive program that taught abstinence plus condom use, a safer-sex program that emphasized condom use, or a health promotion control group. The results reveal that fewer students in the abstinence program became sexually active over a 2-year time span than students in the other three programs. Subsequent analyses reveal that adolescents are more likely to abstain from having sex if they have positive beliefs about abstinence and negative beliefs about having sex during adolescence. In contrast, students who hoped to have sex eventually and who believed that sex is common in their age group are more likely to become sexually active (Zhang, Jemmott, & Jemmott, 2015). Thus, it appears that one successful approach to delaying sexual activity is to focus on the development of positive attitudes about abstinence by emphasizing the gains to be had from delaying the onset of sexual activity, rather than attempting to scare students about the dangers of sex.

■ VIRGINITY PLEDGES

The practice of making a virginity pledge in which an adolescent promises to abstain from sex until marriage began in the early 1990s. Originally sponsored by the Southern Baptist Church, the movement today is a loose collection of religious and secular organizations that includes hundreds of church, school, and college groups. Two of the largest organizations are True Love Waits and The Silver Ring Thing. The True Love Waits pledge states: "Believing that true love waits, I make a commitment to God, myself, my family, my friends, my future mate and my future children to be sexually abstinent from this day until the day I enter a biblical marriage relationship."

The immigrant young woman in the following story describes the pressure her mother put on her to take a virginity pledge. According to the young woman, taking the pledge was embarrassing, and had little or no effect on her behavior.

IN THEIR OWN WORDS

I participated in a virginity pledge with my brother that was hosted by my family's church. My brother and I were made to attend by my mother, who is a devout Christian. At the time, I was 14 and my brother was 17, and we had been in America for 2 years after relocating from Nigeria. I believe the reason that my mother insisted that we take a virginity pledge was because she saw that our previous extremely obedient behavior had started to lean more toward deviance the longer we spent in the United States, and was trying to keep us on the straight and narrow. The entire experience was more embarrassing to me than anything, particularly because my mom and all the parents involved were sitting in a circle watching us take these pledges. We were read bible verses advising chastity and purity, and given pamphlets stating why remaining pure was morally right, after which we pledged our virginity and signed "contracts" of virginity. After the event was over, my mother stuck our virginity pledges on the refrigerator door to remind us every day of the promise we made to God.

I do not think the virginity pledge had much of an effect on my sexual behavior. Despite this, however, I have never had unprotected sex with a partner, although, in my opinion, it is a reflection of my character rather than of my taking the pledge. I believe that a big reason why the pledge did not have an effect on me is because it was based on religion rather than fact. Although I considered myself Christian throughout my childhood, I started to doubt religion around when I hit puberty, and considered myself primarily agnostic by the time I was 14. If I was made to attend an abstinence class based on preventing pregnancy and STDs, it may have had an effect on me.

Adolescents who make a pledge sign a wallet-sized card they can carry with them with the True Love Waits pledge on it. Both organizations sponsor youth rallies with Christian music concerts that provide an opportunity for adolescents to sign pledge cards. It is not known how many adolescents have made a virginity pledge, but one estimate is that the figure is well over three million youth and may be as high as one-fifth of all U.S. adolescents between 12 and 17 years of age (Martino, Elliott, Collins, Kanouse, & Berry, 2008).

Do Virginity Pledges Work?

Could the simple act of uttering the 39 words in the True Love Waits pledge actually lead to a delay in the age of first intercourse? On the face of it, the idea seems preposterous, about as likely to affect behavior as keeping a New Year's resolution to lose weight. However, adolescents who voluntarily make a virginity pledge express a personal intention to remain a virgin until marriage, and become a member of a group of other adolescents who support and reinforce a norm of abstinence—two psychosocial processes more powerful than merely saying a few words.

Pledging for some adolescents is voluntary and a reflection of their personal values, while pledging for others is in response to pressure to sign a pledge card in a health class or youth group. Thus, some youth are enthusiastic supporters of the pledge philosophy, while others who make a pledge have little or no commitment to the pledge. This heterogeneity of commitment makes it difficult to evaluate the impact of virginity pledges on adolescent sexual behavior, since voluntary and involuntary pledgers are fundamentally different in their commitment to their pledge but are treated as a single group. This mixed group is then compared to adolescents who have not made a pledge.

Peter Bearman and Hannah Brückner, social scientists at Columbia University, were the first to evaluate the effect of virginity pledges on adolescent sexual behavior. They found that pledgers are less likely to have sexual intercourse than nonpledgers (Bearman & Brückner, 2001). Pledging is more likely to be associated with virginity during early and middle adolescence when virginity is the norm than during late adolescence when sex becomes more common. Thus, adolescents who take a virginity pledge may not remain virgin until they marry—in fact, they may not remain virgin even through late adolescence, but they are more likely to delay sexual intercourse during early and middle adolescence.

As is often true in the social sciences, there is disagreement and inconsistency in research findings on a question. Using a different study design and another technique of data analyses than that employed by Bearman and Brückner (2001), Janet Rosenbaum (2009) at Harvard University found no differences in the sexual behavior of pledgers and a matched sample of nonpledgers 5 years after making a pledge. The majority of pledgers and nonpledgers reported having sexual intercourse and oral sex. One puzzling finding from this study is that 5 years after making a pledge, 82% of the pledgers reported that they

> *The following young woman describes her experience taking a virginity pledge and her belief that the pledge had little or no effect on her sexual behavior, although she made a pledge to herself to remain a virgin.*

IN THEIR OWN WORDS

My district's policy on sex education was to teach only abstinence-based curriculum. In my class, we were asked to take a pledge that promised to remain a virgin until we found the "right" person. Though I signed the paper, I had already taken a pledge for myself and with my closest friends from church. Even though I clearly did not understand everything about sex, I made up my own mind that I would remain a virgin until marriage. Regardless of my own decision, the piece of paper we were required to turn in to our teacher meant next to nothing to me. I had not done it of my own volition and it was not in the terms that I would have chosen for myself. When I look at my decision to wait on sex until marriage, it is not the pact from health class that I see but the one I made for myself and with true intentions.

do not remember pledging. This finding is consistent with the idea that many pledgers simply say the pledge words but do not commit to the idea of the pledge and, therefore, do not even remember making a pledge.

Do Virginity Pledges Work for Some Adolescents?

Virginity pledges may have little effect on the majority of adolescents, especially if they are pressured to make a pledge, but a virginity pledge may have a modest effect on some adolescents. In one study of young adolescents, findings reveal that making a personal promise or commitment to oneself to remain a virgin reduces the probability of sexual intercourse and oral sex over a 1-year period (Bersamin, Walker, Waiters, Fisher, & Grube, 2005). Similar positive results for private pledges have been found for college males who pledge to remain a virgin while they are in college (Williams & Thompson, 2013). The findings suggest that private pledges may delay the initiation of sexual intercourse because a private pledge is a reflection of one's true value and is an intrinsically motivated commitment to remain a virgin.

One factor related to the effectiveness of a virginity pledge is whether an adolescent is already inclined to delay sexual intercourse (Martino, Elliott, Collins, et al., 2008). More specifically, a pledge may delay the onset of sexual intercourse for teens who do not think that having sex during adolescence will be a positive experience, and who believe that their friends do not approve of premarital sex. Pledging has no effect on adolescents who want to have sex and who believe that their friends are sexually active.

Because virginity pledges are usually, but not always, based on religious teachings about sex and morality, one would expect that virginity pledges would be especially effective for adolescents who are religious. Indeed, that is true (Landor & Simons, 2014). Pledging is associated with an increase in sexual

The following story illustrates the idea that a pledge may reinforce a preexisting belief in the importance of remaining a virgin that, in this young woman's case, was the result of her religious upbringing. It is not possible to determine whether the pledge had any effect on her behavior, even though she remained a virgin throughout high school.

IN THEIR OWN WORDS

As we came to a close on the sex-outside-of-marriage lectures, the sex awareness part of the class ended with the health teacher passing out a purity pledge. This was a non-verbal promise to save ourselves for marriage. It was a document that each person had to sign, promising to stay abstinent until marriage. After we signed the contract, we were given a card made out of thicker paper that we could keep with us at all times. This card stated that we were virgins, or "reclaimed our virginity," and this would not change until we entered into the institution of marriage.

After this class, I still had the same viewpoints as I did prior to taking it. I remained abstinent throughout high school. This abstinence, however, came mostly from my religious beliefs. My parents placed a high emphasis on abstaining from sex; so, this pledge was not the reason for this abstinence.

abstinence for adolescents who have internalized religious beliefs and values, but pledging is ineffective for adolescents who have low religious commitment.

Do Adolescents Who Break Their Pledge Then Engage in Risky Sexual Behavior?

Because virginity pledges have one message and one message only—do not engage in premarital sex—some critics of virginity pledges have proposed that adolescents who break their promise not to have sex are likely to engage in risky sexual behavior, since they do not know much about risky sex and how to avoid it. Findings on this issue are not entirely consistent, but the bulk of the evidence indicates that pledgers who become sexually active are no more likely to engage in risky sexual behavior than nonpledgers (Brückner & Bearman, 2005; Martino, Elliott, Collins, et al., 2008; Rosenbaum, 2009; Williams & Thompson, 2013). Further, the STI rate among pledgers who become sexually active is no greater than sexually active nonpledgers (Brückner & Bearman, 2005; Ford et al., 2005).

■ INTERVENTIONS WITH PARENTS TO REDUCE RISKY ADOLESCENT SEXUAL BEHAVIOR

The majority of programs for parents designed to reduce risky teen sexual behavior focus on enhancing parent communication skills about sex (Silk & Romero, 2014; Wight & Fullerton, 2013). Chapter 4 includes an examination of the effectiveness of many of these programs, which are only briefly summarized in this section. Interventions typically include workshops, role-playing, videos, written material, homework assignments, and support groups.

Do Interventions with Parents Improve the Sexual Health of Adolescents?

Many parenting programs designed to reduce risky adolescent sexual behavior specifically target African American and Hispanic parents and adolescents, because teens in those families are at high risk for unsafe sexual behavior, such as early onset of sexual intercourse and inconsistent condom use. Three features of successful programs emerge from research on interventions targeted at minority parents (Sutton, Lasswell, Lanier, & Miller, 2014). First, successful programs are tailored to a specific racial or ethnic group, and include material on racial and ethnic pride. Second, in successful programs, parents receive specific instruction about adolescent sexual development and STI prevention in order to improve parent knowledge about these topics, and increase the comfort level of parents to talk about these issues. Third, successful programs have joint parent–adolescent sessions in which parents and adolescents can practice what they learn in the presence of a skilled instructor who can offer helpful feedback. In general, parenting programs designed to reduce risky teen sex are associated with improvements in parent–adolescent communication about sex, and some decrease in adolescent risky sexual behavior (Santa Maria et al., 2015).

■ PEER-LED SEX EDUCATION PROGRAMS

What Is Peer-Led Sex Education?

A small number of sex education programs include peer leaders who provide information about sex, STIs, and contraception to other adolescents. Peer-led sex education programs are based on two ideas: teens can more easily talk to other adolescents than to adults about sex, especially about sensitive issues such as oral sex and sexual positions; and peers can have a positive effect on the sexual behavior of other teens.

Peer leaders typically are older than students in the sex education course and are selected on several bases, such as charisma, credibility, and capacity to communicate. The leaders are then given training in sexual content and instructional techniques designed to equip them with the knowledge and skills necessary to teach the material to other students. The training can be extensive as it was for one Italian program that included five full-day training sessions for leaders (Borgia, Marinacci, Schifano, & Perucci, 2005). Peer leaders are then given responsibility for teaching groups of students, usually in classroom settings.

Peer-led sex education may have some advantages over sex education taught by adults, but there are some disadvantages as well, as the following story told by a young woman in college illustrates.

IN THEIR OWN WORDS

We had two college students come into our class and talk to us about love. It was a lot of religious stuff, and after having gone to Catholic school for 9 years I was a little annoyed that this topic was coming up in my public school, but once again I dutifully listened while trying not to zone out too much. Then the students explained what they were really there for—to teach us about how cool abstinence was.

I remember the awkwardness in the classroom as students tried not to laugh when they realized our college presenters were virgins while half of the 14-year-olds in our classroom were not. Regardless of my feelings, I was forced to sign a "Chastity Check Card" at the end of class.

But before the cards came out, the presentation took a different turn where our presenters tried to scare us away from having sex. They explained how condoms aren't very effective because boys keep them in their pockets and they get too hot so if we have sex with a condom, we will most likely still get pregnant. I specifically remember this part because I said something later on to my parents about how condoms aren't worth using because they don't even work and my parents were livid. I got a whole lecture about how what I received in health class was not sex education but abstinence education and they were trying to scare me. I was then given a real explanation of why I should always use condoms.

Does Peer-Led Sex Education Work?

Findings on the effectiveness of peer-led sex education programs have not been impressive. Evaluations of peer-led sex education programs indicate that those programs lead to some improvement in sexual knowledge, especially knowledge about STI transmission and prevention, but have little or no effect on the percentage of students who are sexually active, number of sexual partners, STI rates, or number of pregnancies (Kim & Free, 2008; Tolli, 2012). Some peer interventions do have a positive effect on condom use, although this effect is far from consistent (Maticka-Tyndale & Barnett, 2010).

In general, adult-led sex education courses are more likely to affect adolescent sexual behavior than peer programs. Teens may feel more comfortable discussing some sensitive topics with peers closer to their own age, but there is little evidence that these discussions have an impact on sexual behavior.

■ MEDIA APPROACHES TO SEX EDUCATION

Can the Internet Be Used to Educate Adolescents about Sexual Behavior?

The Internet is already an important technology to deliver information about sexuality to adolescents, and it promises to become even more valuable (Ralph, Berglas, Schwartz, & Brindis, 2011). Between 30 and 40% of U.S. teens have used the Internet to search for information about sex-related topics, primarily STIs, including HIV/AIDS; pregnancy and childbirth; sexual behavior, including oral sex and sexual positions; and contraception (Simon & Daneback, 2013). Several good sites for teens exist such as *www.iwannaknow.org, www.safeteens.org*, and *www.plannedparenthood.org/teens*. Some of the advantages of using the Internet to deliver information about sexuality to teens include the following: it is inexpensive in comparison to face-to-face interactions, it can reach a large audience, it is convenient for users who can access the site any time in multiple settings, and it is an ideal venue for users to get answers to sensitive and embarrassing questions. There are some limitations and disadvantages, however. For example, it can be difficult to find a private location to access sensitive information. Further, the ubiquitous presence of Internet pornography can create problems finding and accessing sites with appropriate information about sexuality. One study found that the majority of sites turned up using keywords related to teen sexuality are sexually explicit sites (Smith, Gertz, Alvarez, & Lurie, 2006). An additional challenge is finding a website with information that is appropriate, teen-friendly, and provides material written at an understandable reading level, since many teens who engage in risky sexual behavior read below their grade level (Marques et al., 2015).

Another problem with using the Internet to find information about sexuality is that sex education sites vary in quality and accuracy, and adolescents have a difficult time distinguishing good from bad sites. Adolescents are frustrated by the amount of contradictory information online and are mistrustful of the health information available to them on the Internet (Jones & Biddlecom, 2011). Many sites contain information that is inaccurate or misleading, and this is especially true for material about contraception and STIs (Buhi et al., 2010). Presently, it is not possible to help adolescents distinguish trustworthy from untrustworthy websites, and teens are left to decide for themselves whether a site provides accurate or inaccurate information.

Several preliminary evaluations of Internet-based sex education sites indicate that adolescents and their parents are enthusiastic about using these sites to obtain sexual health information, although information acquired from the Internet is viewed as less trustworthy than material received from adult teachers (Devine, Bull, Dreisbach, & Shlay, 2014; Guilamo-Ramos et al., 2015).

The Internet can be more than just a venue for obtaining sexual information. One evaluation of an Internet-based sex education program for Mexican adolescents found that the intervention was related to some reduction in self-reported risky sexual behavior (Castillo-Arcos et al., 2016). The development and evaluation of Internet-based sex education interventions is just beginning, but there is hope among sex educators that the vast resources on the Internet can be used in stand-alone programs, or as an adjunct to programs delivered in person.

Can Social Networking Sites Be Used to Influence Adolescent Sexual Behavior?

Social networking sites (SNSs) provide another avenue for youth to access information about sexual issues (Dunne, McIntosh, & Mallory, 2014). In recent years, nonprofit, teen-oriented organizations, such as Sex Etc., have established SNSs where teens can become friends of the organization, post comments, and ask questions of the staff. There are disadvantages to having an online presence, however, which include possible exposure to explicit sexual material and online victimization (Guan & Subrahmanyam, 2009; Ybarra & Mitchell, 2007).

One Facebook page designed to promote condom use delivered prevention messages for 8 weeks to adolescents who agreed to receive news from the page called Just/Us (Bull, Levine, Black, Schmiege, & Santelli, 2012). A mixed set of findings emerge from this study. One important finding is that 2 months after the end of the program adolescents in the intervention group in comparison to youth in a nonintervention group report that they are more likely to use a condom when they have intercourse, a difference that unfortunately vanished at a 6-month assessment. The results suggest that social media can have a short-term effect on condom usage, but the effect disappears over time, underscoring the difficulty of maintaining a prevention effect over a long period of time.

Adolescents report that SNSs are places for learning information about health, including STIs and contraception. Teens indicate that they find the information about sexuality sent to them from SNSs useful, and they want to continue receiving messages about sexual health. User satisfaction of SNSs focused on sexual health is high, and users are satisfied with the messages they receive about STIs and contraception from those sites (Park & Calamaro, 2013).

The use of SNSs to affect the sexual behavior of adolescents is just beginning, and evaluations of these sites are at a preliminary stage. The use of SNSs in sex education is not widespread even in the United States, where most of the sites are located. Further, it appears that most SNSs devoted to sex education are sponsored by organizations with websites that are the basis for the SNS, and there is little attempt to encourage social activity and engagement (Gold et al., 2011). Developers of teen sexual health SNSs need to identify the content, features, and approaches that successfully encourage social engagement and to implement those components into their adolescent sexual health SNS.

What Are the Effects of Computer-Based Instruction on Teen Sexual Behavior?

Is computer-based instruction (CBI) an effective approach to sex education? Three types of CBI have been developed. First, there are programs designed for all adolescents. Second, there are programs with content individually tailored to a specific group, such as young, gay, African American males. Third, there are interactive video interventions that simulate dating and sexual situations, which require users to make choices at various decision points and to view the consequences of their choices.

CBI is a promising new form of information delivery that may replace or augment existing in-person instruction (Noar, 2011). Once developed, CBI is relatively cheap to implement in comparison to the costs of in-person teachers. Also, CBI can be individually tailored to the particular characteristics of users, rather than teaching a common course to all the students in a class. Last, CBI may include interactivity and multimedia material, enhancing the presentation of information, making it more memorable and increasing its impact.

Results from one study indicate that 3 months after the end of a stand-alone interactive video sex education intervention, students are less likely to engage in sexual intercourse, less likely to report an STI, and more likely to use condoms if they become sexually active, than students who receive the same content from a book (Downs et al., 2004).

Reviews of research on sex education programs that use CBI find that it leads to an increase in knowledge about STIs; improvement in attitudes about condoms; and an increase in condom self-efficacy, which is a measure of one's confidence about using a condom (Noar, Pierce, & Black, 2010). Of even more significance are the findings that CBI is related to some increase in condom use, a reduction in number of sexual partners, and a decrease in the frequency of sexual activity (Noar, Black, & Pierce, 2009), although the effects of CBI on adolescent sexual behavior are small (Peskin et al., 2015). These findings show that in general, the use of CBI may lead to an improvement in safer-sex knowledge and attitudes and to some reduction in risky sexual behavior. CBI has about the same impact on adolescents as material delivered in person, making CBI, in the long run, significantly more cost-effective.

Can Computer Technology Augment Traditional Sex Education Classes?

Several traditional school-based sex education courses use computer-based activities as part of the curriculum. Evaluations of these programs show that interactive videos and computer-based activities may enhance traditional sex education classes, facilitating learning and reducing involvement in risky sexual behavior (Hieftje, Edelman, Camenga, & Fiellin, 2013; Roberto et al., 2008). Results from one study reveal that students who complete a course augmented by computer-based activities as part of a sexual risk reduction program are less likely to engage in oral, vaginal, or anal sex in comparison to a nonintervention control group (Tortolero et al., 2010).

New digital media, including the Internet and SNSs, along with the use of computers that allow for multimedia presentations and interactive exercises, are innovative tools for sex education. New media approaches to sex education are only now coming online, but preliminary evidence suggests that these approaches are associated with sex health promotion and sex risk reduction (Guse et al., 2012). New digital media have the potential to augment or replace traditional methods for teaching sex education, perhaps increasing the impact of a sex education course on knowledge and behavior.

■ SCHOOL-BASED HEALTH CLINICS

SBHCs are designed to deliver comprehensive primary health care to youth, especially to those who lack medical coverage and who rarely receive medical attention, even when they need it. SBHCs vary from fully equipped centers that may include a nurse, a physician's assistant, a health educator, and a mental health counselor, to clinics that provide nursing services for only a few hours each week. SBHCs are located in schools or on school grounds.

The prevention and treatment of physical health problems are primary goals of SBHCs, but pregnancy prevention is a top priority. Typical users of SBHCs are females from lower socioeconomic backgrounds who are not doing well in school and who are sexually active (Mason-Jones et al., 2012). The most common reasons students use SBHCs include mental health issues, reproductive health services, and medical exams (Carroll, Lloyd-Jones, Cooke, & Owen, 2012). Most SBHCs offer diagnosis and treatment of STIs. The majority of SBHCs offer pregnancy testing, contraceptive counseling, and follow-up services for contraceptive users, but many SBHCs are prohibited from dispensing contraceptives on-site.

What Can SBHCs Do for Adolescents in the Area of Reproductive Health?

The provision of contraceptive services to minors is a complex issue with an array of local rules, state laws, and federal regulations governing the circumstances under which a minor can receive contraceptive services, which includes counseling. As of 2018, 26 states and the District of Columbia allow minors to consent to contraceptive services without the approval of a parent, 4 states have no policies on the matter, and 20 states allow minors to receive contraceptive services without parental consent only under special circumstances, such as if the minor is married, pregnant, or a parent (Guttmacher Institute, 2018). Even if the law allows minors to receive contraceptive services, many SBHCs are prohibited from providing these services because of clinic rules, or local policies of the school, or the school district (Santelli et al., 2003).

One of the incentives for teens to use an SBHC is to obtain reproductive health services without parent permission or knowledge, but this is not possible in many states and districts. From one perspective, it makes perfect sense that parents should know what health interventions, including prescription drugs, their children are receiving. From another perspective, however, one of the main reasons adolescents give for not seeking health care, including contraceptive services for the prevention or treatment of STIs, is that they fear their parents will find out (Lehrer, Pantell, Tebb, & Shafer, 2007). The need to obtain parental permission to seek contraceptive services is an unfortunate impediment for many adolescents who forgo those services, putting them at risk for an STI or an unplanned pregnancy.

Do SBHCs Have an Impact on Adolescent Sexual Activity?

Evaluations of the relationship between SBHCs and adolescent sexuality are mixed. One recent review of research on SBHCs concludes that in general, the presence of an SBHC does not reduce teen pregnancies (Shackleton et al., 2016). The lack of an effect may be a reflection of the different services available at SBHCs, however. For example, one would not expect an SBHC to have an effect on adolescent contraceptive use if the clinic is not allowed to provide contraceptive services to students in the school. Adolescents in schools with an SBHC that is allowed to provide contraceptives to students are more likely to use contraceptives, with a reduction in unintended pregnancies and STIs than students in schools without an SBHC (Ethier et al., 2011; Minguez, Santelli, Gibson, Orr, & Samant, 2015).

The association between SBHCs and pregnancy prevention is related to the number of hours per week health professionals are available to students using the SBHC. In general, more hours of health care availability is related to a lower number of teen pregnancies (Denny et al., 2012).

Some SBHCs offer programs to teens designed to reduce risky sexual behavior. In one study, a multicomponent intervention called Prime Time was administered through a clinic to girls at high risk for pregnancy. The intervention was a 15-session program designed to improve sexual decision making and contraceptive use, in addition to teaching fundamentals of healthy relationships. Evaluation of the program at 12 months and 24 months revealed an improvement in girls' consistent use of condoms and hormonal contraception (Sieving et al., 2011, 2013). Girls in the program also showed improvement in their confidence that they could refuse unwanted sex. The results reveal that a clinic-based intervention that includes one-on-one visits with a case manager, along with participation in peer-led intervention groups, holds great promise for reducing risky sexual behavior among high-risk girls and, perhaps, boys as well.

Should Schools Give Out Condoms to Students?

One hot-button issue that many high schools and even some middle schools are facing is the advisability of giving condoms to students, either through SBHCs, sex education classes, or in condom dispensers located throughout the school. Some schools even give out condoms at the prom. Emotions run deep on this question and the issues are complex. Courts tend to defer to school boards and allow condom distribution programs to stand where they have been instituted, but legislators tend to restrict the powers of school boards and to prohibit the establishment of these programs. The debate revolves around the needs of adolescents, the responsibilities of parents, and the liability of schools. It also centers on the message these programs send to adolescents. Some parents and others wonder whether the availability of condoms in school encourages students to have sex.

Do Condom Distribution Programs Lead to an Increase in Teen Sexual Behavior?

Assessments of the relationship between condom availability programs and adolescent sexual behavior all point to the same conclusion: there is no evidence that making condoms available to adolescents is associated with an increase in teen sexual activity (Charania et al., 2011). The frequency of sexual intercourse, the age when students first start to have sexual intercourse, and the number of sexual partners students have are not higher in schools with a condom distribution program in comparison to schools without such a program (Kirby, 2002). Condom availability programs are associated with an increase in condom use among students who are already sexually active (Blake et al., 2003; Shackleton et al., 2016). All these findings should be of some consolation to parents who worry that condom distribution in schools might encourage their teens to become sexually active. Whether an adolescent becomes sexually active is dependent on factors other than the easy availability of condoms.

SUMMARY

■ THE HISTORY OF SEX EDUCATION IN THE UNITED STATES

In the United States, and in most of the developed world, school-based sex education is the most common intervention employed to instruct children and adolescents about sexuality. The traditional message of most sex education courses is to "Just say no" to sex before marriage.

Since its beginnings, sex education has been divisive, with the hot-button issue today between those who think sex education should teach adolescents how to practice safe, responsible sex, versus those who believe that sex education should teach abstinence until marriage. The goal of sex education courses is to influence the out-of-school behavior of adolescents over a long period of time, an ambitious goal for any school-based classroom course.

■ COMPREHENSIVE SEX EDUCATION

Some comprehensive sex education programs also promote abstinence, but all include extensive material on condom use for the prevention of STIs and pregnancy. Most evaluations of comprehensive sex education programs report reductions in many risky sexual behaviors, although the effects are modest. Successful programs provide accurate information about how to prevent STIs and pregnancies, and teach adolescents how to correctly use contraceptives, especially condoms. No comprehensive sex education program is associated with an increase in adolescent sexual behavior.

■ ABSTINENCE SEX EDUCATION

Abstinence sex education in the United States has been institutionalized and formalized by the passage of two congressional acts funding abstinence sex education. According to the federal government's definition of abstinence sex education, a true abstinence sex education course adheres to eight specific points that go beyond merely teaching sexual abstinence.

In general, abstinence sex education has little effect on adolescent sexual behavior, although some programs do delay the onset of sexual intercourse. Many programs are not effective, but many programs have not been evaluated. One way to move forward on the issue of the effectiveness of abstinence sex education is for abstinence sex educators to develop and evaluate curricula that build on programs that show some success.

■ VIRGINITY PLEDGES

Adolescents who make a virginity pledge promise to remain sexually abstinent until they marry. Many adolescents make a pledge voluntarily, but some are pressured into making a pledge, undermining the spirit of the pledge, and limiting its effectiveness. Results of evaluations of virginity pledges are inconsistent. Pledges may help some adolescents delay the onset of sexual intercourse if the adolescents are already committed to remaining a virgin, but pledges have little or no effect on adolescents who do not endorse abstinence to begin with. Pledgers who break their promise are not more likely to engage in risky sexual behavior in comparison to adolescents who do not make a pledge.

◾ INTERVENTIONS WITH PARENTS TO REDUCE RISKY ADOLESCENT SEXUAL BEHAVIOR

Parent interventions designed to reduce risky adolescent sexual behavior focus on enhancing parent–adolescent communication about sex. Evaluations of these interventions reveal that some programs lead to an improvement in the ability of parents to talk to their adolescents about sex, which is associated with a reduction in risky adolescent sexual behavior.

◾ PEER-LED SEX EDUCATION PROGRAMS

Peer-led sex education interventions are programs in which adolescents have some responsibility for teaching material on sex education to other adolescents. Peer-led sex education is based on two ideas: adolescents can talk to other adolescents about sex more easily than they can discuss these issues with adults, and peers can be effective agents in reducing risky adolescent sexual behavior. Results from evaluations of peer-led sex education programs are not impressive. Adult-led sex education programs have more of an influence on adolescent sexuality than peer-led programs.

◾ MEDIA APPROACHES TO SEX EDUCATION

Emerging technologies, especially the Internet, provide a new venue for adolescents to learn about sex. Some evidence suggests that information acquired from Internet sites specifically designed to teach sex education can have a positive effect on adolescent sexual behavior. Using social media to teach adolescents about sex is another approach to sex education that may have a positive effect on adolescents. CBI is associated with the development of safer-sex attitudes and some reduction in risky sexual behavior. New technologies are not magic bullets that are going to transform sex education, but they do provide a novel and user-friendly approach to teaching adolescents about sex.

◾ SCHOOL-BASED HEALTH CLINICS

SBHCs housed in school buildings or on school grounds are designed to provide adolescents with comprehensive primary health care, including reproductive health services. Laws and regulations, including policies about parent involvement in the health care of minors, limit the services SBHCs can provide teens. Evaluations of the effects of SBHCs on adolescent sexual behavior are mixed— some find that the presence of a clinic is related to a reduction in risky adolescent sexual behavior while others do not. One factor related to an increase in the use of contraceptives is whether the clinic can provide contraceptive services to students in the school. There is no evidence that access to condoms in schools is associated with an increase in sexual activity among students.

SUGGESTIONS FOR FURTHER READING

Chin, H. B., Sipe, T. A., Elder, R., Mercer, S. L., Chattopadhyay, S. K., Jacob, V., et al. (2012). The effectiveness of group-based comprehensive risk-reduction and abstinence education interventions to prevent or reduce the risk of adolescent pregnancy, human immunodeficiency virus, and sexually transmitted infections. *American Journal of Preventive Medicine, 42,* 272–294.

Gold, J., Pedrana, A. E., Sacks-Davis, R., Hellard, M. E., Chang, S., Howard, S., et al. (2011). A systematic examination of the use of online social networking sites for sexual health promotion. *BMC Public Health, 11,* 583–591.

Moran, J. P. (2000). *Teaching sex: The shaping of adolescence in the 20th century.* Cambridge, MA: Harvard University Press.

Protogerou, C., & Johnson, B. T. (2014). Factors underlying the success of behavioral HIV-prevention interventions for adolescents: A meta-review. *AIDS and Behavior, 18,* 1847–1863.

Reyna, V. F., & Mills, B. A. (2014). Theoretically motivated interventions for reducing sexual risk taking in adolescence: A randomized controlled experiment applying fuzzy-trace theory. *Journal of Experimental Psychology: General, 143,* 1627–1648.

Santa Maria, D., Markham, C., Bluethmann, S., & Mullen, P. D. (2015). Parent-based adolescent sexual health interventions and effect on communication outcomes: A systematic review and meta-analyses. *Perspectives on Sexual and Reproductive Health, 47,* 37–50.

CHAPTER 12

The Sexual Health of Adolescents in the 21st Century

Is sex bad for teens? Is engaging in sexual activity detrimental to the physical, psychological, and social health of adolescents? Most research on teen sexuality emerges from a sex-is-perilous paradigm built on the idea that sexual activity during adolescence is inherently dangerous, likely to result in harm to those youth who engage in it. The purpose of this chapter is to evaluate that idea. The first part of the chapter is a critical examination of the relationship between adolescent sexuality and several problems associated with it, especially pregnancy and STIs, emotional problems including depression, and behavioral difficulties such as substance use. In the second part of the chapter a non-problem-orientated approach to adolescent sexuality is described based on the idea that sexual activity during adolescence is not inherently harmful or injurious to teens.

■ THE TRADITIONAL VIEW OF ADOLESCENT SEXUALITY

The idea that sex is a risky, dangerous activity has shaped thinking about adolescent sexuality among researchers, policymakers, health professionals, and educators, at least from the beginning of the sex education movement in the United States in the early 1900s until today (Schalet, 2011). Research on, and thinking about, adolescent sexuality overwhelmingly focuses on the dark and dangerous aspects of teen sex. There are thousands of studies on teen sexual behavior as it relates to adolescent problems, especially teen pregnancy and STIs. Other research focuses on negative emotions and mental health issues,

A FOCUS ON RESEARCH

It is well-known in the research community that one must be cautious about interpreting a correlation between two variables, but all too often in the popular press and in the minds of many people, finding a significant correlation, for example, between sexual behavior and adolescent problems, such as depression or drug use, is interpreted as indicating that sex is a cause of the problem. It is possible that adolescent sexual behavior may lead to psychological harm and problem behaviors, but there are two other interpretations of a correlation between teen sexual behavior and adolescent problems. Problem behavior may lead to teen sexual activity, or a correlation between teen sexual activity and adolescent problem behavior may be the result of a spurious relationship in which some unidentified third variable is the true cause of the association between sex and problems. For example, sexual activity may lead to depression in some adolescents, depression may lead to sexual activity in other adolescents, or a correlation between sexual activity and depression may exist because some third variable, such as poor parent–adolescent relations, is responsible for the link between teen depression and sexual activity. The idea that teen sex leads to adolescent problems may be more apparent than real for many problems and for many adolescents.

Researchers are well aware of the multiple interpretations of a correlation between two variables and generally do not overinterpret their data by attributing a cause to one variable when only a significant correlation is identified. Demonstrating a cause–effect relationship requires an experimental design in which groups are equal in every way except that one group receives a treatment and another group does not. Such an approach is neither practical nor ethical for most questions about teen sexuality. Instead, the best research on teen sexual behavior is based on a longitudinal design in which variation in one variable at Time 1 is compared to variation in another variable at Time 2. A longitudinal design can be used to establish a temporal relationship between two variables and to show that variation in one variable predicts variation in a second variable, but demonstrating a causal relationship still requires a true experiment.

such as regret, depression, suicidal ideation, and low self-esteem, as reactions to sexual behavior (Oswalt, Cameron, & Koob, 2005). Still other investigations examine adolescent sexuality as part of a general problem behavior syndrome that includes drinking alcohol, using drugs, delinquency, and poor grades in school. Sexual behavior during adolescence is often classified as one of several risky behaviors that are a consequence of poor parent–teen relations and negative peer pressure, and a cause of many undesirable and harmful behaviors that can extend far beyond adolescence, reaching into emerging adulthood and even beyond. Reading the social science literature on adolescent sexuality, one would conclude that teen sex is an intrinsically hazardous activity in the same category as illegal drug use and delinquency.

Is the Only Healthy Sex for Adolescents No Sex at All?

Risky adolescent sexual behavior can lead to the devastating problems of a teen pregnancy or an STI, but the sexual behavior of most teens does not result in those problems. Further, those problems, themselves, emerge from the risky lifestyle and dysfunctional social background of teens who are not representative of adolescents as a group. It is an overgeneralization to portray all teen sexual behavior as dangerous based on the problems experienced by a minority of adolescents who often have preexisting difficulties and poor relations with parents and peers.

Other evidence for the idea that teen sexuality is destructive is the often-found association between adolescent sexual behavior and psychological adjustment difficulties. Two points can be made about that association. First, the correlation between adolescent sexuality and emotional maladjustment is significant but small (e.g., Mendle et al., 2013), indicating that the majority of sexually active teens do not experience any negative effects as a result of their sexual behavior. Second, as discussed in the "A Focus on Research" sidebar in this chapter, there are three possibilities for the correlation between sex and adjustment problems, corresponding to three groups of adolescents. Some teens may be psychologically harmed by their sexual experiences, but the size of this important group is not known, nor are these teens representative of the population of sexually active adolescents. Another group of adolescents with personal problems may be drawn into a sexual relationship. Last, a third group of teens may possess a trait responsible for the link between sexual activity and adjustment problems, such that sexual activity is not the true cause of psychological maladjustment. Thus, the idea that teen sexual behavior is a cause of physical or emotional harm is not true for the large majority of adolescents. In addition, the association between teen sex and emotional maladjustment is open to multiple interpretations, only one of which is that teen sex is a cause of adjustment problems.

Another shortcoming of the teen sex-is-dangerous paradigm is that this view categorizes all teen sex as hazardous and perilous, and fails to distinguish between the responsible sexual behavior practiced by many adolescents and emerging adults, and the irresponsible behavior of some teens. There is a world of difference between the low-risk sexual relations of two older adolescents or emerging adults who use condoms and who are in a long-term monogamous relationship, and the high-risk casual sex between two young adolescents who are inconsistent contraceptive users and involved in several other dangerous activities, such as drug use and delinquency.

An additional problem with the traditional view of adolescent sexuality as dangerous behavior is that a focus on the negative aspects of sexual behavior ignores the normative expression of typical sexuality among the majority of adolescents whose experiences with sex are not negative or associated with adolescent problems (Tolman & McClelland, 2011). That so little is known about the place of sexuality in adolescent psychological and social development is a testament to an understandable, but one-sided emphasis on the dark side of teen sexuality and to an almost complete lack of focus on typical adolescent sexual development. Even less is known about the possibility that sexual activity during adolescence may be associated with positive outcomes for some teens in some contexts, and yet such a possibility exists.

■ SEX AND ADOLESCENT HEALTH

Is Sex Bad for Adolescents?

As discussed in Chapters 9 and 10, teen sexual behavior can be dangerous, especially if the adolescent is young, involved in casual sex with multiple partners, and is an inconsistent contraceptive user. These risky behaviors can lead to an unplanned pregnancy or contracting an STI, and they are associated with depression and problem behaviors. The fact that *some* adolescent sexual behavior can be dangerous has led some abstinent sex educators to the position that *all* sex outside of marriage is harmful, even for older adolescents and emerging adults in a stable relationship who practice safer sex (Vasilenko, Lefkowitz, & Welsh, 2014). Indeed, one of the eight criteria used by the U.S. Department of Health and Human Services (Social Security Act, 2018) to define abstinence sex education is that it is a program teaching that "sexual activity outside of the context of marriage is *likely* [emphasis added] to have harmful psychological and physical effects" (see Chapter 11). Abstinence sex education programs are built on the idea that sex outside of marriage is inherently hazardous to the health of adolescents (Santelli et al., 2006).

In the following story, a college student describes his high school abstinence sex education class, which was different from the sex education class he had in the eighth grade. Note the emphasis on the potential harm of premarital sex as a technique to motivate students to avoid having sexual relations.

IN THEIR OWN WORDS

High school took an opposite approach to the topic of sex. Instead of harmless learning about the biology of sex, we learned about the evil and danger of having sex, and all the consequences that come with it. Sex became more than just something two people do together to procreate, it became an inherent sin than everyone had to hide and keep dormant until marriage. In that aspect, abstinence programs were the focus of every sex ed class in school. Freshman year the "A team" (abstinence team) came to our school and made us do an experiment to show the severity of STDs. Each student was given a clear liquid, some of which had an invisible chemical (an STD), that turned pink when added to water. Students then mixed liquids (had sex) with other students multiple times and then added water to each cup. At the start, four students had the "STD" chemical, and by the end 16 students had the chemical, simulating how fast STDs spread.

The fear tactics only got worse in the following year. In class, we were shown very nasty pictures of STDs, and taught how hard it is to get rid of them, if they even could be rid of. Needless to say, nobody in that class ate lunch that day. After covering STDs, teachers then moved on to teen pregnancy. In this portion of the class, each student was given a mechanical baby to take care of for a week. The baby did everything a normal baby would do: cried, needed changing, needed feeding, woke up during the night, etc. Each student learned the hard way what having a baby entailed, and in turn, what having sex risked.

Physical Health

A teen pregnancy is the primary example of a life-changing negative outcome for the adolescents who experience it and for the children born to teen parents. Any teen may experience a pregnancy, although the probability of a pregnancy is greatly increased if the adolescent engages in risky sex that includes an early sexual debut, multiple partners, and inconsistent contraceptive use. There is no evidence that the majority of teens engage in this type of risky sexual behavior, or that risky sex is typical among most adolescents who are sexually active, however. In fact, the evidence is to the contrary.

The majority of adolescents today are more likely to use a condom, or some other form of birth control, when they have sex than ever before, as discussed in Chapter 9. As a consequence of the increase in responsible sexual behavior among adolescents, the percentage of teens who become pregnant and give birth is decreasing. In 2016, the birth rate was 20.3 births per 1,000 females between 15 and 19 years of age (Hamilton et al., 2017). The approximately 209,480 births to teens in 2016 is the lowest number of teen births in recent U.S. history (National Campaign to Prevent Teen and Unplanned Pregnancy, 2016). Thus, the evidence based on teen birth rates suggests that most sexually active adolescents are responsible users of contraceptives. Further, historical trends in teen pregnancy rates and birth rates indicate that adolescents can learn to be sexually responsible, and more of them have learned that lesson than ever before.

Another physical harm to teens brought on by sexual behavior is contracting an STI. In 2014, the U.S. rate of new cases of chlamydia, the most common STI tracked by the Centers for Disease Control and Prevention (2015) for 15- to 19-year-olds was 1,804.0 per 100,000, and the rate for 20- to 24-year-olds was 2,484.6 per 100,000. These rates are high relative to other age groups, but low on an absolute scale—1.8% of 15- to 19-year-olds and 2.5% of 20- to 24-year-olds contracted chlamydia during 2014 (Braxton et al., 2016). Rates for gonorrhea and syphilis among adolescents and emerging adults are considerably lower. Rates for HPV and herpes are relatively high and increasing, not only among teens and emerging adults but also among all age groups. The STI problem is a serious, growing problem in the United States and around the world among all age groups, especially among the young, and it should not be minimized or discounted when thinking about adolescent sexuality. The good news is that inconsistent condom use, which is the main cause of contracting an STI, is decreasing among adolescents and emerging adults.

It is a mistake to depict the risky sexual behavior that leads to a teen pregnancy or contracting an STI as characteristic of teen sexuality in general, or to use those problems as the primary impetus for research on adolescent sexuality. Focusing on those very real problems and on the patterns of risky sexual behavior associated with them unnecessarily limits our understanding of the place of sexuality in the lives of the millions of sexually active adolescents who engage in responsible sexual activity and do not experience a pregnancy or contract an STI.

Mental Health

The majority of adolescents and emerging adults have positive reactions to their first sexual experience and to casual sex (Heron et al., 2015; Snapp et al., 2015), although a sizable minority of teens, especially young females who have sex in a casual relationship, experience painful memories and negative emotions, such as regret and sadness. In addition, some adolescents, especially young girls, experience serious mental health problems, such as depression and even suicidal ideation, after their first sexual experience if that experience occurs too early, in a casual relationship, or for the wrong reasons, such as curiosity or peer pressure (Deutsch & Slutske, 2015; Kim, 2016; Mendle et al., 2013). Most sexually active adolescents do not experience short- or long-term psychological harm as a result of their sexual activity, however, especially if that sexual activity occurs in a romantic relationship during late adolescence or emerging adulthood (Meier, 2007).

Several studies in the United States and in other countries, such as Brazil, show that sexual initiation at an early age is sometimes associated with depressive symptoms and, more seriously, with a major depressive episode (Gonçalves et al., 2017; Vasilenko, 2017). The association between early sexual initiation and depression is especially strong for females who have sex before their 16th birthday. Cross-cultural research shows that sexual activity at an early age is not always related to poor psychological well-being, however. In one study of Dutch adolescents, early sexual behavior, including intercourse, was unrelated to later psychological well-being (Nogueira Avelar e Silva, van de Bongardt, Baams, & Raat, 2018). The authors suggest that cultural expectancies about the age when sexual intercourse will occur have an influence on the relationship between age of sexual debut and psychological adjustment. In the Netherlands, early sex is common, normalizing what in the United States and Brazil is viewed as problem behavior, revealing that early sex is not inevitably related to psychological adjustment problems.

For some young girls, sexual behavior may trigger emotional reactions these young teens are simply not psychologically equipped to handle, leading to feelings of depression and suicidality, most notably if the two people are not equally invested in the relationship, or when the relationship ends (Hallfors, Waller, Bauer, Ford, & Halpern, 2005). For other adolescents, however, mental health problems are precursors to sexual activity. Findings from longitudinal research suggest that depression is often present prior to first sex (Ethier et al., 2006; Monahan & Lee, 2008). A reciprocal relationship is also possible. Young, depressed girls may be especially vulnerable to sexual coercion from boys who show an interest in them, but then find that casual sex only compounds their unhappiness. Of course, it is also possible that some third variable, such as a poor parent–adolescent relationship, is responsible for both depression and early sexual activity, making sex a marker for depression, but not a cause of it.

Self-Esteem

What is the relationship between sexual activity during adolescence and self-esteem? It turns out there is no consistent relationship between sexual behavior, attitudes, or intentions and global, or overall self-esteem (Goodson, Buhi, & Dunsmore, 2006). Some research on adolescents demonstrates a positive relationship between number of sex partners and high self-esteem (Gentzler & Kerns, 2004), while other research finds a negative relationship between casual sex and self-esteem (Ethier et al., 2006; Fielder, Walsh, Carey, & Carey, 2013; van de Bongardt, Reitz, & Deković, 2016), and still other research finds no relationship between sexual behavior and self-esteem (Kerpelman, McElwain, Pittman, & Adler-Baeder, 2016; Owen et al., 2010). Casual sex is somewhat more likely to be related to high self-esteem among males, but even for males, a high number of sexual partners is not always associated with high self-esteem (Clark, 2006; Ramiro et al., 2013).

All this inconsistency suggests that the association between sexual activity and self-esteem is mediated by other variables. For example, casual sex may be associated with high self-esteem for an adolescent, especially a male, whose self-concept is partly based on his sexual success, while casual sex may be related to low self-esteem among teens who are reluctant participants in a sexual experience they do not want or do not feel ready for. Alternatively, sexual activity may be tied to specific feelings of sexual self-worth, and have little to do with feelings of global self-esteem during adolescence. Indeed, some research on teen girls indicates that sexual activity is related to high sexual self-esteem among girls who have positive beliefs about their sexual behavior, and for whom sex validates a concept of themselves as sexually attractive (Hensel et al., 2011).

Behavioral Problems

Adolescent sexual behavior is positively related to drinking alcohol, experimenting with drugs, delinquency, and poor grades in school, especially when it occurs in early adolescence (Floyd & Latimer, 2010; van Gelder, Reefhuis, Herron, Williams, & Roeleveid, 2011). Indeed, early adolescent sexual activity is part of a problem behavior syndrome that includes substance use, delinquency, and academic difficulties (Jessor, 2014). One must be careful about attributing these behavioral problems to adolescent sexual activity, however. These problems often exist prior to or coexist with sexual activity, rather than being a result of sexual behavior (Bingham & Crockett, 1996). The image of a well-functioning adolescent who becomes sexually active and then goes down a pathway that leads to substance use, delinquency, and poor school performance is not an accurate portrayal of the relationship between sex and problem

In the following example, a college student reflects on her sexual experience and the experiences of her friends, and concludes that involvement with alcohol and drugs preceded sexual activity.

IN THEIR OWN WORDS

For my particular group of friends, a few of them had sex for the first time in middle school. But for the majority, when we got to high school I would definitely say drinking came first, then sex, and then some drug use. I seriously believe that the fact that drinking was the first thing to happen for most of us has something to do with why sex came into the picture at all. A lot of sexual activity tends to happen while already horny teens are under the influence. Same goes for marijuana—high sex is highly preferable as well for some. I feel as though if you were having sex, you were most likely drinking and smoking weed too.

behaviors for most adolescents. Instead, adolescent problem behaviors, including risky sex, are often the result of a long history of poor relations with parents and associating with deviant peers (French & Dishion, 2003).

In Conclusion

The idea that sexual activity outside of marriage ruins lives is not true for the large majority of adolescents and emerging adults. Under some conditions, casual sexual behavior heightens the risk of physical, mental, and behavioral difficulties, especially for females who engage in casual sex at an early age. However, most adolescents and emerging adults do not experience any negative consequences as a result of their sexual activity. Further, when sexual behavior is related to mental health difficulties or behavioral problems the root causes of those difficulties often exist prior to or coexist with sexual activity (Donahue, Lichtenstein, Långström, & D'Onofrio, 2013). Sex is serious business and it should not be taken lightly, but millions of adolescents have safe, responsible sex and do not suffer any negative consequences. The claim that sex outside of marriage is likely to cause physical or psychological harm is simply not true.

■ REASONS FOR HAVING SEX

Why Do Adolescents Have Sex?

Some adolescents have sex for the wrong reasons, which is associated with negative emotional experiences. Three motives for having sex can be especially harmful for adolescents. First, many adolescents report that their first sexual encounter was primarily motivated by curiosity and a desire to experience what can seem like one of life's great mysteries to a sexually inexperienced adolescent (Paradise, Cote, Minsky, Lourenco, & Howland, 2001). Many emerging adults who have not had sex are also curious to experience an event they believe is

In the following story, one young woman writes about her first sexual experience, which was the result of curiosity and a belief that sex would bring her and her boyfriend closer together. The experience was not pleasant, nor did it improve her relationship with her boyfriend. Why do you think the experience ended so badly?

IN THEIR OWN WORDS

When I was 15 years old, I was the last of my friends to still have my virginity. I felt tremendous pressure to change that. Hearing about all my best friends' sexual encounters in the cafeteria at lunch made me envious; they had made it sound so exciting and romantic. Sure, I had fooled around with my boyfriend before, but we had never gone "all the way."

Finally, I had enough. I wanted to know what all the fuss was about, so one afternoon after school while I was hanging out with my boyfriend at the time, I decided it was time. We hadn't been together long, only about a month, and I was already having doubts about our relationship, so along with the curiosity I figured it would bring us closer together as a couple. When I suggested this to him, he was elated. He was a year older than I was, and had already lost his virginity to an ex-girlfriend; I don't think he lost his pants fast enough.

The whole experience was awkward. I wasn't really sure what to do. I kept focusing on trivial things: "What should I do with my hands?"; "Should I tell him he's doing a good job?"; "What if I get pregnant? Condoms aren't always 100% effective!" It was nerve-wracking. I couldn't focus and enjoy myself.

All of my friends also were talking about how good it feels, and honestly, I didn't feel anything. I'm not sure if it was the fact that my mind was racing, or halfway through I just wanted the whole experience to be done.

When it was finally over, all I wanted to do was go home and shower. Even though the whole thing was my idea, I couldn't shake the bad feelings I was having. I was angry at my friends, for lying to me and telling me sex was so amazing. I felt dirty, "slutty," since I had always told myself I was going to wait for marriage, and I hadn't, and most of all, I felt guilty. I had let down my parents—growing up I was taught to wait until marriage and in just a matter of minutes I had ruined that. There is no taking your virginity back.

I was also wrong about the idea that giving my ex-boyfriend my virginity would make our bond as a couple stronger. Just a few weeks later we had broken up, because instead of bringing us together, I feel like having sex pushed us apart. Thankfully, as I grew up and matured I found the "right partner"; I have found sex a more enjoyable experience and realized that maybe my friends weren't lying to me.

important and significant in life. Adolescents whose first sexual experience is motivated by curiosity often report that they later regret their experience and wish they had waited until they were older or for the right person to come along (Levinson, Jaccard, & Beamer, 1995).

A second unhealthy motive for having sex is the belief that sexual activity makes a person popular and attractive, especially to males. Many adolescent boys view sexual activity as a route to popularity among their male peers, while some females believe they will become more accepted by their peers if they are sexually active (Kreager & Staff, 2009). In addition, some females in romantic relationships believe that having sex with their boyfriend is necessary to keep the boyfriend in the relationship, a motive that can lead to regret and disappointment, especially if the relationship ends.

Peer pressure is a third unhealthy reason for having sex. The sexual experiences of most adolescents are typically voluntary, and occur in romantic relationships (Guttmacher Institute, 2016). Sometimes, however, sexual activity is the result of intimidation, coercion, or interpersonal pressure (Collibee & Furman, 2014). One 17-year-old girl from California described the explicit pressure her boyfriend put on her to have sex and on her later feelings about having sex with him:

> " . . . like he was my first sexual relationship. And I was like—I told him no but he kept telling me, 'Come on, come on, let's do it.' And like I guess—I guess I felt that pressure and I was like: Oh, my God. And I can't even say no. Like it was hard for me to say no. And like to this day I feel—I feel sad about it you know. I wish he wasn't the first guy. . . . I still feel like he shouldn't have been my first." (Suleiman & Deardorff, 2015, p. 770)

Many females experience interpersonal pressure to put their partner's desires above their own and have sex to please their boyfriend. Some males also report that their early sexual activity was at least partly due to pressure from

---

The following story illustrates the idea that having sex with a popular boy made this young woman feel prettier and increased her social status, all of which came crashing down when her relationship ended.

IN THEIR OWN WORDS

When he told me that I was beautiful in 11th grade, I believed him. Until that point, I'd always doubted it. I was never convinced by the idea. He was an attractive, popular boy in school with all of the latest clothes, and friends in the highest social group. Of all of the girls in our grade, he'd chosen me. Well, sort of. He also had a girlfriend that lived in another state. I fought the idea of a relationship with him at first, but soon his infatuation with me was reciprocated. I soon expected his presence. I knew that he would walk me to class every day and that we would go home after school together. We had a routine, and I liked it. I gained friends in his peer group—people that I would not have talked to before, as they were more popular than I was. Things went well for a while, until the day that he broke up with his girlfriend. After 2 years of a relationship with her, he was excited to have his freedom, leaving our pseudo-relationship hanging in the balance.

Drastically, our relationship changed. He always sat with me before school started, but he stopped. I'd leave sixth period, expecting to see him at my locker, but he wasn't there. I didn't receive text messages from him after his baseball practice anymore. After a week of this I began to understand that he and I were no longer. There was no closure, and no discussion of how I felt. I simply turned inward, blaming myself and citing my carelessness as the reason for this situation.

In dating X, I gained a new group of peers, who occupied a higher social position. Many of the athletes and popular girls became acquaintances of mine. My initial reason for agreeing to date X was because of his impact on my perception of self-worth and attractiveness. His words impacted those aspects of my self-evaluation the most, so his absence precipitated feelings of diminished beauty.

male peers to have sex. Peer pressure can subvert the personal desires of both females and males, and lead adolescents down a pathway they later wish they had not followed.

Some adolescents have sex for the wrong reasons and many of those adolescents, especially girls, experience regret and depression afterward. This is an important finding that could be of great value to many adolescents who are only dimly aware of their motives for having sex and end up regretting the decision they make. A good sex education program might allow adolescents to explore their reasons for wanting to have sex, which may help them avoid sex tied to unhealthy motives likely to lead to regret and disappointment.

■ ADOLESCENTS AND RESPONSIBLE SEXUAL BEHAVIOR

One common justification for why teens should remain sexually abstinent is that adolescents are cognitively, emotionally, and socially immature—too young to control their own sexual impulses and incapable of managing the powerful emotions associated with sexual activity. Adolescents are seen as the victims of their own age, incapable of engaging in responsible sexual behavior, and recklessly acting on their impulses and making bad decisions. There certainly is some validity to this idea, especially for teens who are young and cognitively or emotionally immature, but it is more difficult to apply this idea of immaturity to older adolescents and emerging adults. The idea that adolescents should not engage in sex because they are immature and irresponsible underestimates the ability of youth, especially older adolescents and emerging adults, to make mature decisions about their sexual behavior and to act responsibly.

Three lines of evidence point to the conclusion that most adolescents are capable of managing their sexual emotions and acting sexually responsible. First, the evidence on condom use among adolescents, discussed in Chapter 10, reveals that about 60% of U.S. teens report they used a condom the last time they had sexual intercourse, and an additional 15% indicate that they used some form of birth control. Data on condom usage in the United States indicate that teens will use condoms, given the right education at home and school and the availability of condoms (Fortenberry et al., 2010).

A second line of evidence that adolescents are capable of sexual responsibility is the increase in the use of condoms and other forms of birth control that has occurred over the past several decades in the United States. Only a minority of adolescents used some form of contraception the last time they had intercourse in the early 1980s and before, compared to a majority of adolescents who used some form of contraception the last time they had intercourse in the mid-2000s and beyond (Kann, McManus, et al., 2016). The message that condoms prevent pregnancies and protect against acquiring an STI, a message that is fundamental in comprehensive sex education courses is having an increasing effect on adolescents.

Third, cross-cultural research demonstrates that adolescents can be taught to act sexually responsible. One of the most impressive examples of teen sexual responsibility is the Netherlands, where over 90% of adolescents as young as 15 years of age report using some form of contraception the last time they had sexual intercourse, indicating that even young adolescents can act sexually responsible if they are given the message at home and school to practice safer sex, and if contraceptives are easily available (Godeau et al., 2008). All of these findings point to the conclusion that adolescents are not intrinsically sexually irresponsible. Instead, the evidence on contraception use reveals that sexual responsibility can be taught and that adolescents are capable of acting in a sexually prudent manner.

■ A SEX-POSITIVE APPROACH TO ADOLESCENT SEXUALITY

Recently, some social scientists have challenged the disease model of adolescent sexuality and proposed that sex is a natural part of development for most adolescents and may even contribute to psychological growth and social maturity (Diamond, 2014; Harden, 2014b). A sexual health approach to the study of adolescent sexuality has been referred to as a "sex-positive" or "sexual well-being" framework and includes several points (Fortenberry, 2016; Harden, 2014b). First, for many, if not most, adolescents, sex is not associated with negative experiences but is a normal developmental occurrence advanced by puberty and reflective of larger processes that include the development of autonomy from parents, an orientation toward peers, and the establishment of a romantic relationship. Second, abstinence is not the only form of healthy, responsible sexual behavior for adolescents. The opposite of abstinence is not necessarily risky sex but can be safe, responsible sex based on good decision making and reliable use of contraception. Third, research on adolescent sexuality needs to focus not only on possible negative consequences but also on how sex might contribute to positive development, including personal growth and interpersonal intimacy. Fourth, research on adolescent sexuality needs to move beyond only examining contrasting "good/bad" dichotomies—such as virgin/nonvirgin, non-STI/STI, and nonpregnant/pregnant—to studies of variation in sexuality among the majority of adolescents who do not experience problems related to their sexual behavior.

A sex-positive approach to teen sex can be traced back to the sex-positive movement articulated by Wilhelm Reich as early as 1945, who argued that sexual abstinence during adolescence mainly serves to repress what is natural and normal. Reich and his followers accepted sexual pleasure and experimentation as long as it is safe and consensual (Reich, 1986). Sex positivity is contrasted with antisexualism, or sex negativity, which emphasizes the idea that the only acceptable form of sexual expression is between married heterosexuals and that all other forms of sexual expression are wrong and immoral.

Some health educators have called for an approach to sex education that emphasizes sexual health in contrast to both abstinence sex education, which stresses abstaining from all sexual activity until marriage, and safer-sex education that narrowly focuses on the prevention of pregnancies and STIs through the use of condoms (Cameron-Lewis & Allen, 2013; Rohrbach et al., 2015). A sex education program based on a sexual health model portrays sexual behavior as a normal part of growing up and addresses issues such as understanding and accepting one's own sexual desires, developing a personal ethic to guide sexual behavior, giving and getting sexual consent, negotiating contraceptive use, setting and respecting boundaries, and coping with relationship issues (Arbeit, 2014; McFarland & Williams, 2016).

Is Sex Good for Adolescents?

Recent research on adolescents' reactions to their first sexual experience illustrates the difference between a traditional approach to the study of adolescent sexuality that focuses on negative reactions to sexual behavior and a sex-positive approach. Consider reactions to first sexual experience. One consistent finding in the literature is that more young females have negative reactions to their first sexual experience than do young males. For example, college women are more likely to report that their first sexual experience left them feeling unsatisfied, disappointed, guilty, and regretful in comparison to the experiences of young men (Sprecher, 2014). In contrast to an approach that focuses on gender differences in negative reactions to first sexual experiences, a sex-positive approach focuses on factors related to positive reactions to first sexual experiences for each gender. Such an approach reveals that many young women have positive first sexual experiences, especially when the experience is planned, occurs in a long-term relationship, takes place when the adolescents are older, and includes the use of contraception (Smiler, Ward, Caruthers, & Merriwether, 2005). Many of these same findings are echoed in the accounts of young men who report that their first sexual experience was positive when it was planned, in a long-term relationship, and included the use of protection. Sex need not be a negative experience, even for young women, but can be a positive experience, especially when sex occurs between two adolescents who act responsibly and are in a long-term romantic relationship.

One factor highly related to having a positive sexual debut is the age of the adolescent. For example, results from one study reveal that adolescents who have sexual intercourse around the 12th grade, or after graduation from high school, report few psychological problems (Golden, Furman, & Collibee, 2016). In contrast, adolescents with an early sexual debut before the 10th grade report more depression, anxiety, externalizing behaviors, substance use, and lower global self-worth. The findings show the advantages of late-occurring sexual intercourse, which can be related to good mental health, and the disadvantages of early intercourse. Other research also finds that having first sex later rather than earlier is associated with good psychological adjustment, especially for girls (Vasilenko, 2017; Vrangalova & Savin-Williams, 2011). What these studies demonstrate is that positive adjustment during late adolescence is not confined to adolescents who are sexually abstinent, but also includes sexually active adolescents who decide to wait until late adolescence to have sex.

Results from another study of girls between ages 14 and 17 years reveal that sex in a satisfying romantic relationship, in comparison to casual sex, is associated with few depressive symptoms, less frequent alcohol and marijuana use, and low delinquency (Hensel, Nance, & Fortenberry, 2016). Findings from this study demonstrate the importance of a good romantic relationship as a context for healthy sexual activity. Most sexually active girls in this type of relationship are well-adjusted and avoid risky, unhealthy behaviors, in general.

Other findings indicate that the quality of the parent–adolescent relationship is associated with the quality of adolescent sexual behavior. Adolescents with parents who are emotionally supportive are more likely to have sexual experiences that are satisfying, safer, and occur within a romantic relationship, while teens who perceive their parents to be unsupportive are more likely to have sex that is unsatisfactory and occurs in a casual relationship (Parkes, Henderson, Wight, & Nixon, 2011). Thus, an emotionally supportive parent–adolescent relationship not only protects teens from involvement in risky, dangerous behaviors such as substance use and delinquency but is also a context for a safe, high-quality sexual relationship.

Another study of the parent–adolescent relationship examines the association between parent emotional support and the sexual activity and psychosocial adjustment of LGB youth. Results reveal that lesbian and bisexual girls with emotionally supportive parents are more likely to be sexually active, have lower levels of depression, and lower internalized homophobia than lesbian and bisexual girls with unsupportive parents (Dickenson & Huebner, 2016). Unexpectedly, the pattern of these results was not found for sexual-minority males. Thus, parent emotional support is related to sexual exploration and psychosexual health among lesbian and bisexual girls, but may be less essential for the psychosocial adjustment of gay and bisexual males.

Other research reveals that among heterosexual adults there is a strong association between the frequency and quality of sexual intercourse, especially when it occurs in a long-term relationship, and better mental and physical health (Brody, 2010; Schmiedeberg, Huyer-May, Castiglioni, & Johnson, 2017). Of course, it is not possible to generalize from adults to adolescents, but the findings for adults indicate that a link exists between sexuality and health, a link that may first appear during emerging adulthood (Vasilenko, Lefkowitz, & Maggs, 2012).

In conclusion, it is too early to identify the conditions under which sexual behavior might be a positive experience for adolescents or lead to positive development, but the results from studies thus far suggest some tentative conclusions. First, positive sexual experiences generally are not spontaneous or risky but are planned, take place in a long-term romantic relationship, and include the use of some form of protection. Second, positive sexual experiences are more likely to occur during late adolescence or emerging adulthood, and are less common in early adolescence. Third, positive sexual experiences are associated with a supportive parent–adolescent relationship. These tentative findings indicate that adolescents, especially older adolescents who have good relations with their parents, are capable of making good decisions about their sexuality, which is associated with positive sexual experiences and psychological health.

The experience of sexuality during adolescence is a natural part of growing up for millions of adolescents. For the majority of teens, sexuality is part of a normal developmental process that is transformed by puberty, endorsed by peers, and practiced in a social context that typically emerges from friendship and romance. It is important to continue to attempt to understand the causes of the very real problems some adolescents have as a result of their sexual behavior in order to develop interventions that might prevent or alleviate those difficulties, but it is important to also examine the developmental significance of the usual sexual behavior of adolescents who practice safer sex and are not negatively affected by their sexual activity.

SUMMARY

■ THE TRADITIONAL VIEW OF ADOLESCENT SEXUALITY

Thinking about adolescent sexuality by sex educators, health professionals, policymakers, and researchers has focused on sex as a dangerous activity, emphasizing teen pregnancy and contracting an STI. Although these are very real problems, a narrow focus on the dark side of adolescent sexuality has limited our understanding of teen sex, and ignores sex as normative experience that is not associated with negative outcomes for millions of adolescents.

■ SEX AND ADOLESCENT HEALTH

Sex during adolescence can lead to a pregnancy or an STI for some adolescents. Further, risky sex is related to adolescent mental health difficulties, such as depression and behavioral problems, including substance use and delinquency for some teens. These problems are not usually the result of sexual activity, however, but have their origins in poor parent–child relations and associating with deviant peers. Many teens, especially older adolescents, are capable of making mature judgments about their sexual activity, avoiding the problems that can be associated with risky teen sexuality.

■ REASONS FOR HAVING SEX

Several unhealthy reasons for having sex have been identified that are associated with negative emotional outcomes. Having sex because one is curious about the experience can lead to regret later on. Another unhealthy reason for having sex is the belief that it will lead to popularity and an increase in attractiveness, especially to males. Peer pressure can also lead to a sexual experience that is disappointing and unfulfilling.

◾ ADOLESCENCE AND RESPONSIBLE SEXUAL BEHAVIOR

Many people believe that adolescents are immature and unable to control their sexual impulses. Three lines of evidence suggest that adolescents can make responsible decisions about their sexual behavior. First, the majority of adolescents currently use some form of birth control when they have sex, a percentage that should increase with better sex education and easy access to condoms. Second, adolescents have been learning the importance of using condoms when they have sex, and more than ever before they are using them. Third, cross-cultural evidence shows that even young adolescents can be taught to use condoms when they have sexual intercourse.

◾ A SEX-POSITIVE APPROACH TO ADOLESCENT SEXUALITY

Another paradigm called a "sex-positive," or "sexual well-being" approach to adolescent sexuality has emerged recently that focuses on sexual activity as a normal part of adolescent development with potentially positive consequences for teens. Several tentative conclusions emerge from this framework. Positive sexual behavior generally follows from sexual experiences that are planned, occur in a romantic relationship, and include the use of contraception. In addition, positive sexual experiences are more common when they occur during late adolescence in the context of supportive relations with parents.

SUGGESTIONS FOR FURTHER READING

Diamond, L. M. (2014). Expanding the scope of a dynamic perspective on positive adolescent sexual development. *Human Development, 57,* 292–304.

Goodson, P., Buhi, E. R., & Dunsmore, S. C. (2006). Self-esteem and adolescent sexual behaviors, attitudes, and intentions: A systematic review. *Journal of Adolescent Health, 38,* 310–319.

Harden, K. P. (2014b). A sex-positive framework for research on adolescent sexuality. *Perspectives on Psychological Science, 9,* 455–469.

Tolman, D. L., & McClelland, S. I. (2011). Normative sexuality development in adolescence: A decade in review, 2000–2009. *Journal of Research on Adolescence, 21,* 242–255.

References

Abbott, D. A., & Dalla, R. L. (2008). "It's a choice, simple as that": Youth reasoning for sexual abstinence or activity. *Journal of Youth Studies, 11,* 629–649.

Abma, J. C., & Sonenstein, F. L. (2001). Sexual activity and contraceptive practices among teenagers in the United States, 1988 and 1995. *Vital Health Statistics, 21,* 1–79.

Abreu, A. P., Dauber, A., Macedo, D. B., Noel, S. D., Brito, V. N., Gill, J. C., et al. (2013). Central precocious puberty caused by mutations in the imprinted gene *MKRN3. New England Journal of Medicine, 368,* 2467–2475.

Abreu, R. L., & Kenny, M. C. (2018). Cyberbullying and LGBTQ youth: A systematic literature review and recommendations for prevention and intervention. *Journal of Child and Adolescent Trauma, 11,* 81–97.

Adshade, M. (2013). *Dollars and sex: How economics influences sex and love.* San Francisco: Chronicle Books.

Ajilore, O. (2015). Identifying peer effects using spatial analysis: The role of peers on risky sexual behavior. *Review of Economics of the Household, 13,* 635–652.

Ajzen, I. (2012). The theory of planned behavior. In P. A. M. Van Lange, A. W. Kruglanski, & E. T. Higgins (Eds.), *Handbook of theories of social psychology* (Vol. 1, pp. 438–459). London: SAGE.

Akers, A. Y., Holland, C. L., & Bost, J. (2011). Interventions to improve parental communication about sex: A systematic review. *Pediatrics, 127,* 494–510.

Akinbami, L. J., Cheng, T. L., & Kornfeld, D. (2001). A review of teen–tot programs: Comprehensive clinical care for young parents and their children. *Adolescence, 36,* 381–393.

Albarracin, D., Johnson, B. T., Fishbein, M., & Muellerleile, P. A. (2001). Theories of reasoned action and planned behavior as models of condom use: A meta-analysis. *Psychological Bulletin, 127,* 142–161.

Albert, B. (2012, August). *With One Voice 2012: Highlights from a survey of teens and adults about teen pregnancy and related issues.* Washington, DC: National Campaign to Prevent Teen and Unplanned Pregnancy. Retrieved July 10, 2016, from *http://thenationalcampaign.org/resource/one-voice-2012.*

Alexander, M. G., & Fisher, T. D. (2003). Truth and consequences: Using the bogus pipeline to examine sex differences in self-reported sexuality. *Journal of Sex Research, 40,* 27–35.

Ali, M. M., & Dwyer, D. S. (2011). Estimating peer effects in sexual behavior among adolescents. *Journal of Adolescence, 34,* 183–190.

Allard-Hendren, R. (2000). Alcohol use and adolescent pregnancy. *MCN: American Journal of Maternal Child Nursing, 25,* 159–162.

Allison, R., & Risman, B. J. (2013). A double standard for "hooking up": How far have we come toward gender equality? *Social Science Research, 42,* 1191–1206.

Almeida, J., Johnson, R. M., Corliss, H. L., Molnar, B. E., & Azrael, D. (2009). Emotional distress among LGBT youth: The influence of perceived discrimination based on sexual orientation. *Journal of Youth and Adolescence, 38,* 1001–1014.

Amato, P. R., & Kane, J. B. (2011). Parents' marital distress, divorce, and remarriage: Links with daughters' early family formation transitions. *Journal of Family Issues, 32,* 1073–1103.

Amu, E. O., & Adegun, P. T. (2015). Awareness and knowledge of sexually transmitted infections among secondary school adolescents in Ado Ekiti, South Western Nigeria. *Journal of Sexually Transmitted Diseases, 2015,* 260126.

Anatale, K., & Kelly, S. (2015). Factors influencing adolescent girls' sexual behavior: A secondary analysis of the 2011 Youth Risk Behavior Survey. *Issues in Mental Health Nursing, 36,* 217–221.

Arbeit, M. R. (2014). What does healthy sex look like among youth?: Towards a skills-based model for promoting adolescent sexuality development. *Human Development, 57,* 259–286.

Armstrong, E. A., England, P., & Fogarty, A. C. (2012). Accounting for women's orgasm and sexual enjoyment in college hook-ups and relationships. *American Sociological Review, 77,* 435–462.

Arnarsson, A., Sveinbjornsdottir, S., Thorsteinsson, E. B., & Bjarnason, T. (2015). Suicidal risk and sexual orientation in adolescence: A population-based study in Iceland. *Scandinavian Journal of Public Health, 43,* 497–505.

Arrington-Sanders, R., Harper, G. W., Morgan, A., Ogunbajo, A., Trent, M., & Fortenberry, J. D. (2015). The role of sexually explicit material in the sexual development of same-sex-attracted black adolescent males. *Archives of Sexual Behavior, 44,* 597–608.

Ashenhurst, J. R., Wilhite, E. R., Harden, K. P., & Fromme, K. (2017). Number of sexual partners and relationship status are associated with unprotected sex across emerging

adulthood. *Archives of Sexual Behavior, 46,* 419–432.

Aspy, C. B., Vesely, S. K., Oman, R. F., Rodine, S., Marshall, L., & McLeroy, K. (2007). Parental communication and youth sexual behaviour. *Journal of Adolescence, 30,* 449–466.

Assini-Meytin, L. C., & Green, K. M. (2015). Long-term consequences of adolescent parenthood among African-American urban youth: A propensity score matching approach. *Journal of Adolescent Health, 56,* 529–535.

Astone, N. M., & McLanahan, S. (1994). Family structure, residential mobility, and school report: A research note. *Demography, 31,* 575–584.

Atienzo, E. E., Campero, L., Herrera, C., & Lozada, A. L. (2015). Family formation expectations and early pregnancy in Mexican adolescents. *Journal of Child and Family Studies, 24,* 2509–2520.

Atienzo, E. E., Ortiz-Panozo, E., & Campero, L. (2015). Congruence in reported frequency of parent–adolescent sexual health communication: A study from Mexico. *International Journal of Adolescent Medicine and Health, 27,* 275–283.

Aubrey, J. S., Harrison, K., Kramer, L., & Yellin, J. (2003). Variety versus timing: Gender differences in college students' sexual expectations as predicted by exposure to sexually oriented television. *Communication Research, 30,* 432–460.

Augustine, J. M., Nelson, T. J., & Edin, K. (2009). Why do poor men have children?: Fertility intentions among low-income unmarried U.S. fathers. *Annals of the American Academy of Political and Social Science, 626,* 99–117.

Auslander, B. A., Biro, F. M., Succop, P. A., Short, M. B., & Rosenthal, S. L. (2009). Racial/ethnic differences in patterns of sexual behavior and STI risk among sexually experienced adolescent girls. *Journal of Pediatric and Adolescent Gynecology, 22,* 33–39.

Averett, P., Moore, A., & Price, L. (2014). Virginity definitions and meaning among the LGBT community. *Journal of Gay and Lesbian Social Services, 26,* 259–278.

Ayalew, M., Mengistie, B., & Semahegn, A.

(2014). Adolescent–parent communication on sexual and reproductive health issues among high school students in Dire Dawa, Eastern Ethiopia: A cross sectional study. *Reproductive Health, 11,* 77.

Baams, L., Bos, H. M. W., & Jonas, K. J. (2014). How a romantic relationship can protect same-sex attracted youth and young adults from the impact of expected rejection. *Journal of Adolescence, 37,* 1293–1302.

Baams, L., Dubas, J. S., Overbeek, G., & van Aken, M. A. (2015). Transitions in body and behavior: A meta-analytic study on the relationship between pubertal development and adolescent sexual behavior. *Journal of Adolescent Health, 56,* 586–598.

Baams, L., Overbeek, G., Dubas, J. S., Doornwaard, S. M., Rommes, E., & van Aken, M. A. (2015). Perceived realism moderates the relation between sexualized media consumption and permissive sexual attitudes in Dutch adolescents. *Archives of Sexual Behavior, 44,* 743–754.

Baams, L., Overbeek, G., van de Bongardt, D., Reitz, E., Dubas, J. S., & van Aken, M. A. (2015). Adolescents' and their friends' sexual behavior and intention: Selection effects of personality dimensions. *Journal of Research in Personality, 54,* 2–12.

Bachanas, P. J., Morris, M. K., Lewis-Gess, J. K., Sarett-Cuasay, E. J., Sirl, K., Ries, J. K., et al. (2002). Predictors of risky sexual behavior in African American adolescent girls: Implications for prevention interventions. *Journal of Pediatric Psychology, 27,* 519–530.

Balter, A. S., van Rhijn, T. M., & Davies, A. W. J. (2016). The development of sexuality in childhood in early learning settings: An exploration of early childhood educators' perceptions. *Canadian Journal of Human Sexuality, 25,* 30–40.

Bámaca-Colbert, M. Y., Greene, K. M., Killoren, S. E., & Noah, A. J. (2014). Contextual and developmental predictors of sexual initiation timing among Mexican-origin girls. *Developmental Psychology, 50,* 2353–2359.

Bankole, A., Biddlecom, A., Guiella, G., & Singh, S. (2007). Sexual behavior, knowledge and information sources of very young adolescents in four sub-Saharan African countries. *African Journal of Reproductive Health, 11,* 28–43.

Barczyk, A. N., Duzinski, S. V., Brown, J. M., & Lawson, K. A. (2015). Perceptions of injury prevention and familial adjustment among mothers of teen parents. *Journal of Safety Research, 52,* 15–21.

Barr, A. B., Simons, R. L., Simons, L. G., Gibbons, F. X., & Gerrard, M. (2013). Teen motherhood and pregnancy prototypes: The role of social context in changing young African American mothers' risk images and contraceptive expectations. *Journal of Youth and Adolescence, 42,* 1884–1897.

Batchelor, S. A., Kitzinger, J., & Burtney, E. (2004). Representing young people's sexuality in the "youth" media. *Health Education Research: Theory and Practice, 19,* 669–676.

Bauermeister, J. A., Zimmerman, M. A., & Caldwell, C. H. (2011). Neighborhood disadvantage and changes in condom use among African American adolescents. *Journal of Urban Health, 88,* 66–83.

Baumeister, R. F., Catanese, K. R., & Vohs, K. D. (2001). Is there a gender difference in strength of sex drive?: Theoretical views, conceptual distinctions, and a review of relevant evidence. *Personality and Social Psychology Review, 5,* 242–273.

Bayatpour, M., Wells, R. D., & Holford, S. (1992). Physical and sexual abuse as predictors of substance use and suicide among pregnant teenagers. *Journal of Adolescent Health, 13,* 128–132.

Bearman, P. S., & Brückner, H. (2001). Promising the future: Virginity pledges and first intercourse. *American Journal of Sociology, 106,* 859–912.

Beers, L. A. S., & Hollo, R. E. (2009). Approaching the adolescent-headed family: A review of teen parenting. *Current Problems in Pediatric and Adolescent Health Care, 39,* 216–233.

Bell, D. L., Rosenberger, J. G., & Ott, M. A. (2015). Masculinity in adolescent males' early romantic and sexual heterosexual relationships. *American Journal of Men's Health, 9,* 201–208.

Belsky, J., Schlomer, G. L., & Ellis, B. J. (2012). Beyond cumulative risk: Distinguishing harshness and unpredictability as determinants of parenting and early life history strategy. *Developmental Psychology, 48,* 662–673.

Belsky, J., Steinberg, L., & Draper, P. (1991). Childhood experience, interpersonal development, and reproductive strategy: An evolutionary theory of socialization. *Child Development, 62,* 647–670.

Belsky, J., Steinberg, L., Houts, R. M., Friedman, S. L., DeHart, G., Cauffman, E., et al. (2007). Family rearing antecedents of pubertal timing. *Child Development, 78,* 1302–1321.

Belsky, J., Steinberg, L., Houts, R. M., & Halpern-Felsher, B. L. (2010). The development of reproductive strategy in females: Early maternal harshness → earlier menarche → increased sexual risk taking. *Developmental Psychology, 46,* 120–128.

Bennett, S. E., & Assefi, N. P. (2005). School-based teenage pregnancy prevention programs: A systematic review of randomized controlled trials. *Journal of Adolescent Health, 36,* 72–81.

Bergström, M., Fransson, E., Modin, B., Berlin, M., Gustafsson, P. A., & Hjern, A. (2015). Fifty moves a year: Is there an association between joint physical custody and psychosomatic problems in children? *Journal of Epidemiology and Community Health, 69,* 769–774.

Bermudez, M. P., Castro, A., & Buela-Casal, G. (2011). Psychosocial correlates of condom use and their relationship with worry about STI and HIV in native and immigrant adolescents in Spain. *Spanish Journal of Psychology, 14,* 746–754.

Berndt, T. J. (1996). Transitions in friendship and friends' influence. In J. A. Graber, J. Brooks-Gunn, & A. C. Petersen (Eds.), *Transitions through adolescence: Interpersonal domains and context* (pp. 57–84). Mahwah, NJ: Erlbaum.

Bersamin, M. M., Walker, S., Fisher, D. A., & Grube, J. W. (2006). Correlates of oral sex and vaginal intercourse in early and middle adolescence. *Journal of Research on Adolescence, 16,* 59–68.

Bersamin, M. M., Walker, S., Waiters, E. D., Fisher, D. A., & Grube, J. W. (2005). Promising to wait: Virginity pledges and adolescent sexual behavior. *Journal of Adolescent Health, 36,* 428–436.

Bersamin, M. M., Zamboanga, B. L., Schwartz, S. J., Donnellan, M. B., Hudson, M., Weisskirch, R. S., et al. (2014). Risky business: Is there an association between casual sex and mental health among emerging adults? *Journal of Sex Research, 51,* 43–51.

Bhana, D. (2016). Virginity and virtue: African masculinities and femininities in the making of teenage sexual cultures. *Sexualities, 19,* 465–481.

Biblarz, T. J., & Stacey, J. (2010). How does the gender of parents matter? *Journal of Marriage and the Family, 72,* 3–22.

Billy, J. O. G., Brewster, K. L., & Grady, W. R. (1994). Contextual effects on the sexual behavior of adolescent women. *Journal of Marriage and the Family, 56,* 387–404.

Bingham, C. R., & Crockett, L. J. (1996). Longitudinal adjustment patterns of boys and girls experiencing early, middle, and late sexual intercourse. *Developmental Psychology, 32,* 647–658.

Birkett, M., Espelage, D. L., & Koenig, B. (2009). LGB and questioning students in schools: The moderating effects of homophobic bullying and school climate on negative outcomes. *Journal of Youth and Adolescence, 38,* 989–1000.

Birkett, M., Newcomb, M. E., & Mustanski, B. (2015). Does it get better?: A longitudinal analysis of psychological distress and victimization in lesbian, gay, bisexual, transgender, and questioning youth. *Journal of Adolescent Health, 56,* 280–285.

Birkett, M., Russell, S. T., & Corliss, H. L. (2014). Sexual-orientation disparities in school: The mediational role of indicators of victimization in achievement and truancy because of feeling unsafe. *American Journal of Public Health, 104,* 1124–1128.

Bisson, M. A., & Levine, T. R. (2009). Negotiating a friends with benefits relationship. *Archives of Sexual Behavior, 38,* 66–73.

Black, M. M., Ricardo, I. B., & Stanton, B. (1997). Social and psychological factors associated with AIDS risk behaviors among low-income, urban, African American adolescents. *Journal of Research on Adolescence, 7,* 173–195.

Blake, S. M., Ledsky, R., Goodenow, C., Sawyer, R., Lohrmann, D., & Windsor, R. (2003). Condom availability programs in Massachusetts high schools: Relationships with condom use and sexual behavior. *American Journal of Public Health, 93,* 955–962.

Blank, H. (2007). *Virgin: The untouched history.* New York: Bloomsbury.

Bleakley, A., Hennessy, M., & Fishbein, M. (2011). A model of adolescents' seeking of sexual content in their media choices. *Journal of Sex Research, 48,* 309–315.

Bleakley, A., Hennessy, M., Fishbein, M., & Jordan, A. (2009). How sources of sexual information relate to adolescents' beliefs about sex. *American Journal of Health Behavior, 33,* 37–48.

Bleakley, A., Hennessy, M., Fishbein, M., & Jordan, A. (2011). Using the integrative model to explain how exposure to sexual media content influences adolescent sexual behavior. *Health Education and Behavior, 38,* S30–S40.

Bleakley, A., Romer, D., & Jamieson, P. E. (2014). Violent film characters' portrayal of alcohol, sex, and tobacco-related behaviors. *Pediatrics, 133,* 71–77.

Boden, J. M., Fergusson, D. M., & Horwood, L. J. (2008). Early motherhood and subsequent life outcomes. *Journal of Child Psychology and Psychiatry, 49,* 151–160.

Bogle, K. A. (2008). *Hooking up: Sex, dating, and relationships on campus.* New York: NYU Press.

Boislard, M.-A. P., Dussault, F., Brendgen, M., & Vitaro, F. (2013). Internalizing and externalizing behaviors as predictors of sexual onset in early adolescence. *Journal of Early Adolescence, 33,* 920–945.

Boislard, M.-A. P., Poulin, F., Kiesner, J., & Dishion, T. J. (2009). A longitudinal examination of risky sexual behaviors among Canadian and Italian adolescents: Considering individual, parental, and friend characteristics. *International Journal of Behavioral Development, 33,* 265–276.

Bond, B. J. (2015). The mediating role of self-discrepancies in the relationship between media exposure and well-being among lesbian, gay, and bisexual adolescents. *Media Psychology, 18,* 51–73.

Bontempo, D. E., & D'Augelli, A. R. (2002). Effects of at-school victimization and sexual orientation on lesbian, gay, bisexual youths' health risk behavior. *Journal of Adolescent Health, 30,* 364–374.

Boonstra, H. D. (2014, Summer). What is behind the declines in teen pregnancy rates? *Guttmacher Policy Review, 17.* Retrieved July 24, 2016, from *www.guttmacher.org/sites/default/files/article_files/gpr170315.pdf.*

Bordini, G. S., & Sperb, T. M. (2013). Sexual double standard: A review of the literature between 2001 and 2010. *Sexuality and Culture, 17,* 686–704.

Borgia, P., Marinacci, C., Schifano, P., & Perucci, C. A. (2005). Is peer education the best approach for HIV prevention in schools?: Findings from a randomized controlled trial. *Journal of Adolescent Health, 36,* 508–516.

Bos, H. M. W., Sandfort, T. G. M., de Bruyn, E. H., & Hakvoort, E. M. (2008). Same-sex attraction, social relationships, psychosocial functioning, and school performance in early adolescence. *Developmental Psychology, 44,* 59–68.

Bos, H., van Beusekom, G., & Sandfort, T. (2016). Drinking motives, alcohol use, and sexual attraction in youth. *Journal of Sex Research, 53,* 309–312.

Bostwick, W. B., Meyer, I., Aranda, F., Russell, S., Hughes, T., Birkett, M., et al. (2014). Mental health and suicidality among racially/ethnically diverse sexual minority youths. *American Journal of Public Health, 104,* 1129–1136.

Bouris, A., Guilamo-Ramos, V., Jaccard, J., Ballan, M., Lesesne, C. A., & Gonzalez, B. (2012). Early adolescent romantic relationships and maternal approval among inner city Latino families. *AIDS and Behavior, 16,* 1570–1583.

Braithwaite, S. R., Coulson, G., Keddington, K., & Fincham, F. D. (2015). The influence of pornography on sexual scripts and hooking up among emerging adults in college. *Archives of Sexual Behavior, 44,* 111–123.

Braje, S. E., Eddy, J. M., & Hall, G. C. N. (2016). A comparison of two models of risky sexual behavior during late adolescence. *Archives of Sexual Behavior, 45,* 73–83.

Braun-Courville, D. K., & Rojas, M. (2009). Exposure to sexually explicit web sites and adolescent sexual attitudes and behaviors. *Journal of Adolescent Health, 45,* 156–162.

Brawner, B. M., Gomes, M. M., Jemmott, L. S., Deatrick, J. A., & Coleman, C. L. (2012). Clinical depression and HIV risk-related sexual behaviors among African-American adolescent females: Unmasking the numbers. *AIDS Care, 24,* 618–625.

Braxton, J., Carey, D., Davis, D., Flagg, E., Footman, A., & Grier, L., et al. (2016). *Sexually transmitted disease surveillance 2015.* Atlanta, GA: Centers for Disease Control and Prevention. Retrieved November 2, 2016, from *www.cdc.gov/std/stats15/std-surveillance-2015-print.pdf.*

Brechwald, W. A., & Prinstein, M. J. (2011). Beyond homophily: A decade of advances in understanding peer influence processes. *Journal of Research on Adolescence, 21,* 166–179.

Brewster, K. L., & Tillman, K. H. (2008). Who's doing it?: Patterns and predictors of youths' oral sexual experiences. *Journal of Adolescent Health, 42,* 73–80.

Brinkley, D. Y., Ackerman, R. A., Ehrenreich, S. E., & Underwood, M. K. (2017). Sending and receiving text messages with sexual content: Relations with early sexual activity and borderline personality features in late adolescence. *Computers in Human Behavior, 70,* 119–130.

Brody, S. (2010). The relative health benefits of different sexual activities. *Journal of Sexual Medicine, 7,* 1336–1361.

Bronfenbrenner, U. (1979). *The ecology of human development.* Cambridge, MA: Harvard University Press.

Brook, D. W., Morojele, N. K., Zhang, C., & Brook, J. S. (2006). South African adolescents: Pathways to risky sexual behavior. *AIDS Education and Prevention, 18,* 259–272.

Brotto, L. A., Chik, H. M., Ryder, A. G., Gorzalka, B. B., & Seal, B. N. (2005). Acculturation and sexual function in Asian women. *Archives of Sexual Behavior, 34,* 613–626.

Brown, D. L., Rosnick, C. B., Webb-Bradley, T., & Kirner, J. (2014). Does daddy know best?: Exploring the relationship between paternal sexual communication and safe sex practices among African-American women. *Sex Education, 14,* 241–256.

Brown, J. D., & L'Engle, K. L. (2009). X-rated: Sexual attitudes and behaviors associated with U.S. early adolescents' exposure to sexually explicit media. *Communication Research, 36,* 129–151.

Brown, J. D., L'Engle, K. L., Pardun, C. J., Guo, G., Kenneavy, K., & Jackson, C. (2006). Sexy media matter: Exposure to sexual content in music, movies, television, and magazines predicts black and white adolescents' sexual behavior. *Pediatrics, 117,* 1018–1027.

Brown, L. K., DiClemente, R., Crosby, R., Fernandez, M. I., Pugatch, D., Cohn, S., et al. (2008). Condom use among high-risk adolescents: Anticipation of partner disapproval and less pleasure associated with not using condoms. *Public Health Reports, 123,* 601–607.

Browning, C. R., Burrington, L. A., Leventhal, T., & Brooks-Gunn, J. (2008). Neighborhood structural inequality, collective efficacy, and sexual risk behavior among urban youth. *Journal of Health and Social Behavior, 49,* 269–285.

Bruce, D., Harper, G. W., Fernández, M. I., & Jamil, O. B. (2012). Age-concordant and age-discordant sexual behavior among gay and bisexual male adolescents. *Archives of Sexual Behavior, 41,* 441–448.

Brückner, H., & Bearman, P. (2005). After the promise: The STD consequences of adolescent virginity pledges. *Journal of Adolescent Health, 36,* 271–278.

Brückner, H., Martin, A., & Bearman, P. S. (2004). Ambivalence and pregnancy: Adolescents' attitudes, contraceptive use and pregnancy. *Perspectives on Sexual and Reproductive Health, 36,* 248–257.

Bryan, A. D., Schmiege, S. J., & Magnan, R. E. (2012). Marijuana use and risky sexual behavior among high-risk adolescents: Trajectories, risk factors, and event-level relationships. *Developmental Psychology, 48,* 1429–1442.

Buchanan, C. M., Eccles, J. S., & Becker, J. B. (1992). Are adolescents the victims of raging hormones?: Evidence for activational effects of hormones on moods and behavior at adolescence. *Psychological Bulletin, 111,* 62–107.

Buhi, E. R., Daley, E. M., Oberne, A., Smith, S. A., Schneider, T., & Fuhrmann, H. J. (2010). Quality and accuracy of sexual health information web sites visited by young people. *Journal of Adolescent Health, 47,* 206–208.

Buhi, E. R., & Goodson, P. (2007). Predictors of adolescent sexual behavior and intention: A theory-guided systematic review. *Journal of Adolescent Health, 40,* 4–21.

Bulcroft, R. A. (1991). The value of physical change in adolescence: Consequences for the parent–adolescent exchange relationship. *Journal of Youth and Adolescence, 20,* 89–104.

Bull, S. S., Levine, D. K., Black, S. R., Schmiege, S. J., & Santelli, J. (2012). Social media-delivered sexual health intervention: A cluster randomized controlled trial. *American Journal of Preventive Medicine, 43,* 467–474.

Bunting, L., & McAuley, C. (2004). Teenage pregnancy and parenthood: The role of fathers. *Child and Family Social Work, 9,* 295–303.

Burgard, S. A., & Lee-Rife, S. M. (2009). Community characteristics, sexual initiation, and condom use among young black South Africans. *Journal of Health and Social Behavior, 50,* 293–309.

Burns, M. N., Ryan, D. T., Garofalo, R., Newcomb, M. E., & Mustanski, B. (2015). Mental health disorders in young urban sexual minority men. *Journal of Adolescent Health, 56,* 52–58.

Burrington, L. A., Kreager, D. A., & Haynie, D. L. (2011, January). *Negotiating desire: Gender, intercourse, and depression in adolescent romantic couples.* Paper presented at the annual meeting of the American Sociological Association, Las Vegas, NV.

Burton, C. M., Marshal, M. P., Chisolm, D. J., Sucato, G. S., & Friedman, M. S. (2013). Sexual minority-related victimization as a mediator of mental health disparities in sexual minority youth: A longitudinal analysis. *Journal of Youth and Adolescence, 42,* 394–402.

Busby, D. M., Carroll, J. S., & Willoughby, B. J. (2010). Compatibility or restraint: The effects of sexual timing on marriage relationships. *Journal of Family Psychology, 24,* 766–774.

Buss, D. M. (2016). *The evolution of desire: Strategies of human mating.* New York: Basic Books.

Busse, P., Fishbein, M., Bleakley, A., & Hennessy, M. (2010). The role of communication with friends in sexual initiation. *Communication Research, 37,* 239–255.

Byers, E. S., & Sears, H. A. (2012). Mothers who do and do not intend to discuss sexual health with their young adolescents. *Family Relations, 61,* 851–863.

Byers, E. S., Sears, H. A., & Hughes, K. (2017). Predicting mother–adolescent sexual communication using the integrative model of behavioral prediction. *Journal of Family Issues, 39,* 1213–1235.

Byne, W., Bradley, S. J., Coleman, E., Eyler, A. E., Green R., Menvielle, E. J., et al. (2012). Report of the American Psychiatric Association task force on treatment of gender identity disorder. *Archives of Sexual Behavior, 41,* 759–796.

Cabral, P., Wallander, J. L., Song, A. V., Elliott, M. N., Tottolero, S. R., Reisner, S. L., et al. (2017). Generational status and social factors predicting initiation of partnered sexual activity among Latino/a youth. *Health Psychology, 36,* 169–178.

Caldini, R. B., & Trost, M. R. (1998). Social influence: Social norms, conformity, and compliance. In D. T. Gilbert, S. T. Fiske, & G. Lindzey (Eds.), *The handbook of social psychology* (Vol. 2, 4th ed., pp. 151–192). New York: Oxford University Press.

Callister, M., Coyne, S. M., Stern, L. A., Stockdale, L., Miller, M. J., & Wells, B. M. (2012). A content analysis of the prevalence and portrayal of sexual activity in adolescent literature. *Journal of Sex Research, 49,* 477–486.

Callister, M., Stern, L. A., Coyne, S. M., Robinson, T., & Bennion, E. (2011). Evaluation of sexual content in teen-centered films from 1980 to 2007. *Mass Communication and Society, 14,* 454–474.

Cameron-Lewis, V., & Allen, L. (2013). Teaching pleasure *and* danger in sexuality education. *Sex Education, 13,* 121–132.

Cancian, M., Meyer, D., Brown, P., & Cook, S. (2014). Who gets custody now?: Dramatic changes in children's living arrangements after divorce. *Demography, 51,* 1381–1396.

Capaldi, D. M., Crosby, L., & Stoolmiller, M. (1996). Predicting the timing of first sexual intercourse for at-risk adolescent males. *Child Development, 67,* 344–359.

Capaldi, D. M., Stoolmiller, M., Clark, S., & Owen, L. D. (2002). Heterosexual risk behaviors in at-risk young men from early adolescence to young adulthood: Prevalence, prediction, and association with STD contraction. *Developmental Psychology, 38,* 394–406.

Carlson, M. D., Mendle, J., & Harden, K. P. (2014). Early adverse environments and genetic influences on age at first sex: Evidence for gene × environment interaction. *Developmental Psychology, 50,* 1532–1542.

Carlsund, Å., Eriksson, U., Löfstedt, P., & Sellström, E. (2012). Risk behaviour in Swedish adolescents: Is shared physical custody after divorce a risk or a protective factor? *European Journal of Public Health, 23,* 3–8.

Caron, S. L., & Hinman, S. P. (2013). "I took his V-card": An exploratory analysis of college student stories involving male virginity loss. *Sexuality and Culture, 17,* 525–539.

Carpenter, L. M. (2002). Gender and the meaning and experience of virginity loss in the contemporary United States. *Gender and Society, 16,* 345–365.

Carpenter, L. M. (2005). *Virginity lost: An intimate portrait of first sexual experiences.* New York: NYU Press.

Carroll, C., Lloyd-Jones, M., Cooke, J., & Owen, J. (2012). Reasons for the use and non-use of school sexual health services: A systematic review of young people's views. *Journal of Public Health, 34,* 403–410.

Carroll, J. S., Padilla-Walker, L. M., Nelson, L. J., Olson, C. D., Barry, C. M., & Madsen, S. D. (2008). Generation XXX: Pornography acceptance and use among emerging adults. *Journal of Adolescent Research, 23,* 6–30.

Carter, J. B. (2001). Birds, bees, and venereal disease: Toward an intellectual history of sex education. *Journal of the History of Sexuality, 10,* 213–249.

Carvajal, S. C., Parcel, G. S., Basen-Engquist, K., Banspach, S. W., Coyle, K. K., Kirby, D., et al. (1999). Psychosocial predictors of delay of first sexual intercourse by adolescents. *Health Psychology, 18,* 443–452.

Carver, K., Joyner, K., & Udry, J. R. (2003). National estimates of adolescent romantic relationships. In P. Florsheim (Ed.), *Adolescent romantic relations and sexual behavior* (pp. 23–56). Mahwah, NJ: Erlbaum.

Casey, B. J. (2015). Beyond simple models of self-control to circuit-based accounts of adolescent behavior. *Annual Review of Psychology, 66,* 295–319.

Casey, B. J., Getz, S., & Galvan, A. (2008). The adolescent brain. *Developmental Review, 28,* 62–77.

Casey, B. J., Jones, R. M., & Hare, T. A. (2008). The adolescent brain. *Annals of the New York Academy of Science, 1124,* 111–126.

Caspi, A. M., & Moffitt, T. E. (1991). Individual differences are accentuated during periods of social change: The sample case of girls at puberty. *Journal of Personality and Social Psychology, 61,* 157–168.

Cass, V. C. (1979). Homosexual identity formation: A theoretical model. *Journal of Homosexuality, 4,* 219–235.

Cass, V. C. (1984). Homosexual identity formation: Testing a theoretical model. *Journal of Sex Research, 20,* 143–167.

Castillo-Arcos, L. C., Benavides-Torres, R. A., López-Rosales, F., Onofre-Rodriguez, D. J., Valdez-Montero, C., & Maas-Gongóra, L. (2016). The effect of an Internet-based intervention designed to reduce HIV/AIDS sexual risk among Mexican adolescents. *AIDS Care, 28,* 191–196.

Castrucci, B. C., Clark, J., Lewis, K., Samsel, R., & Mirchandani, G. (2010). Prevalence and risk factors for adult paternity among adolescent females ages 14 through 16 years. *Maternal and Child Health Journal, 14,* 895–900.

Cederbaum, J. A., Rodriguez, A. J., Sullivan, K., & Gray, K. (2017). Attitudes, norms, and the effect of social connectedness on adolescent sexual risk intention. *Journal of School Health, 87,* 575–583.

Centers for Disease Control and Prevention. (2009, July 17). Sexual and reproductive health of persons aged 10–24 years: United States, 2002–2007. *Morbidity and Mortality Weekly Report, 58.* Retrieved July 11, 2016, from *www.cdc.gov/mmwr/pdf/ss/ss5806.pdf.*

Centers for Disease Control and Prevention. (2011). *1991–2011 High School Youth Risk Behavior Survey data.* Atlanta, GA: U.S. Department of Health and Human Services. Retrieved July 10, 2016, from *http://apps.nccd.cdc.gov/youthonline.*

Centers for Disease Control and Prevention. (2013). *HIV among gay and bisexual men.* Atlanta, GA: U.S. Department of Health and Human Services. Retrieved November 30, 2016, from *www.cdc.gov/hiv/group/msm/index.html.*

Centers for Disease Control and Prevention. (2015). *Sexually transmitted disease surveillance 2014.* Atlanta, GA: U.S. Department of Health and Human Services. Retrieved December 27, 2016, from *www.cdc.gov/std/stats14/surv-2014-print.pdf.*

Chambers, W. C. (2007). Oral sex: Varied behaviors and perceptions in a college population. *Journal of Sex Research, 44,* 28–42.

Chan, S. M., & Chan, K. W. (2011). Adolescents' susceptibility to peer pressure: Relations to parent–adolescent relationship and adolescents' emotional autonomy from parents. *Youth and Society, 45,* 286–302.

Chandra, A., Martino, S. C., Collins, R. L., Elliott, M. N., Berry, S. H., Kanouse, D. E., et al., (2008). Does watching sex on television predict teen pregnancy?: Findings from a national longitudinal survey of youth. *Pediatrics, 122,* 1047–1054.

Chandra-Mouli, V., Camacho, A. V., & Michaud, P. A. (2013). WHO guidelines on preventing early pregnancy and poor reproductive outcomes among adolescents in developing countries. *Journal of Adolescent Health, 52,* 517–522.

Charania, M. R., Crepaz, N., Guenther-Gray, C., Henny, K., Liau, A., Willis, L. A., et al. (2011). Efficacy of structural-level condom distribution interventions: A meta-analysis of U.S. and international studies, 1998–2007. *AIDS Behavior, 15,* 1283–1297.

Charmaraman, L., & McKamey, C. (2011). Urban early adolescent narratives on sexuality: Accidental and intentional influences of family, peers, and the media. *Sexuality Research and Social Policy, 8,* 253–266.

Charnigo, R., Garnett, C., Crosby, R.,

Palmgreen, P., & Zimmerman, R. S. (2013). Sensation seeking and impulsivity: Combined associations with risky sexual behavior in a large sample of young adults. *Journal of Sex Research, 50,* 480–488.

Chein, J., Albert, D., O'Brien, L., Uckeert, K., & Steinberg, L. (2011). Peers increase adolescent risk taking by enhancing activity in the brain's reward circuitry. *Developmental Science, 14,* F1–F10.

Chen, C.-W., Tsai, C.-Y., Sung, F.-C., Lee, Y.-Y., Lu, T.-H., Li, C.-Y., et al. (2009). Adverse birth outcomes among pregnancies of teen mothers: Age-specific analysis of national data in Taiwan. *Child: Care, Health and Development, 36,* 232–240.

Chen, M., Fuqua, J., & Eugster, E. A. (2016). Characteristics of referrals for gender dysphoria over a 13-year period. *Journal of Adolescent Health, 58,* 369–371.

Cherie, A., & Berhane, Y. (2012). Knowledge of sexually transmitted infections and barriers to seeking health services among high school adolescents in Addis Ababa, Ethiopia. *Journal of AIDS and Clinical Research, 3,* 5.

Chesson, H. W., Gift, T. L., Owusu-Edusei, K., Tao, G., Johnson, A. P., & Kent, C. K. (2011). A brief review of the estimated economic burden of sexually transmitted diseases in the United States: Inflation-adjusted updates of previously published cost studies. *Sexually Transmitted Diseases, 38,* 889–891.

Child Trends. (2015a, November). *Oral sex behaviors among teens.* Child Trends Data Bank. Retrieved November 30, 2016, from *www.childtrends.org/wp-content/uploads/2013/12/95_Oral_Sex_1.pdf.*

Child Trends. (2015b, December). *Dating: Indicators on children and youth.* Child Trends Data Bank. Retrieved July 10, 2016, from *www.childtrends.org/?indicators=dating.*

Chin, H. B., Sipe, T. A., Elder, R., Mercer, S. L., Chattopadhyay, S. K., Jacob, V., et al. (2012). The effectiveness of group-based comprehensive risk-reduction and abstinence education interventions to prevent or reduce the risk of adolescent pregnancy, human immunodeficiency virus, and sexually transmitted infections. *American Journal of Preventive Medicine, 42,* 272–294.

Chirinda, W., & Peltzer, K. (2014). Correlates of inconsistent condom use among youth aged 18–24 years in South Africa. *Journal of Child and Adolescent Mental Health, 26,* 75–82.

Christenson, P. G., & Roberts, D. F. (1998). *It's not only rock & roll: Popular music in the lives of adolescents.* Cresskill, NJ: Hampton Press.

Clark, A. P. (2006). Are the correlates of socio-sexuality different for men and women? *Personality and Individual Differences, 41,* 1321–1327.

Clark, L. R., Jackson, M., & Allen-Taylor, L. (2002). Adolescent knowledge about sexually transmitted diseases. *Sexually Transmitted Diseases, 29,* 436–443.

Clark, T. C., Lucassen, M. F. G., Bullen, P., Denny, S. J., Fleming, T. M., Robinson, E. M., et al. (2014). The health and well-being of transgender high school students: Results from the New Zealand adolescent health survey (Youth '12). *Journal of Adolescent Health, 55,* 93–99.

Clawson, C. L., & Reese-Weber, M. (2003). The amount and timing of parent–adolescent sexual communication as predictors of late adolescent sexual risk-taking behaviors. *Journal of Sex Research, 40,* 256–265.

Cleveland, H. H. (2003). The influence of female and male risk on the occurrence of sexual intercourse within adolescent relationships. *Journal of Research on Adolescence, 13,* 81–112.

Cleveland, H. H., & Gilson, M. (2004). The effects of neighborhood proportion of single-parent families and mother–adolescent relationships on adolescents' number of sexual partners. *Journal of Youth and Adolescence, 33,* 319–329.

Coetzee, J., Dietrich, J., Otwombe, K., Nkala, B., Khunwane, M., van der Watt, M., et al. (2014). Predictors of parent–adolescent communication in post-apartheid South Africa: A protective factor in adolescent sexual and reproductive health. *Journal of Adolescence, 37,* 313–324.

Cohen-Kettenis, P. T., Delemarre-van de Waal, H. A., & Gooren, L. J. G. (2008). The treatment of adolescent transsexuals: Changing insights. *Journal of Sexual Medicine, 5,* 1892–1897.

Cohen-Kettenis, P. T., Schagen, S. E. E., Steensma, T. D., de Vries, A. L. C., & Delemarre-van de Waal, H. A. (2011). Puberty suppression in a gender-dysphoric adolescent: A 22 year follow-up. *Archives of Sexual Behavior, 40,* 843–847.

Colebunders, B., De Cuypere, G., & Monstrey, S. (2015). New criteria for sex reassignment surgery: WPATH Standards of Care, Version 7, revisited. *International Journal of Transgenderism, 16,* 222–233.

Coley, R. L., Lombardi, C. M., Lynch, A. D., Mahalik, J. R., & Sims, J. (2013). Sexual partner accumulation from adolescence through early adulthood: The role of family, peer, and school social norms. *Journal of Adolescent Health, 53,* 91–97.

Coley, R. L., Medeiros, B. L., & Schindler, H. S. (2008). Using sibling differences to estimate effects of parenting on adolescent sexual risk behaviors. *Journal of Adolescent Health, 43,* 133–140.

Coley, R. L., Votruba-Drzal, E., & Schindler, H. S. (2009). Fathers' and mothers' parenting predicting and responding to adolescent sexual risk behaviors. *Child Development, 80,* 808–827.

Collado, A., Johnson, P. S., Loya, J. M., Johnson, M. W., & Yi, R. (2017). Discounting of condom-protected sex as a measure of high risk for sexually transmitted infection among college students. *Archives of Sexual Behavior, 46,* 2187–2195.

Collibee, C., & Furman, W. (2014). Impact of sexual coercion on romantic experiences of adolescents and young adults. *Archives of Sexual Behavior, 43,* 1431–1441.

Collier, K. L., van Beusekom, G., Bos, H. M. W., & Sandfort, T. G. M. (2013). Sexual orientation and gender identity/expression related peer victimization in adolescence: A systematic review of associated psychosocial and health outcomes. *Journal of Sex Research, 50,* 299–317.

Collins, R. L., Elliott, M. N., Berry, S. H., Kanouse, D. E., Kunkel, D., Hunter, S. B., et al. (2004). Watching sex on TV predicts adolescent initiation of sexual behavior. *Pediatrics, 114,* e280–e289.

Collins, W. A., & van Dulmen, M. (2014).

"The course of true love(s) . . .": Origins and pathways in the development of romantic relationships. In A. C. Crouter & A. Booth (Eds.), *Romance and sex in adolescence and emerging adulthood: Risks and opportunities* (pp. 63–86). New York: Psychology Press.

Collins, W. A., Welsh, D. P., & Furman, W. (2009). Adolescent romantic relationships. *Annual Review of Psychology, 60*, 631–652.

Comings, D. E., Muhleman, D., Johnson, J. P., & MacMurray, J. P. (2002). Parent–daughter transmission of the androgen receptor gene as an explanation of the effect of father absence on age of menarche. *Child Development, 73*, 1046–1051.

Connolly, J., Craig, W., Goldberg, A., & Pepler, D. (1999). Conceptions of cross-sex friendships and romantic relationships in early adolescence. *Journal of Youth and Adolescence, 28*, 481–494.

Connolly, M. D., Zervos, M. J., Barone, C. J., II, Johnson, C. C., & Joseph, C. L. M. (2016). The mental health of transgender youth: Advances in understanding. *Journal of Adolescent Health, 59*, 489–495.

Conradt, E., Lagasse, L. L., Shankaran, S., Bada, H., Bauer, C. R., Whitaker, T. M., et al. (2014). Physiological correlates of neurobehavioral disinhibition that relate to drug use and risky sexual behavior in adolescents with prenatal substance exposure. *Developmental Neuroscience, 36*, 306–315.

Cooksey, E. C., Mott, F. L., & Neubauer, S. A. (2002). Friendships and early relationships: Links to sexual initiation among American adolescents born to young mothers. *Perspectives on Sexual and Reproductive Health, 34*, 118–126.

Cooper, K., Quayle, E., Jonsson, L., & Svedin, C. G. (2016). Adolescents and self-taken sexual images: A review of the literature. *Computers in Human Behavior, 55*, 706–716.

Copeland, W., Shanahan, L., Miller, S., Costello, E. J., Angold, A., & Maughan, B. (2010). Outcomes of early pubertal timing in young women: A prospective population-based study. *American Journal of Psychiatry, 167*, 1218–1225.

Copen, C. E., Chandra, A., & Martinez, G. (2012, August). *Prevalence and timing of oral sex with opposite-sex partners among females and males aged 15–24 years: United States, 2007–2010* (National Health Statistics Report No. 56). Hyattsville, MD: National Center for Health Statistics.

Corcoran, J., & Pillai, V. K. (2007). Effectiveness of secondary pregnancy prevention programs: A meta-analysis. *Research on Social Work Practice, 17*, 5–18.

Corliss, H. L., Rosario, M., Birkett, M. A., Newcomb, M. E., Buchting, F. O., & Matthews, A. K. (2014). Sexual orientation disparities in adolescent cigarette smoking: Intersections with race/ethnicity, gender, and age. *American Journal of Public Health, 104*, 1137–1147.

Corliss, H. L., Rosario, M., Wypij, D., Wylie, S. A., Frazier, A. L., & Austin, B. (2010). Sexual orientation and drug use in a longitudinal cohort study of U.S. adolescents. *Addictive Behaviors, 35*, 517–521.

Cornell, J. L., & Halpern-Felsher, B. L. (2006). Adolescents tell us why teens have oral sex. *Journal of Adolescent Health, 38*, 299–301.

Cox, R. B., Shreffler, K. M., Merten, M. J., Gallus, K. L. S., & Dowdy, J. L. (2015). Parenting, peers, and perceived norms: What predicts attitudes toward sex among early adolescents? *Journal of Early Adolescence, 35*, 30–53.

Coyne, C. A., Fontaine, N. M. G., Långström, N., Lichtenstein, P., & D'Onofrio, B. M. (2013). Teenage childbirth and young adult criminal convictions: A quasi-experimental study of criminal outcomes for teenage mothers. *Journal of Criminal Justice, 41*, 318–323.

Coyne, C. A., Långström, N., Lichtenstein, P., & D'Onofrio, B. M. (2013). The association between teenage motherhood and poor offspring outcomes: A national cohort study across 30 years. *Twin Research and Human Genetics, 16*, 679–689.

Coyne, S. M., & Padilla-Walker, L. M. (2015). Sex, violence, & rock 'n' roll: Longitudinal effects of music on aggression, sex, and prosocial behavior during adolescence. *Journal of Adolescence, 41*, 96–104.

Crandall, A., Magnusson, B. M., Novilla, M. L., Novilla, L. K. B., & Dyer, W. J. (2017). Family financial stress and adolescent sexual risk-taking: The role of self-regulation. *Journal of Youth and Adolescence, 46*, 45–62.

Crawford, M., & Popp, D. (2003). Sexual double standards: A review and methodological critique of two decades of research. *Journal of Sex Research, 40*, 13–26.

Crittenden, C. P., Boris, N. W., Rice, J. C., Taylor, C. A., & Olds, D. (2009). The role of mental health factors, behavioral factors, and past experiences in the prediction of rapid repeat pregnancy in adolescence. *Journal of Adolescent Health, 44*, 25–32.

Crockett, L. J., Bingham, C. R., Chopak, J. S., & Vicary, J. R. (1996). Timing of first sexual intercourse: The role of social control, social learning, and problem behavior. *Journal of Youth and Adolescence, 25*, 89–111.

Crosby, R., Charnigo, R. A., Weathers, C., Caliendo, A. M., & Shrier, L. A. (2012). Condom effectiveness against non-viral sexually transmitted infections: A prospective study using electronic daily diaries. *Sexually Transmitted Infections, 88*, 484–489.

Crosby, R. A., DiClemente, R. J., Wingood, G. M., Lang, D. L., & Harrington, K. (2003). Infrequent parental monitoring predicts sexually transmitted infections among low-income African American female adolescents. *Archives of Pediatrics and Adolescent Medicine, 157*, 169–173.

Crosby, R., Shrier, L. A., Charnigo, R., Sanders, S. A., Graham, C. A., Milhausen, R., et al. (2013). Negative perceptions about condom use in a clinic population: Comparisons by gender, race and age. *International Journal of STD and AIDS, 24*, 100–105.

Crosnoe, R., & McNeely, C. (2008). Peer relations, adolescent behavior, and public health research and practice. *Family and Community Health, 31*, S71–S80.

Crowder, K., & Teachman, J. (2004). Do residential conditions explain the relationship between living arrangements and adolescent behavior? *Journal of Marriage and the Family, 66*, 721–738.

Crugnola, C. R., Ierardi, E., Gazzotti, S., & Albizzati, A. (2014). Motherhood in adolescent mothers: Maternal attachment, mother–infant styles of interaction and emotion regulation at three months. *Infant Behavior and Development, 37*, 44–56.

Cubbin, C., Brindis, C. D., Jain, S., Santelli, J., & Braveman, P. (2010). Neighborhood poverty, aspirations and expectations, and initiation of sex. *Journal of Adolescent Health, 47*, 399–406.

Dalla, R. L., & Kennedy, H. R. (2015). "I want to leave—go far away—I don't want to get stuck on the res[ervation]": Developmental outcomes of adolescent-aged children of Navajo Native American teen mothers. *Journal of Adolescent Research, 30*, 113–139.

Dariotis, J. K., & Johnson, M. W. (2015). Sexual discounting among high-risk youth ages 18–24: Implications for sexual and substance use risk behaviors. *Experimental and Clinical Psychopharmacology, 23*, 49–58.

Dariotis, J. K., Pleck, J. H., Astone, N. M., & Sonenstein, F. L. (2011). Pathways of early fatherhood, marriage, and employment: A latent class growth analysis. *Demography, 48*, 593–623.

Das, A. (2007). Masturbation in the United States. *Journal of Sex and Marital Therapy, 33*, 301–317.

D'Augelli, A. R., Hershberger, S. L., & Pilkington, N. W. (1998). Lesbian, gay, and bisexual youth and their families: Disclosure of sexual orientation and its consequences. *American Journal of Orthopsychiatry, 68*, 361–371.

Davila, J., Stroud, C. B., Starr, L. R., Miller, M. R., Yoneda, A., & Hershenberg, R. (2009). Romantic and sexual activities, parent-adolescent stress, and depressive symptoms among early adolescent girls. *Journal of Adolescence, 32*, 909–924.

Davis, K. C., Evans, D., & Kamyab, K. (2012). Effectiveness of a national media campaign to promote parent–child communication about sex. *Health Education and Behavior, 40*, 97–106.

Dawson, S. J., & Chivers, M. L. (2014). Gender differences and similarities in sexual desire. *Current Sexual Health Reports, 6*, 211–219.

Day, N. (2013, June 21). How to address the masturbating child. *The Atlantic*. Retrieved July 10, 2016, from *www.theatlantic.com/health/archive/2013/06/how-to-address-the-masturbating-child/277026*.

De Bruyn, E. H., Cillessen, A. H. N., & Weisfeld, G. E. (2012). Dominance-popularity status, behavior, and the emergence of sexual activity in young adolescents. *Evolutionary Psychology, 10,* 296–319.

De Genna, N. M., & Cornelius, M. D. (2015). Maternal drinking and risky sexual behavior in offspring. *Health Education and Behavior, 42,* 185–193.

De Genna, N. M., Goldschmidt, L., & Cornelius, M. D. (2015). Maternal patterns of marijuana use and early sexual behavior in offspring of teenage mothers. *Maternal and Child Health Journal, 19,* 626–634.

De Genna, N. M., Larkby, C., & Cornelius, M. D. (2011). Pubertal timing and early sexual intercourse in the offspring of teenage mothers. *Journal of Youth and Adolescence, 40,* 1315–1328.

de Graaf, H., & Rademakers, J. (2006). Sexual development of prepubertal children. *Journal of Psychology and Human Sexuality, 18,* 1–21.

de Graaf, H., van de Schoot, R., Woertman, L., Hawk, S. T., & Meeus, W. (2012). Family cohesion and romantic and sexual initiation: A three wave longitudinal study. *Journal of Youth and Adolescence, 41,* 583–592.

de Graaf, H., Vanwesenbeeck, I., Woertman, L., Keijsers, L., Maijer, S., & Meeus, W. (2010). Parental support and knowledge and adolescents' sexual health: Testing two mediational models in a national Dutch sample. *Journal of Youth and Adolescence, 39,* 189–198.

de Graaf, H., Vanwesenbeeck, I., Woertman, L., & Meeus, W. (2011). Parenting and psychosexual development in adolescence: A literature review. *European Psychologist, 16,* 21–31.

De Looze, M., Constantine, N. A., Jerman, P., Vermeulen-Smit, E., & ter Bogt, T. (2015). Parent–adolescent sexual communication and its association with adolescent sexual behaviors: A nationally representative analysis in the Netherlands. *Journal of Sex Research, 52,* 257–268.

Dearden, K., Hale, C. G., & Woolley, T. (1995). The antecedents of teen fatherhood: A retrospective case-control study of Great British young. *American Journal of Public Health, 85,* 551–554.

Deardorff, J., Gonzales, N. A., Christopher, S., Roosa, M. W., & Millsap, R. E. (2005).

Early puberty and adolescent pregnancy: The influence of alcohol use. *Pediatrics, 116,* 1451–1456.

Defoe, I. N., Dubas, J. S., Figner, B., & van Aken, M. A. (2015). A meta-analysis on age differences in risky decision making: Adolescents versus children and adults. *Psychological Bulletin, 141,* 48–84.

Dehne, K. L., & Riedner, G. (2005). *Sexually transmitted infections among adolescents: The need for adequate health services.* Geneva, Switzerland: World Health Organization. Retrieved July 25, 2016, from *http://apps.who.int/iris/bitstream/10665/43221/1/9241562889.pdf.*

Dekker, A., & Schmidt, G. (2003). Patterns of masturbatory behaviour: Changes between the sixties and the nineties. *Journal of Psychology and Human Sexuality, 14,* 35–48.

DeLeire, T., & Kalil, A. (2002). Good things come in threes: Single-parent multigenerational family structure and adolescent development. *Demography, 39,* 393–413.

Denny, S., Robinson, E., Lawler, C., Bagshaw, S., Farrant, B., Bell, F., et al. (2012). Association between availability and quality of health services in schools and reproductive health outcomes among students: A multilevel observational study. *American Journal of Public Health, 102,* e14–e20.

Deptula, D. P., Henry, D. B., & Schoeny, M. E. (2010). How can parents make a difference?: Longitudinal associations with adolescent sexual behavior. *Journal of Family Psychology, 24,* 731–739.

Dermody, S. S., Marshal, M. P., Cheong, J., Burton, C., Hughes, T., Aranda, F., et al. (2014). Longitudinal disparities of hazardous drinking between sexual minority and heterosexual individuals from adolescence to young adulthood. *Journal of Youth and Adolescence, 43,* 30–39.

DeRosa, C. J., Ethier, K. A., Kim, D. H., Cumberland, W. G., Afifi, A. A., Kotlerman, J., et al. (2010). Sexual intercourse and oral sex among public middle school students: Prevalence and correlates. *Perspectives on Sexual and Reproductive Health, 42,* 197–205.

Deutsch, A. R., & Crockett, L. J. (2016). Gender, generational status, and parent–adolescent sexual communication: Implications for Latino/a adolescent sexual behavior. *Journal of Research on Adolescence, 26,* 300–315.

Deutsch, A. R., & Slutske, W. S. (2015). A noncausal relation between casual sex in adolescence and early adult depression and suicidal ideation: A longitudinal discordant twin study. *Journal of Sex Research, 52,* 770–780.

Devine, S., Bull, S., Dreisbach, S., & Shlay, J. (2014). Enhancing a teen pregnancy prevention program with text messaging: Engaging minority youth to develop TOP plus text. *Journal of Adolescent Health, 54,* S78–S83.

DeWitt, S. J., Aslan, S., & Filbey, F. M. (2014). Adolescent risk-taking and resting state functional connectivity. *Psychiatry Research: Neuroimaging, 222,* 157–164.

Diamond, L. M. (2003). Was it a phase?: Young women's relinquishment of lesbian/bisexual identities over a 5-year-period. *Journal of Personality and Social Psychology, 84,* 352–364.

Diamond, L. M. (2014). Expanding the scope of a dynamic perspective on positive adolescent sexual development. *Human Development, 57,* 292–304.

Diamond, L. M., & Rosky, C. J. (2016). Scrutinizing immutability: Research on sexual orientation and U.S. legal advocacy for sexual minorities. *Journal of Sex Research, 53,* 363–391.

Diamond, L. M., Savin-Williams, R. C., & Dubé, E. M. (1999). Sex, dating, passionate friendships, and romance: Intimate peer relations among lesbian, gay, and bisexual adolescents. In W. Furman, B. B. Brown, & C. Feiring (Eds.), *The development of romantic relationships in adolescence* (pp. 175–210). New York: Cambridge University Press.

Dickenson, J. A., & Huebner, D. M. (2016). The relationship between sexual activity and depressive symptoms in lesbian, gay, and bisexual youth: Effects of gender and family support. *Archives of Sexual Behavior, 45,* 671–681.

Dickson, N., van Roode, T., Cameron, C., & Paul, C. (2013). Stability and change in same-sex attraction, experience, and identity by sex and age in a New Zealand birth cohort. *Archives of Sexual Behavior, 42,* 753–763.

DiClemente, R. J., Salazar, L. F., Crosby, R. A., & Rosenthal, S. L. (2005). Prevention and control of sexually transmitted infections among adolescents: The importance of a socio-ecological perspective—a commentary. *Public Health, 119,* 825–836.

DiClemente, R. J., Wingood, G. M., Crosby, R. A., Sionean, C., Cobb, B. K., Harrington, K., et al. (2001). Parental monitoring: Association with adolescents' risk behaviors. *Pediatrics, 107,* 1363–1368.

DiClemente, R. J., Wingood, G. M., Crosby, R. A., Sionean, C., Cobb, B. K., Harrington, K., et al. (2002). Sexual risk behaviors associated with having older sex partners. *Sexually Transmitted Diseases, 29,* 20–24.

Diiorio, C., Pluhar, E., & Belcher, L. (2003). Parent–child communication about sexuality: A review of the literature from 1980–2002. *Journal of HIV/AIDS Prevention and Education for Adolescents and Children, 5,* 7–32.

Dir, A. L., Coskunpinar, A., & Cyders, M. A. (2014). A meta-analytic review of the relationship between adolescent risky sexual behavior and impulsivity across gender, age, and race. *Clinical Psychology Review, 34,* 551–562.

Dishion, T. J., Ha, T., & Véronneau, M. H. (2012). An ecological analysis of the effects of deviant peer clustering on sexual promiscuity, problem behavior, and childbearing from early adolescence to adulthood: An enhancement of the life history framework. *Developmental Psychology, 48,* 703–717.

Dittus, P., & Jaccard, J. (2000). Adolescents' perceptions of maternal disapproval of sex: Relationships to sexual outcomes. *Journal of Adolescent Health, 26,* 268–278.

Dodge, B., Herbenick, D., Fu, T. C., Schick, V., Reece, M., Sanders, S., et al. (2016). Sexual behaviors of U.S. men by self-identified sexual orientation: Results from the 2012 National Survey of Sexual Health and Behavior. *Journal of Sexual Medicine, 13,* 637–649.

Donahue, K. L., D'Onofrio, B. M., Bates, J. E., Lansford, J. E., Dodge, K. A., & Pettit, G. S. (2010). Early exposure to parents' relationship instability: Implications for sexual behavior and depression in adolescence. *Journal of Adolescent Health, 47,* 547–554.

Donahue, K. L., Lichtenstein, P., Långström, N., & D'Onofrio, B. M. (2013). Why does early sexual intercourse predict subsequent maladjustment?: Exploring potential familial confounds. *Health Psychology, 32,* 180–189.

Donaldson, A. A., Lindberg, L. D., Ellen, J. M., & Marcell, A. V. (2013). Receipt of sexual health information from parents, teachers, and healthcare providers by sexually experienced U.S. adolescents. *Journal of Adolescent Health, 53,* 235–240.

Donohew, L., Zimmerman, R., Cupp, P., Novak, S., Colon, S., & Abell, R. (2000). Sensation seeking, impulsive decision-making, and risky sex: Implications for risk-taking and design of interventions. *Personality and Individual Differences, 28,* 1079–1091.

Doornwaard, S. M., Bickham, D. S., Rich, M., ter Bogt, T. F. M., & van den Eijnden, R. J. J. M. (2015). Adolescents' use of sexually explicit Internet material and their sexual attitudes and behavior: Parallel development and directional effects. *Developmental Psychology, 51,* 1476–1488.

Doornwaard, S. M., Moreno, M. A., van den Eijnden, R. J. J. M., Vanwesenbeeck, I., & ter Bogt, T. F. M. (2014). Young adolescents' sexual and romantic reference displays on Facebook. *Journal of Adolescent Health, 55,* 535–541.

Doornwaard, S. M., van den Eijnden, R. J. J. M., Baams, L., Vanwesenbeeck, I., & ter Bogt, T. F. M. (2016). Lower psychological well-being and excessive sexual interest predict symptoms of compulsive use of sexually explicit Internet material among adolescent boys. *Journal of Youth and Adolescence, 45,* 73–84.

Doornwaard, S. M., van den Eijnden, R. J. J. M., Overbeek G., & ter Bogt, T. F. M. (2015). Differential developmental profiles of adolescents using sexually explicit Internet material. *Journal of Sex Research, 52,* 269–281.

Dorn, L. D., & Biro, F. M. (2011). Puberty and its measurement: A decade in review. *Journal of Research on Adolescence, 21,* 180–195.

Downs, J. S., Bruine de Bruin, W., Murray, P. J., & Fischhoff, B. (2006). Specific STI knowledge may be acquired too late. *Journal of Adolescent Health, 38,* 65–67.

Downs, J. S., Murray, P. J., Bruine de Bruin, W., Penrose, J., Palmgren, C., & Fishhoff, B. (2004). Interactive video behavioral intervention to reduce adolescent females' STD risk: A randomized controlled trial. *Social Science and Medicine, 59,* 1561–1572.

Dreyfuss, M., Caudle, K., Drysdale, A. T., Johnston, N. E., Cohen, A. O., Somerville, L. H., et al. (2014). Teens impulsively react rather than retreat from threat. *Developmental Neuroscience, 36,* 220–227.

Drigotas, S. M., & Udry, J. R. (1993). Biosocial models of adolescent problem behavior: Extension to panel design. *Social Biology, 40,* 1–7.

Drouin, M., & Tobin, E. (2014). Unwanted but consensual sexting among young adults: Relations with attachment and sexual motivations. *Computers in Human Behavior, 31,* 412–418.

Drouin, M., Vogel, K. N., Surbey, A., & Stills, J. R. (2013). Let's talk about sexting, baby: Computer-mediated sexual behaviors among young adults. *Computers in Human Behavior, 29,* A25–A30.

Dufur, M. J., Hoffmann, J. P., & Erickson, L. D. (2018). Single parenthood and adolescent sexual outcomes. *Journal of Child and Family Studies, 27,* 802–815.

Dunne, A., McIntosh, J., & Mallory, D. (2014). Adolescents, sexually transmitted infections, and education using social media: A review of the literature. *Journal for Nurse Practitioners, 10,* 401–408.

Dyer, T. P., Regan, R., Pacek, L. R., Acheampong, A., & Khan, M. R. (2015). Psychosocial vulnerability and HIV-related sexual risk among men who have sex with men and women in the United States. *Archives of Sexual Behavior, 44,* 429–441.

East, L., Jackson, D., Peters, K., & O'Brien L. (2010). Disrupted sense of self: Young women and sexually transmitted infections. *Journal of Clinical Nursing, 19,* 1995–2003.

East, P. L. (1998). Impact of adolescent childbearing on families and younger siblings: Effects that increase younger siblings' risk for early pregnancy. *Applied Developmental Science, 2,* 62–74.

Eaton, A. A., Rose, S. M., Interligi, C., Fernandez, K., & McHugh, M. (2016). Gender and ethnicity in dating, hanging out,

and hooking up: Sexual scripts among Hispanic and white young adults. *Journal of Sex
Research, 53,* 788–804.

Ebrahim, S. H., & Gfroerer, J. (2003).
Pregnancy-related substance use in the
United States during 1996–1998. *Obstetrics
and Gynecology, 101,* 374–379.

Eckstrand, K. L., Choukas-Bradley, S.,
Mohanty, A., Cross, M., Allen, N. B., Silk,
J. S., et al. (2017). Heightened activity in
social reward networks is associated with
adolescents' risky sexual behaviors. *Developmental Cognitive Neuroscience, 27,* 1–9.

Eder, D. (1995). *School talk: Gender and adolescent
culture.* New Brunswick, NJ: Rutgers University Press.

Edin, K., & Kefalas, M. (2005). *Promises I can
keep: Why poor women put motherhood before
marriage.* Berkeley: University of California
Press.

Eisenberg, M. E., Ackard, D. M., Resnick, M.
D., & Neumark-Sztainer, D. (2009). Casual
sex and psychological health among young
adults: Is having "friends with benefits"
emotionally damaging? *Perspectives on Sexual
and Reproductive Health, 41,* 231–237.

Ekéus, C., & Christensson, K. (2003). Socioeconomic characteristics of fathers of children born to teenage mothers in Stockholm,
Sweden. *Scandinavian Journal of Public Health,
31,* 73–76.

Eliason, M. J. (1996). Identity formation for
lesbian, bisexual, and gay persons: Beyond a
"minoritizing" view. *Journal of Homosexuality, 30,* 31–58.

Elkington, K. S., Bauermeister, J. A., & Zimmerman, M. A. (2010). Psychological distress, substance use, and HIV/STI risk
behaviors among youth. *Journal of Youth and
Adolescence, 39,* 514–527.

Elkington, K. S., Bauermeister, J. A., & Zimmerman, M. A. (2011). Do parents and peers
matter?: A prospective socio-ecological
examination of substance use and sexual risk
among African American youth. *Journal of
Adolescence, 34,* 1035–1047.

Elliott, S. (2012). *Not my kid: What parents
believe about the sex lives of their teenagers.* New
York: NYU Press.

Ellis, B. J. (2013). The hypothalamic–
pituitary–gonadal axis: A switch-controlled,
condition-sensitive system in the regulation
of life history strategies. *Hormones and Behavior, 64,* 215–225.

Ellis, B. J., Bates, J. E., Dodge, K. A., Fergusson, D. M., Horwood, L. J., Pettit, G. S., et
al. (2003). Does father absence place daughters at special risk for early sexual activity
and teenage pregnancy? *Child Development,
74,* 801–821.

Ellis, B. J., Schlomer, G. L., Tilley, E. H., &
Butler, E. A. (2012). Impact of fathers on
risky sexual behavior in daughters: A genetically and environmentally controlled sibling
study. *Development and Psychopathology, 24,*
317–332.

Eltahawy, M. (2016). *Headscarves and hymens:
Why the Middle East needs a sexual revolution.*
New York: Farrar, Straus & Giroux.

Emerson, S., & Rosenfeld, C. (1996). Stages
of adjustment in family members of transgender individuals. *Journal of Family Psychotherapy, 7,* 1–12.

Emmerink, P. M. J., Vanwesenbeeck, I., van
den Eijnden, R. J. J. M., & ter Bogt, T. F.
M. (2016). Psychosexual correlates of sexual
double standard endorsement in adolescent
sexuality. *Journal of Sex Research, 53,* 286–
297.

Epstein, M., Bailey, J. A., Manhart, L. E., Hill,
K. G., Hawkins, J. D., Haggerty, K. P., et
al. (2014). Understanding the link between
early sexual initiation and later sexually
transmitted infection: Test and replication in
two longitudinal studies. *Journal of Adolescent
Health, 54,* 435–441.

Epstein, M., & Ward, L. M. (2008). "Always
use protection": Communication boys
receive about sex from parents, peers, and
the media. *Journal of Youth and Adolescence,
37,* 113–126.

Escobar-Chaves, S. L., Tortolero, S. R.,
Markham, C. M., Low, B. J., Eitel, P., &
Thickstun, P. (2005). Impact of the media
on adolescent sexual attitudes and behaviors.
Pediatrics, 116, 303–326.

Escribano, S., Espada, J. P., Morales, A., &
Orgilés, M. (2015). Mediation analysis of
an effective sexual health promotion intervention for Spanish adolescents. *AIDS and
Behavior, 19,* 1850–1859.

Eshbaugh, E. M., & Gute, G. (2008). Hookups

and sexual regret among college women. *Journal of Social Psychology, 148,* 77–89.

Espinosa-Hernández, G., Bissell-Havran, J., & Nunn, A. (2015). The role of religiousness and gender in sexuality among Mexican adolescents. *Journal of Sex Research, 52,* 887–897.

Espinosa-Hernández, G., & Vasilenko, S. A. (2015). Patterns of relationship and sexual behaviors in Mexican adolescents and associations with well-being: A latent class approach. *Journal of Adolescence, 44,* 280–290.

Ethier, K. A., Dittus, P. J., DeRosa, C. J., Chung, E. Q., Martinez, E., & Kerndt, P. R. (2011). School-based health center access, reproductive health care, and contraceptive use among sexually experienced high school students. *Journal of Adolescent Health, 48,* 562–565.

Ethier, K. A., Harper, C. R., Hoo, E., & Dittus, P. J. (2016). The longitudinal impact of perceptions of parental monitoring on adolescent initiation of sexual activity. *Journal of Adolescent Health, 59,* 570–576.

Ethier, K. A., Kershaw, T. S., Lewis, J. B., Milan, S., Niccolai, L. M., & Ickovics, J. R. (2006). Self-esteem, emotional distress and sexual behavior among adolescent females: Inter-relationships and temporal effects. *Journal of Adolescent Health, 38,* 268–274.

Ethier, K. A., Kershaw, T., Niccolai, L., Lewis, J. B., & Ickovics, J. R. (2003). Adolescent women underestimate their susceptibility to sexually transmitted infections. *Sexually Transmitted Infections, 79,* 408–411.

Evans, W. D., Davis, K. C., Ashley, O. S., & Khan, M. (2012). Effects of media messages on parent–child sexual communication. *Journal of Health Communication, 17,* 498–514.

Everett, B. G., Talley, A. E., Hughes, T. L., Wilsnack, S. C., & Johnson, T. P. (2016). Sexual identity mobility and depressive symptoms: A longitudinal analysis of moderating factors among sexual minority women. *Archives of Sexual Behavior, 45,* 1731–1744.

Ewing, S. W. F., & Bryan A. D. (2015). A question of love and trust?: The role of relationship factors in adolescent sexual decision making. *Journal of Developmental and Behavioral Pediatrics, 36,* 628–634.

Eyal, K., & Kunkel, D. (2008). The effects of sex in television drama shows on emerging adults' sexual attitudes and moral judgments. *Journal of Broadcasting and Electronic Media, 52,* 161–181.

Eyal, K., Kunkel, D., Biely, E., & Finnerty, K. (2007). Sexual socialization messages on television programs most popular among teens. *Journal of Broadcasting and Electronic Media, 51,* 316–336.

Eyal, K., Raz, Y., & Levi, M. (2014). Messages about sex on Israeli television: Comparing local and foreign programming. *Journal of Broadcasting and Electronic Media, 58,* 42–58.

Eyre, S. L., Milbrath, C., & Peacock, B. (2007). Romantic relationships trajectories of African American gay/bisexual adolescents. *Journal of Adolescent Research, 22,* 107–131.

Farrell, C. T., Clyde, A., Katta, M., & Bolland, J. (2017). The impact of sexuality concerns on teenage pregnancy: A consequence of heteronormativity? *Culture, Health, and Sexuality, 19,* 135–149.

Fasula, A. M., Miller, K. S., & Wiener, J. (2007). The sexual double standard in African American adolescent women's sexual risk reduction socialization. *Women and Health, 46,* 3–21.

Feldman, S. S., & Rosenthal, D. A. (2000). The effect of communication characteristics on family members' perceptions of parents as sex educators. *Journal of Research on Adolescence, 10,* 119–150.

Feldman, S. S., Rosenthal, D. R., Brown, N. L., & Canning, R. D. (1995). Predicting sexual experience in adolescent boys from peer rejection and acceptance during childhood. *Journal of Research on Adolescence, 5,* 387–411.

Feldstein Ewing, S. W., Ryman, S. G., Gillman, A. S., Weiland, B. J., Thayer, R. E., & Bryan, A. D. (2016). Developmental cognitive neuroscience of adolescent sexual risk and alcohol use. *AIDS and Behavior, 20,* S97–S108.

Felson, R. B., & Haynie, D. L. (2002). Pubertal development, social factors, and delinquency among adolescent boys. *Criminology, 40,* 967–988.

Fergusson D. M., McLeod, G. F. H., & Horwood, J. (2014). Parental separation/divorce in childhood and partnership outcomes at age 30. *Journal of Child Psychology and Psychiatry, 55,* 352–360.

Fielder, R. L., & Carey, M. P. (2010). Predictors and consequences of sexual "hookups" among college students: A short-term prospective study. *Archives of Sexual Behavior, 39,* 1105–1119.

Fielder, R. L., Walsh, J. L., Carey, K. B., & Carey, M. P. (2013). Predictors of sexual hookups: A theory-based, prospective study of first-year college women. *Archives of Sexual Behavior, 42,* 1425–1441.

Fielder, R. L., Walsh, J. L., Carey, K. B., & Carey, M. P. (2014). Sexual hookups and adverse health outcomes: A longitudinal study of first-year college women. *Journal of Sex Research, 51,* 131–144.

Fine, M., & McClelland, S. I. (2006). Sexuality education and desire: Still missing after all these years. *Harvard Educational Review, 76,* 297–338.

Finer, L. B., & Philbin, J. M. (2013). Sexual initiation, contraceptive use, and pregnancy among young adolescents. *Pediatrics, 131,* 886–891.

Finkelhor, D. (1980). Sex among siblings: A survey of prevalence, variety, and effects. *Archives of Sexual Behavior, 9,* 171–194.

Fish, J. N., & Russell, S. T. (2017). Have mischievous responders misidentified sexual minority youth disparities in the National Longitudinal Study of Adolescent to Adult Health? *Archives of Sexual Behavior, 47,* 1053–1067.

Fisher, M. L., Worth, K., Garcia, J. R., & Meredith, T. (2012). Feelings of regret following uncommitted sexual encounters in Canadian university students. *Culture, Health and Sexuality, 14,* 45–57.

Flack, W. F., Daubman, K. A., Caron, M. L., Asadorian, J. A., D'Aureli, N. R., Gigliotti, S. N., et al. (2007). Risk factors and consequences of unwanted sex among university students: Hooking up, alcohol, and stress response. *Journal of Interpersonal Violence, 22,* 139–157.

Fletcher, J. M., & Wolfe, B. L. (2012). The effects of teenage fatherhood on young adult outcomes. *Economic Inquiry, 50,* 182–201.

Flood, M. (2007). Exposure to pornography among youth in Australia. *Journal of Sociology, 43,* 45–60.

Floyd, L. J., & Latimer, W. (2010). Adolescent sexual behaviors at varying levels of substance use frequency. *Journal of Child and Adolescent Substance Abuse, 19,* 66–77.

Ford, C. A., Pence, B. W., Miller, W. C., Resnick, M. D., Bearinger, L. H., Pettingell, S., et al. (2005). Predicting adolescents' longitudinal risk for sexually transmitted infection: Results from the National Longitudinal Study of Adolescent Health. *Archives of Pediatrics and Adolescent Medicine, 159,* 657–664.

Forhan, S. E., Gottlieb, S. L., Sternberg, M. R., Xu, F., Datta, S. D., McQuillan, G. M., et al. (2009). Prevalence of sexually transmitted infections among female adolescents aged 14 to 19 in the United States. *Pediatrics, 124,* 1505–1512.

Forrester, K. (2016, September 26). Lights. Camera. Action. *The New Yorker,* pp. 64–68. Retrieved November 11, 2016, from *www.newyorker.com/magazine/2016/09/26/making-sense-of-modern-pornography.*

Fortenberry, J. D. (2016). Adolescent sexual well-being in the 21st century. *Journal of Adolescent Health, 58,* 1–2.

Fortenberry, J. D., & Hensel, D. J. (2011). The association of sexual interest and sexual behaviors among adolescent women: A daily diary perspective. *Hormones and Behavior, 59,* 739–744.

Fortenberry, J. D., Schick, V., Herbenick, D., Sanders, S. A., Dodge, B., & Reece, M. (2010). Sexual behaviors and condom use at last vaginal intercourse: A national sample of adolescents ages 14 to 17 years. *Journal of Sexual Medicine, 7,* 305–314.

Fortunato, L., Young, A. M., Boyd, C. J., & Fons, C. E. (2010). Hook-up sexual experiences and problem behaviors among adolescents. *Journal of Child and Adolescent Substance Abuse, 19,* 261–278.

Foxman, B., Newman, M., Percha, B., Holmes, K. K., & Aral, S. O. (2006). Measures of sexual partnerships: Lengths, gaps, overlaps, and sexually transmitted infection. *Sexually Transmitted Diseases, 33,* 209–214.

Freitas, D. (2013). *The end of sex: How hookup*

culture is leaving a generation unhappy, sexually unfulfilled, and confused about intimacy. New York: Basic Books.

French, D. C., & Dishion, T. J. (2003). Predictors of early initiation of sexual intercourse among high-risk adolescents. *Journal of Early Adolescence, 23,* 295–315.

Friedlander, L. J., Connolly, J. A., Pepler, D. J., & Craig, W. M. (2007). Biological, familial, and peer influences on dating in early adolescence. *Archives of Sexual Behavior, 36,* 821–830.

Friedman, M. S., Marshal, M. P., Guadamuz, T. E., Wei, C., Wong, C. F., Saewyc, E. M., et al. (2011). A meta-analysis of disparities in childhood sexual abuse, parental physical abuse, and peer victimization among sexual minority and sexual nonminority individuals. *American Journal of Public Health, 101,* 1481–1494.

Friedrich, W. N., Fisher, J., Broughton, D., Houston, M., & Shafran, C. R. (1998). Normative sexual behavior in children: A contemporary sample. *Pediatrics, 101,* E9.

Friedrich, W. N., Fisher, J. L., Dittner, C. A., Acton, R., Butler, J., Damon, L., et al. (2001). Child Sexual Behavior Inventory: Normative, psychiatric, and sexual abuse comparisons. *Child Maltreatment, 6,* 37–49.

Friedrich, W. N., Grambsch, P., Damon, L., Hewitt, S. K., Koverola, C., Lang, R. A., et al. (1992). Child Sexual Behavior Inventory: Normative and clinical comparisons. *Psychological Assessment, 4,* 303–311.

Friedrich, W. N., Sandfort, T. G. M., Oostveen, J., & Cohen-Kettenis, P. T. (2000). Cultural differences in sexual behavior: 2–6 year old Dutch and American children. *Journal of Psychology and Human Sexuality, 12,* 117–129.

Frison, E., Vandenbosch, L., Trekels, J., & Eggermont, S. (2015). Reciprocal relationships between music television exposure and adolescents' sexual behaviors: The role of perceived peer norms. *Sex Roles, 72,* 183–197.

Frontline WBGH. (1999). *The lost children of Rockdale County* [Television broadcast]. Boston: Public Broadcasting Service.

Furman, W., & Shaffer, L. (2011). Romantic partners, friends, friends with benefits, and casual acquaintances as sexual partners. *Journal of Sex Research, 48,* 554–564.

Furstenberg, F. F., Jr. (2003). Teenage childbearing as a public issue and private concern. *Annual Review of Sociology, 29,* 23–39.

Garcia, J. R., Reiber, C., Massey, S. G., & Merriwether, A. M. (2012). Sexual hookup culture: A review. *Review of General Psychology, 16,* 161–176.

Garfield, C. F., Duncan, G., Peters, S., Rutsohn, J., McDade, T. W., Adam, E. K., et al. (2016). Adolescent reproductive knowledge, attitudes, and beliefs and future fatherhood. *Journal of Adolescent Health, 58,* 497–503.

Garneau, C., Olmstead, S. B., Pasley, K., & Fincham, F. D. (2013). The role of family structure and attachment in college student hookups. *Archives of Sexual Behavior, 42,* 1473–1486.

Garofalo, R., Wolf, R. C., Kessel, S., Palfrey, J., & DuRant, R. H. (1998). The association between health risk behaviors and sexual orientation among a school-based sample of adolescents. *Pediatrics, 101,* 895–902.

Gaudie, J., Mitrou, F., Lawrence, D., Stanley, F. J., Silburn, S. R., & Zubrick, S. R. (2010). Antecedents of teenage pregnancy from a 14-year follow-up using data linkage. *BMC Public Health, 10,* 63.

Ge, X., Natsuaki, M. N., Neiderhiser, J. M., & Reiss, D. (2007). Genetic and environmental influences on pubertal timing: Results from two national sibling studies. *Journal of Research on Adolescence, 17,* 767–788.

Gelbal, S., Duyan, V., & Öztürk, A. B. (2008). Gender differences in sexual information sources, and sexual attitudes and behaviors of university students in Turkey. *Social Behavior and Personality: An International Journal, 36,* 1035–1052.

Gentzler, A. L., & Kerns, K. A. (2004). Associations between insecure attachment and sexual experiences. *Personal Relationships, 11,* 249–265.

Gerressu, M., Mercer, C. H., Graham, C. A., Wellings, K., & Johnson, A. M. (2008). Prevalence of masturbation and associated factors in a British national probability sample. *Archives of Sexual Behavior, 37,* 266–278.

Gibbs, C. M., Wendt, A., Peters, S., & Hogue,

C. J. (2012). The impact of early age at first childbirth on maternal and infant health. *Paediatric and Perinatal Epidemiology, 26,* 259–284.

Gillmore, M. R., Chen, A. C., Haas, S. A., Kopak, A. M., & Robillard, A. G. (2011). Do family and parenting factors in adolescence influence condom use in early adulthood in a multiethnic sample of young adults? *Journal of Youth and Adolescence, 40,* 1503–1518.

Giordano, P. C., Manning, W. D., & Longmore, M. A. (2014). Adolescent romantic relationships: An emerging portrait of their nature and developmental significance. In A. C. Crouter & A. Booth (Eds.), *Romance and sex in adolescence and emerging adulthood: Risks and opportunities* (pp. 127–150). New York: Psychology Press.

Glassman, J. R., Potter, S. C., Baumier, E. R., & Coyle, K. K. (2015). Estimates of intraclass correlation coefficients from longitudinal group-randomized trials of adolescent HIV/STI/pregnancy prevention programs. *Health Education and Behavior, 42,* 545–553.

Glenn, N., & Marquardt, E. (2001). *Hooking up, hanging out, and hoping for Mr. Right: College women on dating and mating today.* New York: Institute for American Values.

Godeau, E., Nic Gabhainn, S., Vignes, C., Ross, J., Boyce, W., & Todd, J. (2008). Contraceptive use by 15-year-old students at their last sexual intercourse: Results from 24 countries. *Archives of Pediatrics and Adolescent Medicine, 162,* 66–73.

Goesling, B., Colman, S., Trenholm, C., Terzian, M., & Moore, K. (2014). Programs to reduce teen pregnancy, sexually transmitted infections, and associated sexual risk behaviors: A systematic review. *Journal of Adolescent Health, 54,* 499–507.

Gold, J., Pedrana, A. E., Sacks-Davis, R., Hellard, M. E., Chang, S., Howard, S., et al. (2011). A systematic examination of the use of online social networking sites for sexual health promotion. *BMC Public Health, 11,* 583–591.

Goldbach, J. T., Tanner-Smith, E. E., Bagwell, M., & Dunlap, S. (2014). Minority stress and substance use in sexual minority adolescents: A meta-analysis. *Prevention Science, 15,* 350–363.

Goldberg, S. K., Reese, B. M., & Halpern, C. T. (2016). Teen pregnancy among sexual minority women: Results from the National Longitudinal Study of Adolescent to Adult Health. *Journal of Adolescent Health, 59,* 429–437.

Golden, R. L., Furman, W., & Collibee, C. (2016). The risks and rewards of sexual debut. *Developmental Psychology, 52,* 1913–1925.

Goldenberg, D., Telzer, E. H., Lieberman, M. D., Fuligni, A., & Galván, A. (2013). Neural mechanisms of impulse control of sexually risky adolescents. *Developmental Cognitive Neuroscience, 6,* 23–29.

Goldman, J. D. G., & Bradley, G. L. (2001). Sexuality education across the lifestyle in the new millennium. *Sex Education, 1,* 198–217.

Goldstein, S. E., Davis-Kean, P. E., & Eccles, J. S. (2005). Parents, peers, and problem behavior: A longitudinal investigation of the impact of relationship perceptions and characteristics on the development of adolescent problem behavior. *Developmental Psychology, 41,* 401–413.

Gonçalves, H., Gonçalves Soares, A. L., Bierhals, I. O., Machado, A. K. F., Fernandes, M. P., Hirschmann, R., et al. (2017). Age of sexual initiation and depression in adolescents: Data from the 1993 Pelotas (Brazil) birth cohort. *Journal of Affective Disorders, 221,* 259–266.

González-Ortega, E., Vicario-Molina, I., Martinez, J. L., & Orgaz, B. (2015). The Internet as a source of sexual information in a sample of Spanish adolescents: Associations with sexual behavior. *Sexuality Research and Social Policy, 12,* 290–300.

Goodrum, N. M., Armistead, L. P., Tully, E. C., Cook, S. L., & Skinner, D. (2017). Parenting and youth sexual risk in context: The role of community factors. *Journal of Adolescence, 57,* 1–12.

Goodson, P., Buhi, E. R., & Dunsmore, S. C. (2006). Self-esteem and adolescent sexual behaviors, attitudes, and intentions: A systematic review. *Journal of Adolescent Health, 38,* 310–319.

Gordon, A. R., Conron, K. J., Calzo, J. P., Reisner, S. L., & Austin, S. B. (2016). Nonconforming gender expression is a predictor of bullying and violence victimization among high school students in four U.S. school districts. *Journal of Adolescent Health, 58*, S1–S2.

Gray, P. B., Garcia, J. R., Crosier, B. S., & Fisher, H. E. (2015). Dating and sexual behavior among single parents of young children in the United States. *Journal of Sex Research, 52*, 121–128.

Green, K. E., & Feinstein, B. A. (2012). Substance use in lesbian, gay, and bisexual populations: An update on empirical research and implications for treatment. *Psychology of Addictive Behavior, 26*, 265–278.

Greenberg, D. S. (1994). Out goes the surgeon general. *Lancet, 344*, 1760.

Greene, G. J., Andrews, R., Kuper, L., & Mustanski, B. (2014). Intimacy, monogamy, and condom problems drive unprotected sex among young men in serious relationships with other men: A mixed methods dyadic study. *Archives of Sexual Behavior, 43*, 73–87.

Greenwald, E., & Leitenberg, H. (1989). Long-term effects of sexual experiences with siblings and nonsiblings during childhood. *Archives of Sexual Behavior, 18*, 389–399.

Grossman, A. H., & D'Augelli, A. R. (2007). Transgender youth and life-threatening behaviors. *Suicide and Life-Threatening Behavior, 37*, 527–537.

Grossman, J. M., Charmaraman, L., & Erkut, S. (2016). Do as I say, not as I did: How parents talk with early adolescents about sex. *Journal of Family Issues, 37*, 177–197.

Grossman, J. M., Tracy, A. J., Richer, A. M., & Erkut, S. (2015). The role of extended family in teen sexual health. *Journal of Adolescent Research, 30*, 31–56.

Guan, S. A., & Subrahmanyam, K. (2009). Youth Internet use: Risks and opportunities. *Current Opinion in Psychiatry, 22*, 351–356.

Guilamo-Ramos, V., Jaccard, J., & Dittus, P. (Eds.). (2010). *Parental monitoring of adolescents: Current perspectives for researchers and practitioners.* New York: Columbia University Press.

Guilamo-Ramos, V., Lee, J. J., Kantor, L. M., Levine, D. S., Baum, S., & Johnsen, J. (2015). Potential for using online and mobile education with parents and adolescents to impact sexual and reproductive health. *Prevention Science, 16*, 53–60.

Guillamon, A., Junque, C., & Gómez-Gil, E. (2016). A review of the status of brain structure research in transsexualism. *Archives of Sexual Behavior, 45*, 1615–1648.

Gunasekera, H., Chapman, S., & Campbell, S. (2005). Sex and drugs in popular movies: An analysis of the top 200 films. *Journal of the Royal Society of Medicine, 98*, 464–470.

Guse, K., Levine, D., Martins, S., Lira, A., Gaarde, J., Westmorland, W., et al. (2012). Interventions using new digital media to improve adolescent sexual health: A systematic review. *Journal of Adolescent Health, 51*, 535–543.

Guttmacher Institute. (2016, June). Fact sheet: American teens' sexual and reproductive health. Retrieved July 28, 2016, from *www.guttmacher.org/fact-sheet/american-teens-sexual-and-reproductive-health.*

Guttmacher Institute. (2018, April). An overview of minors' consent law. Retrieved April 29, 2018, from *www.guttmacher.org/state-policy/explore/overview-minors-consent-law.*

Haas, A. P., Eliason, M., Mayes, V. M., Mathy, R. M., Cochran, S. D., D'Augelli, A. R., et al. (2011). Suicide and suicide risk in lesbian, gay, bisexual, and transgender populations: Review and recommendations. *Journal of Homosexuality, 58*, 10–51.

Haberland, N., & Rogow, D. (2015). Sexuality education: Emerging trends in evidence and practice. *Journal of Adolescent Health, 56*, S15–S21.

Hadley, W., Houck, C. D., Barker, D., & Senocak, N. (2015). Relationships of parental monitoring and emotion regulation with early adolescents' sexual behaviors. *Journal of Developmental and Behavioral Pediatrics, 36*, 381–388.

Hadley, W., Lansing, A., Barker, D. H., Brown, L. K., Hunter, H., Donenberg, G., et al. (2018). The longitudinal impact of a family-based communication intervention on observational and self-reports of sexual communication. *Journal of Child and Family Studies, 27,* 1098–1109.

Hald, G. M., Kuyper, L., Adam, P. C. G., & de Wit, J. B. F. (2013). Does viewing explain doing?: Assessing the association between sexually explicit materials use and sexual behaviors in a large sample of Dutch adolescents and young adults. *Journal of Sexual Medicine, 10,* 2986–2995.

Halkitis, P. N., & Parsons, J. T. (2002). Recreational drug use and HIV-risk sexual behavior among men frequenting gay social venues. *Journal of Gay and Lesbian Social Services, 14,* 19–39.

Hall, K., Kusunoki, Y., Gatny, H., & Barber, J. (2015). Social discrimination, stress, and risk of unintended pregnancy among young women. *Journal of Adolescent Health, 56,* 330–337.

Hall, P. C., West, J. H., & Hill, S. (2012). Sexualization in lyrics of popular music from 1959 to 2009: Implications for sexuality educators. *Sexuality and Culture, 16,* 103–117.

Halley, A. C., Boretsky, M., Puts, D. A., & Shriver, M. (2016). Self-reported sexual behavioral interests and polymorphisms in the dopamine receptor D4 (DRD4) exon III VNTR in heterosexual young adults. *Archives of Sexual Behavior, 45,* 2091–2100.

Hallfors, D. D., Waller, M. W., Bauer, D., Ford, C. A., & Halpern, C. T. (2005). Which comes first in adolescence: Sex and drugs or depression? *American Journal of Preventive Medicine, 29,* 163–170.

Halpern, C. T. (2006). Integrating hormones and other biological factors into a developmental systems model of adolescent female sexuality. In L. M. Diamond (Ed.), *Rethinking positive adolescent female sexual development* (pp. 9–22). San Francisco: Jossey-Bass.

Halpern, C. T., & Haydon, A. A. (2012). Sexual timetables for oral–genital, vaginal, and anal intercourse: Sociodemographic comparisons in a nationally representative sample of adolescents. *American Journal of Public Health, 102,* 1221–1228.

Halpern, C. T., Udry, J. R., Campbell, B., & Suchindran, C. (1993). Testosterone and pubertal development as predictors of sexual activity: A panel analysis of adolescent males. *Psychosomatic Medicine, 55,* 436–447.

Halpern, C. T., Udry, J. R., Campbell, B., & Suchindran, C. (1999). Effects of body fat on weight concerns, dating, and sexual activity: A longitudinal analysis of black and white adolescent girls. *Developmental Psychology, 35,* 721–736.

Halpern, C. T., Udry, J. R., Campbell, B., Suchindran, C., & Mason, G. A. (1994). Testosterone and religiosity as predictors of sexual attitudes and activity among adolescent males: A biosocial model. *Journal of Biosocial Science, 26,* 217–234.

Halpern, C. T., Udry, J. R., & Suchindran, C. (1997). Testosterone predicts initiation of coitus in adolescent females. *Psychosomatic Medicine, 59,* 161–171.

Halpern, C. T., Udry, J. R., & Suchindran, C. (1998). Monthly measures of salivary testosterone predict sexual activity in adolescent males. *Archives of Sexual Behavior, 27,* 445–465.

Halpern, C. T., Udry, J. R., Suchindran, C., & Campbell, B. (2000). Adolescent males' willingness to report masturbation. *Journal of Sex Research, 37,* 327–332.

Hamilton, B. E., Martin, J. A., Osterman, M. J. K., Driscoll, A. K., & Rossen, L. M. (2017, June). *Births: Provisional data for 2016* (Vital Statistics Rapid Release Report No. 002). Hyattsville, MD: National Center for Health Statistics. Retrieved August 13, 2017, from *www.cdc.gov/nchs/data/vsrr/report002.pdf.*

Hammen, C., Brennan, P. A., & Le Brocque, R. (2011). Youth depression and early childrearing: Stress generation and intergenerational transmission of depression. *Journal of Consulting and Clinical Psychology, 79,* 353–363.

Handelsman, C. D., Cabral, R. J., & Weisfeld, G. E. (1987). Sources of information and adolescent sexual knowledge and behavior. *Journal of Adolescent Research, 2,* 455–463.

Handsfield, H. H. (2015). Sexually transmitted diseases, infections, and disorders: What's in a name? *Sexually Transmitted Diseases, 42,* 169.

Hans, J. D., Gillen, M., & Akande, K. (2010). Sex redefined: The reclassification of oral–genital contact. *Perspectives on Sexual and Reproductive Health, 42,* 74–78.

Harden, A., Brunton, G., Fletcher, A., &

Oakley, A. (2009). Teenage pregnancy and social disadvantage: Systematic review integrating controlled trials and qualitative studies. *BMJ Research, 339,* b4254.

Harden, K. P. (2012). True love waits?: A sibling-comparison study of age at first sexual intercourse and romantic relationships in young adulthood. *Psychological Science, 23,* 1324–1336.

Harden, K. P. (2014a). Genetic influences on adolescent sexual behavior: Why genes matter for environmentally oriented researchers. *Psychological Bulletin, 140,* 434–465.

Harden, K. P. (2014b). A sex-positive framework for research on adolescent sexuality. *Perspectives on Psychological Science, 9,* 455–469.

Harden, K. P., Lynch, S. K., Turkheimer, E., Emery, R. E., D'Onofrio, B. M., Slutske, W. S., et al. (2007). A behavior genetic investigation of adolescent motherhood and offspring mental health problems. *Journal of Abnormal Psychology, 116,* 667–683.

Hardy, J. B., Astone, N. M., Brooks-Gunn, J., Shapiro, S., & Miller, T. L. (1998). Like mother, like child: Intergenerational patterns of age at first birth and associations with childhood and adolescent characteristics and adult outcomes in the second generation. *Developmental Psychology, 34,* 1220–1232.

Hardy, M. S. (2001). Physical aggression and sexual behavior among siblings: A retrospective study. *Journal of Family Violence, 16,* 255–268.

Harris, J. A., Vernon, P. A., & Boomsma, D. I. (1998). The heritability of testosterone: A study of Dutch adolescent twins and their parents. *Behavior Genetics, 28,* 165–171.

Harris, J. R. (1998). *The nurture assumption: Why children turn out the way they do.* New York: Free Press.

Harrison, A., Smit, J., Hoffman, S., Nzama, T., Leu, C. S., Mantell, J., et al. (2012). Gender, peer and partner influences on adolescent HIV risk in rural South Africa. *Sexual Health, 9,* 178–186.

Hatzenbuehler, M. L. (2009). How does sexual minority stigma "get under the skin"?: A psychological mediation framework. *Psychological Bulletin, 135,* 707–730.

Hatzenbuehler, M. L., McLaughlin, K. A., & Xuan, Z. (2012). Social networks and risk for depressive symptoms in a national sample of sexual minority youth. *Social Science and Medicine, 75,* 1184–1191.

Haurin, R. J., & Mott, F. L. (1990). Adolescent sexual activity in the family context: The impact of older siblings. *Demography, 27,* 537–557.

Haydon, A. A., Herring, A. H., Prinstein, M. J., & Halpern, C. T. (2012). Beyond age at first sex: Patterns of emerging sexual behavior in adolescence and young adulthood. *Journal of Adolescent Health, 50,* 456–463.

Hayter, M., Jones, C., Owen, J., & Harrison, C. (2016). A qualitative evaluation of home-based contraceptive and sexual health care for teenage mothers. *Primary Health Care Research and Development, 17,* 287–297.

Heins, M. (2007). *Not in front of the children: Indecency, censorship, and the innocence of youth* (2nd ed.) New Brunswick, NJ: Rutgers University Press.

Henry, D. B., Deptula, D. P., & Schoeny, M. E. (2012). Sexually-transmitted infections and unintended pregnancy: A longitudinal analysis of risk transmission through friends and attitudes. *Social Development, 21,* 195–214.

Henry, D. B., Schoeny, M. E., Deptula, D. P., & Slavick, J. T. (2007). Peer selection and socialization effects on adolescent intercourse without a condom and attitudes about the costs of sex. *Child Development, 78,* 825–838.

Hensel, D. J., Fortenberry, J. D., O'Sullivan, L. F., & Orr, D. P. (2011). The developmental association of sexual self-concept with sexual behavior among adolescent women. *Journal of Adolescence, 34,* 675–684.

Hensel, D. J., Hummer, T. A., Acrurio, L. R., James, T. W., & Fortenberry, D. (2015). Feasibility of functional neuroimaging to understand adolescent women's sexual decision making. *Journal of Adolescent Health, 56,* 389–395.

Hensel, D. J., Nance, J., & Fortenberry, J. D. (2016). The association between sexual health and physical, mental, and social health in adolescent women. *Journal of Adolescent Health, 59,* 416–421.

Herbenick, D., Reece, M., Schick, V.,

Sanders, S. A., Dodge, B., & Fortenberry, J. D. (2010). Sexual behavior in the United States: Results from a national probability sample of men and women ages 14–94. *Journal of Sexual Medicine, 7,* 255–265.

Heron, J., Low, N., Lewis, G., Macleod, J., Ness, A., & Waylen, A. (2015). Social factors associated with readiness for sexual activity in adolescents: A population-based cohort study. *Archives of Sexual Behavior, 44,* 669–678.

Herrman, J. W. (2014). Adolescent girls who experience abuse or neglect are at an increased risk of teen pregnancy. *Evidence Based Nursing, 17,* 79.

Hetherington, E. M., & Kelly, J. (2003). *For better or for worse: Divorce reconsidered.* New York: Norton.

Heywood, W., Patrick, K., Pitts, M., & Mitchell, A. (2016). "Dude, I'm seventeen. . . . It's okay not to have sex by this age": Feelings, reasons, pressures, and intentions reported by adolescents who have not had sexual intercourse. *Journal of Sex Research, 53,* 1207–1214.

Hieftje, K., Edelman, J., Camenga, D. R., & Fiellin, L. E. (2013). Electronic media-based health interventions promoting behavior change in youth: A systematic review. *JAMA Pediatrics, 167,* 574–580.

Hodgkinson, S., Beers, L., Southammakosane, C., & Lewin, A. (2014). Addressing the mental health needs of pregnant and parenting adolescents. *Pediatrics, 133,* 114–122.

Hoekstra, R. A., Bartels, M., & Boomsma, D. I. (2006). Heritability of testosterone levels in 12-year-old twins and its relation to pubertal development. *Twin Research and Human Genetics, 9,* 558–565.

Hoffman, J. (2016, April 7). The persistent myth about oral sex. *New York Times.* Retrieved November 30, 2016, from *www.nytimes.com/2016/04/07/health/misconceptions-oral-sex-stds.html?_r=0.*

Hogan, D. P., Sun, R., & Cornwell, G. T. (2000). Sexual and fertility behaviors of American females aged 15–19 years: 1985, 1990, and 1995. *American Journal of Public Health, 90,* 1421–1425.

Hokororo, A., Kihunrwa, A., Hoekstra, P., Kalluvya, S. E., Changalucha, J. M., Fitzgerald, D. W., et al. (2015). High prevalence of sexually transmitted infections in pregnant adolescent girls in Tanzania: A multi-community cross-sectional study. *Sexually Transmitted Infections, 91,* 473–478.

Hollenstein, T., & Lougheed, J. P. (2013). Beyond storm and stress: Typicality, transactions, timing, and temperament to account for adolescent change. *American Psychologist, 68,* 444–454.

Holman, A., & Kellas, J. K. (2015). High school adolescents' perceptions of the parent–child sex talk: How communication, relational, and family factors relate to sexual health. *Southern Communication Journal, 80,* 388–403.

Holway, G. V. (2015). Vaginal and oral sex initiation timing: A focus on gender and race/ethnicity. *International Journal of Sexual Health, 27,* 351–367.

Horan, S. M., & Cafferty, L. A. (2017). Condom communication: Reports of sexually active young adults' recent messages with new partners. *Journal of Health Communication, 22,* 763–771.

Hoskins, D. H., & Simons, L. G. (2015). Predicting the risk of pregnancy among African American youth: Testing a social contextual model. *Journal of Child and Family Studies, 24,* 1163–1174.

Houck, C. D., Barker, D., Rizzo, C., Hancock, E., Norton, A., & Brown, L. K. (2014). Sexting and sexual behavior in at-risk adolescents. *Pediatrics, 133,* e276–e282.

Hu, Y., Wong, M. L., Prema, V., Wong, M. L., Fong, N. P., Tsai, F. F., et al. (2012). Do parents talk to their adolescent children about sex?: Findings from a community survey in Singapore. *Annals of the Academy of Medicine, Singapore, 41,* 239–246.

Hu, Y., Xu, Y., & Tornello, S. L. (2016). Stability of self-reported same-sex and both-sex attraction from adolescence to young adulthood. *Archives of Sexual Behavior, 45,* 651–659.

Huang, D. Y. C., Murphy, D. A., & Hser, Y. I. (2011). Parental monitoring during early adolescence deters adolescent sexual initiation: Discrete-time survival mixture analysis. *Journal of Child and Family Studies, 20,* 511–520.

Hughes, G., Brady, A. R., Catchpole, M. A., Fenton, K. A., Rogers, P. A., Kinghorn, G. R., et al. (2001). Characteristics of those who repeatedly acquire sexually transmitted infections: A retrospective cohort study of attendees at three urban sexually transmitted disease clinics in England. *Sexually Transmitted Diseases, 28*, 379–386.

Humphreys, T. P. (2013). Cognitive frameworks of virginity and first intercourse. *Journal of Sex Research, 50*, 664–675.

Hyde, A., Drennan, J., Howlett, E., & Brady, D. (2008). Heterosexual experiences of secondary school pupils in Ireland: Sexual coercion in context. *Culture, Health and Sexuality, 10*, 479–493.

Igartua, K., Thombs, B. D., Burgos, G., & Montoro, R. (2009). Concordance and discrepancy in sexual identity, attraction, and behavior among adolescents. *Journal of Adolescent Health, 45*, 602–608.

Impett, E. A., & Tolman, D. L. (2006). Late adolescent girls' sexual experiences and sexual satisfaction. *Journal of Adolescent Research, 21*, 628–646.

Ivanova, K., Mills, M., & Veenstra, R. (2011). The initiation of dating in adolescence: The effect of parental divorce: The TRAILS study. *Journal of Research on Adolescence, 21*, 769–775.

Ivanova, K., Veenstra, R., & Mills, M. (2012). Who dates?: The effects of temperament, puberty, and parenting on early adolescent experience with dating: The TRAILS study. *Journal of Early Adolescence, 32*, 340–363.

Jaccard, J., Blanton, H., & Dodge, T. (2005). Peer influences on risk behavior: An analysis of the effects of a close friend. *Developmental Psychology, 41*, 135–147.

Jaccard, J., Dittus, P. J., & Gordon, V. V. (1998). Parent–adolescent congruency in reports of adolescent sexual behavior and in communications about sexual behavior. *Child Development, 69*, 247–261.

Jaccard, J., Dittus, P. J., & Gordon, V. V. (2000). Parent–teen communication about premarital sex: Factors associated with the extent of communication. *Journal of Adolescent Research, 15*, 187–208.

Jaccard, J., Dodge, T., & Dittus, P. (2003). Do adolescents want to avoid pregnancy?: Attitudes toward pregnancy as predictors of pregnancy. *Journal of Adolescent Health, 33*, 79–83.

Jacobellis v. Ohio, 378 U.S. 184 (1964). Retrieved April 22, 2018, from *https://supreme.justia.com/cases/federal/us/378/184/case.html.*

Jacobs, J., & Mollborn, S. (2012). Early motherhood and the disruption in significant attachments: Autonomy and reconnection as a response to separation and loss among African American and Latina teen mothers. *Gender and Society, 26*, 922–944.

Jaffee, S., Caspi, A., Moffitt, T. E., Belsky, J., & Silva, P. (2001). Why are children born to teen mothers at risk for adverse outcomes in young adulthood?: Results from a 20-year longitudinal study. *Development and Psychopathology, 13*, 377–397.

Jaffee, S. R., Caspi, A., Moffitt, T. E., Taylor, A., & Dickson, N. (2001). Predicting early fatherhood and whether young fathers live with their children: Prospective findings and policy reconsiderations. *Journal of Child Psychology and Psychiatry, 42*, 803–815.

James, E. L. (2012). *Fifty shades of grey.* New York: Vintage Books.

James, J., Ellis, B. J., Schlomer, G. L., & Garber, J. (2012). Sex-specific pathways to early puberty, sexual debut, and sexual risk taking: Tests of an integrated evolutionary-developmental model. *Developmental Psychology, 48*, 667–702.

Jemmott, J. B., Jemmott, L. S., & Fong, G. T. (2010). Efficacy of a theory-based abstinence-only intervention over 24 months. *Archives of Pediatrics and Adolescent Medicine, 164*, 152–159.

Jemmott, L. S., & Jemmott, J. B. (1992). Family structure, parental strictness, and sexual behavior among inner-city black male adolescents. *Journal of Adolescent Research, 7*, 192–207.

Jennings, J. M., Taylor, R., Iannacchione, V. G., Rogers, S. M., Chung, S. E., Huettner, S., et al. (2010). The available pool of sex partners and risk for a current bacterial sexually transmitted infection. *Annals of Epidemiology, 20*, 532–538.

Jerman, P., & Constantine, N. A. (2010). Demographic and psychological predictors of parent–adolescent communication about sex: A representative statewide analysis. *Journal of Youth and Adolescence, 39,* 1164–1174.

Jessor, R. (2014). Problem behavior theory: A half century of research on adolescent behavior and development. In R. M. Lerner, A. C. Petersen, R. K. Silbereisen, & J. Brooks-Gunn (Eds.), *The developmental science of adolescence: History through autobiography* (pp. 239–256). New York: Psychology Press.

Johnson, B. T., Scott-Sheldon, L. J., Huedo-Medina, T. B., & Carey, M. P. (2011). Interventions to reduce sexual risk for human immunodeficiency virus in adolescents: A meta-analysis of trials, 1985–2008. *Archives of Pediatrics and Adolescent Medicine, 165,* 77–84.

Johnson, M. D., & Chen, J. (2015). Blame it on the alcohol: The influence of alcohol consumption during adolescence, the transition to adulthood, and young adulthood on one-time sexual hookups. *Journal of Sex Research, 52,* 570–579.

Johnson-Baker, K. A., Markham, C., Baumler, E., Swain, H., & Emery, S. (2016). Rap music use, perceived peer behavior, and sexual initiation among ethnic minority youth. *Journal of Adolescent Health, 58,* 317–322.

Jonason, P. K., Li, N. P., & Richardson, J. (2011). Positioning the booty-call relationship on the spectrum of relationships: Sexual but more emotional than one-night stands. *Journal of Sex Research, 48,* 486–495.

Jones, A., Robinson, E., Oginni, O., Rahman, Q., & Rimes, K. A. (2017). Anxiety disorders, gender nonconformity, bullying and self-esteem in sexual minority adolescents: Prospective birth cohort study. *Journal of Child Psychology and Psychiatry, 58,* 1201–1209.

Jones, C. J., Smith, H., & Llewellyn, C. (2014). Evaluating the effectiveness of health belief model interventions in improving adherence: A systematic review. *Health Psychology Review, 8,* 253–269.

Jones, R. K., & Biddlecom, A. E. (2011). Is the Internet filling the sexual health information gap for teens?: An exploratory study. *Journal of Health Communication, 16,* 112–123.

Jones, R., Biddlecom, A., Hebert, L., & Mellor, R. (2011). Teens reflect on their sources of contraceptive information. *Journal of Adolescent Research, 26,* 423–446.

Josephs, L. (2015). How children learn about sex: A cross-species and cross-cultural analysis. *Archives of Sexual Behavior, 44,* 1059–1069.

Jovic, S., Delpierre, C., Ehlinger, V., Sentenac, M., Young, H., Arnaud, C., et al. (2014). Associations between life contexts and early sexual initiation among young women in France. *Perspectives on Sexual and Reproductive Health, 46,* 31–39.

Jozkowski, K. N., & Satinsky, S. A. (2013). A gender discrepancy analysis of heterosexual sexual behaviors in two university samples. *Journal of Community Health, 38,* 1157–1165.

Kaiser Family Foundation. (2003). *National survey of adolescents and young adults: Sexual health knowledge, attitudes, and experiences.* Menlo Park, CA. Retrieved December 2, 2016, from *http://kff.org/hivaids/report/national-survey-of-adolescents-and-young-adults.*

Kalil, A., Ziol-Guest, K. M., & Coley, R. L. (2005). Perceptions of father involvement patterns in teenage-mother families: Predictors and links to mothers' psychological adjustment. *Family Relations, 54,* 197–211.

Kalish, R., & Kimmel, M. (2011). Hooking up: Hot hetero sex or the new numb normative? *Australian Feminist Studies, 26,* 137–151.

Kane, E. W. (2006). "No way my boys are going to be like that!": Parents' responses to children's gender nonconformity. *Gender and Society, 20,* 149–176.

Kann, L., McManus, T., Harris, W. A., Shanklin, S. L., Flint, K. H., Hawkins, J., et al. (2016, June 10). Youth risk behavior surveillance: United States, 2015. *Morbidity and Mortality Weekly Report, 65.* Retrieved September 21, 2016, from *www.cdc.gov/healthyyouth/data/yrbs/pdf/2015/ss6506_updated.pdf.*

Kann, L., Olsen, E. O., McManus, T., Harris, W. A., Shanklin, S. L., Flint, K. H., et al. (2016, August 12). Sexual identity, sex of sexual contacts, and health-related behaviors among students in grades 9–12: United States and selected sites, 2015. *Morbidity and Mortality Weekly Report, 65.* Retrieved November 21, 2016, from *www.cdc.gov/mmwr/volumes/65/ss/pdfs/ss6509.pdf.*

Kao, T.-S. A., & Carter, W. A. (2013). Family influences on adolescent sexual activity and alcohol use. *Open Family Studies Journal, 5,* 10–18.

Kao, T.-S. A., & Martyn, K. K. (2014, April–June). Comparing white and Asian American adolescents' perceived parental expectations and their sexual behaviors. *Sage Open,* 1–16. Retrieved July 10, 2016, from *http://sgo.sage-pub.com/content/4/2/2158244014535411.*

Kapadia, F., Bub, K., Barton, S., Stults, C. B., & Halkitis, P. N. (2015). Longitudinal trends in sexual behaviors without a condom among sexual minority youth: The P18 Cohort Study. *AIDS and Behavior, 19,* 2152–2161.

Kapadia, F., Frye, V., Bonner, S., Emmanuel, P. J., Samples, C. L., & Latka, M. H. (2012). Perceived peer safer sex norms and sexual risk behaviors among substance-using Latino adolescents. *AIDS Education and Prevention, 24,* 27–40.

Kaplowitz, P. B. (2008). Link between body fat and the timing of puberty. *Pediatrics, 121,* S208–S217.

Kapungu, C. T., Baptiste, D., Holmbeck, G., McBride, C., Robinson-Brown, M., Sturdivant, A., et al. (2010). Beyond the "birds and the bees": Gender differences in sex-related communication among urban African-American adolescents. *Family Process, 49,* 251–264.

Karoly, H. C., Callahan, T., Schmiege, S. J., & Feldstein Ewing, S. W. (2016). Evaluating the Hispanic paradox in the context of adolescent risky sexual behavior: The role of parent monitoring. *Journal of Pediatric Psychology, 41,* 429–440.

Kauffman, L., Orbe, M. P., Johnson, A. L., & Cooke-Jackson, A. (2013). Memorable familial messages about sex: A qualitative content analysis of college student narratives. *Electronic Journal of Human Sexuality, 16.*

Kawachi, I., & Berkman, L. F. (2003). *Neighborhoods and health.* New York: Oxford University Press.

Kaye, K., Suellentrop, K., & Sloup, C. (2009). *The fog zone: How misperceptions, magical thinking, and ambivalence put young adults at risk for unplanned pregnancy.* Washington, DC: National Campaign to Prevent Teen and Unplanned Pregnancy. Retrieved November 30, 2016, from *http://thenationalcampaign.org/resource/fog-zone.*

Kearney, M. S., & Levine, P. B. (2012). Why is the teen birth rate in the United States so high and why does it matter? *Journal of Economic Perspectives, 26,* 141–166.

Kearney, M. S., & Levine, P. B. (2014, January). Media influences on social outcomes: The impact of MTV's *16 and Pregnant* on teen childbearing (NBER Working Paper No. 19759). Retrieved July 11, 2016, from *www.nber.org/papers/w19795.*

Kelleher, C. (2009). Minority stress and health: Implications for lesbian, gay, bisexual, transgender, and questioning (LGBTQ) young people. *Counseling Psychology Quarterly, 22,* 373–379.

Keller, S. N., & Brown, J. D. (2002). Media interventions to promote responsible sexual behavior. *Journal of Sex Research, 39,* 67–72.

Kelley, S. S., Borawski, E. A., Flocke, S. A., & Keen K. J. (2003). The role of sequential and concurrent sexual relationships in the risk of sexually transmitted diseases among adolescents. *Journal of Adolescent Health, 32,* 296–305.

Kellogg, N. D. (2009). Clinical report: The evaluation of sexual behaviors in children. *Pediatrics, 124,* 992–998.

Kenny, M. C., & Wurtele, S. K. (2013). Child Sexual Behavior Inventory: A comparison between Latino and normative samples of preschoolers. *Journal of Sex Research, 50,* 449–457.

Kerpelman, J. L., McElwain, A. D., Pittman, J. F., & Adler-Baeder, F. M. (2016). Engagement in risky sexual behavior: Adolescents' perceptions of self and the parent–child relationship matter. *Youth and Society, 48,* 101–125.

Kerr, D. C. R., Washburn, I. J., Morris, M. K., Lewis, K. A. G., & Tiberio, S. S. (2015). Event-level associations of marijuana and heavy alcohol use with intercourse and condom use. *Journal of Studies of Alcohol and Drugs, 76,* 733–737.

Khan, M. R., Berger, A. T., Wells, B. E., & Cleland, C. M. (2012). Longitudinal associations between adolescent alcohol use and adulthood sexual risk behavior and sexually transmitted infection in the United States: Assessment of differences by race. *American Journal of Public Health, 102,* 867–876.

Khashan, A. S., Baker, P. N., & Kenny, L. C. (2010). Preterm birth and reduced birthweight in first and second teenage pregnancies: A register-based cohort study. *BMC Pregnancy and Childbirth, 10,* 36.

Khurana, A., & Cooksey, E. C. (2012). Examining the effect of maternal sexual communication and adolescents' perceptions of maternal disapproval on adolescent risky sexual involvement. *Journal of Adolescent Health, 51,* 557–565.

Khurana, A., Romer, D., Betancourt, L. M., Brodsky, N. L., Giannetta, J. M., & Hurt, H. (2015). Stronger working memory reduces sexual risk taking in adolescents, even after controlling for parental influences. *Child Development, 86,* 1125–1141.

Kiefer, A. K., & Sanchez, D. T. (2007). Scripting sexual passivity: A gender role perspective. *Personal Relationships, 14,* 269–290.

Killoren, S. E., Updegraff, K. A., Christopher, F. S., & Umaña-Taylor, A. J. (2011). Mothers, fathers, peers, and Mexican-origin adolescents' sexual intentions. *Journal of Marriage and the Family, 73,* 209–220.

Kim, C. R., & Free, C. (2008). Recent evaluations of the peer-led approach in adolescent sexual health education: A systematic review. *Perspectives on Sexual and Reproductive Health, 40,* 144–151.

Kim, H. S. (2016). Sexual debut and mental health among South Korean adolescents. *Journal of Sex Research, 53,* 313–320.

Kim, J. L., & Ward, L. M. (2007). Silence speaks volumes. *Journal of Adolescent Research, 22,* 3–31.

Kincaid, C., Jones, D. J., Sterrett, E., & McKee, L. (2012). A review of parenting and adolescent sexual behavior: The moderating role of gender. *Clinical Psychology Review, 32,* 177–188.

King, K. A., Vidourek, R. A., & Singh, A. (2014). Condoms, sex, and sexually transmitted diseases: Exploring sexual health issues among Asian-Indian college students. *Sexuality and Culture, 18,* 649–663.

Kinsey, A. C., Pomeroy, W. B., & Martin, C.

E. (1948). *Sexual behavior in the human male.* New York: Saunders.

Kinsey, A. C., Pomeroy, W. B., Martin, C. E., & Gebhard, P. H. (1953). *Sexual behavior in the human female.* New York: Saunders.

Kinsman, S. B., Romer, D., Furstenberg, F. F., & Schwarz, D. F. (1998). Early sexual initiation: The role of peer norms. *Pediatrics, 102,* 1185–1192.

Kipke, M. D., Weiss, G., Ramirez, M., Dorey, R., Ritt-Olson, A., Iverson, E., et al. (2007). Club drug use in Los Angeles among young men who have sex with men. *Substance Use and Misuse, 42,* 1723–1743.

Kirby, D. B. (2002). The impact of schools and school programs upon adolescent sexual behavior. *Journal of Sex Research, 39,* 27–33.

Kirby, D. B. (2008). The impact of abstinence and comprehensive sex and STD/HIV education programs on adolescent sexual behavior. *Sexuality Research and Social Policy, 5,* 18–27.

Kirby, D., & Laris, B. A. (2009). Effective curriculum-based sex and STD/HIV education programs for adolescents. *Child Development Perspectives, 3,* 21–29.

Kirkman, M., Rosenthal, D. A., & Feldman, S. S. (2002). Talking to a tiger: Fathers reveal difficulties in communicating about sexuality. In S. S. Feldman & D. A. Rosenthal (Eds.), *Talking sexuality: Parent–adolescent communication* (pp. 57–74). San Francisco: Jossey-Bass.

Klink, D., & Den Heijer, M. (2014). Genetic aspects of gender identity development and gender dysphoria. In B. P. C. Kreukels, T. D. Steensma, & A. L. C. de Vries (Eds.), *Gender dysphoria and disorders of sex development* (pp. 25–51). New York: Springer.

Kneale, D., Fletcher, A., Wiggins, R., & Bonell, C. (2013). Distribution and determinants of risk of teenage motherhood in three British longitudinal studies: Implications for targeted prevention interventions. *Journal of Epidemiology and Community Health, 67,* 48–55.

Kogan, S. M., Cho, J., Simons, L. G., Allen, K. A., Beach, S. R. H., Simons, R. L., et al. (2015). Pubertal timing and sexual risk behaviors among rural African American male youth: Testing a model based on life history theory. *Archives of Sexual Behavior, 44,* 609–618.

Kogan, S. M., Yu, T., Allen, K. A., Pocock, A. M., & Brody, G. H. (2015). Pathways from racial discrimination to multiple sexual partners among male African American adolescents. *Psychology of Men and Masculinity, 16,* 218–228.

Kohler, P. K., Manhart, L. E., & Lafferty, W. E. (2008). Abstinence-only and comprehensive sex education and the initiation of sexual activity and teen pregnancy. *Journal of Adolescent Health, 42,* 344–351.

Kok, G., & Akyuz, A. (2015). Evaluation of effectiveness of parent health education about the sexual developments of adolescents with intellectual disabilities. *Sexuality and Disability, 33,* 157–174.

Koletić, G. (2017). Longitudinal associations between the use of sexually explicit material and adolescents' attitudes and behaviors: A narrative review of studies. *Journal of Adolescence, 57,* 119–133.

Kontula, O., & Haavio-Mannila, E. (2002). Masturbation in a generational perspective. *Journal of Psychology and Human Sexuality, 14,* 49–83.

Koo, H. P., Rose, A., Bhaskar, B., & Walker, L. R. (2012). Relationships of pubertal development among early adolescents to sexual and nonsexual risk behaviors and caregivers parenting behaviors. *Journal of Early Adolescence, 32,* 589–614.

Kosciw, J. G., Greytak, E. A., Palmer, N. A., & Boesen, M. J. (2014). *The 2013 National School Climate Survey: The experiences of lesbian, gay, bisexual and transgender youth in our nation's schools.* New York: GLSEN. Retrieved July 13, 2016, from *www.glsen. org/sites/default/files/2013%20National%20 School%20Climate%20Survey%20Full%20 Report_0.pdf.*

Kosciw, J. G., Palmer, N. A., & Kull, R. M. (2015). Reflecting resiliency: Openness about sexual orientation and/or gender identity and its relationship to well-being and educational outcomes for LGBT students. *American Journal of Community Psychology, 55,* 167–178.

Kost, K., Maddow-Zimet, I., & Arpala, A. (2017, September). *Pregnancies, births and abortions among adolescents and young women in the United States, 2013: National and state trends by age, race and ethnicity.* New York: Guttmacher Institute. Retrieved December 5, 2017, from *www.guttmacher.org/sites/ default/files/report_pdf/us-adolescent-pregnancy-trends-2013.pdf.*

Kotva, H. J., & Schneider, H. G. (1990). Those "talks": General and sexual communication between mothers and daughters. *Journal of Social Behavior and Personality, 5,* 603–613.

Kreager, D. A., & Staff, J. (2009). The sexual double standard and adolescent peer acceptance. *Social Psychology Quarterly, 72,* 143–164.

Kreager, D. A., Staff, J., Gauthier, R., Lefkowitz, E. S., & Feinberg, M. E. (2016). The double standard at sexual debut: Gender, sexual behavior and adolescent peer acceptance. *Sex Roles, 75,* 377–392.

Kreukels, B. P. C., Steensma, T. D., & de Vries, A. L. C. (Eds.). (2014). *Gender dysphoria and disorders of sex development.* New York: Springer.

Krienert, J. L., & Walsh, J. A. (2011). Sibling sexual abuse: An empirical analysis of offender, victim, and event characteristics in National Incident-Based Reporting System (NIBRS) data, 2000–2007. *Journal of Child Sexual Abuse, 20,* 353–372.

Ku, L. F., Sonenstein, L., Lindberg, L. D., Bradner, C. H., Boggess, S., & Pleck, J. H. (1998). Understanding changes in sexual activity among young metropolitan men: 1979–1995. *Family Planning Perspectives, 30,* 256–262.

Ku, L. F., Sonenstein, L., & Pleck, J. H. (1993). Factors influencing first intercourse for teenage men. *Public Health Reports, 108,* 680–694.

Kubicek, K., Beyer, W. J., Weiss, G., Iverson, E., & Kipke, M. D. (2010). In the dark: Young men's stories of sexual initiation in the absence of relevant sexual health information. *Health Education and Behavior, 37,* 243–263.

Kunkel, D., Eyal, K., Biely, E., Donnerstein, E., & Rideout, V. (2007). Sexual socialization messages on entertainment television:

Comparing content trends 1997–2002, *Media Psychology, 9,* 595–622.

Kuper, L. E., Coleman, B. R., & Mustanski, B. S. (2014). Coping with LGBT and racial-ethnic-related stressors: A mixed-methods study of LGBT youth of color. *Journal of Research on Adolescence, 24,* 703–719.

Kuperberg, A., & Padgett, J. E. (2017). Partner meeting contexts and risky behavior in college students' other-sex and same-sex hook-ups. *Journal of Sex Research, 54,* 55–72.

Kuyper, L., & Bos, H. (2016). Mostly heterosexual and lesbian/gay young adults: Differences in mental health and substance use and role of minority stress. *Journal of Sex Research, 53,* 731–741.

Kuyper, L., de Roos, S., Iedema, J., & Stevens, G. (2016). Growing up with the right to marry: Sexual attraction, substance use, and well-being of Dutch adolescents. *Journal of Adolescent Health, 59,* 276–282.

La Greca, A. M., Prinstein, M. J., & Fetter, M. D. (2001). Adolescent peer crowd affiliation: Linkages with health-risk behaviors and close friendships. *Journal of Pediatric Psychology, 26,* 131–143.

LaBrie, J. W., Hummer, J. F., Ghaidarov, T. M., Lac, A., & Kenney, S. R. (2014). Hooking up in the college context: The event-level effects of alcohol use and partner familiarity on hookup behaviors and contentment. *Journal of Sex Research, 51,* 62–73.

Ladapo, J. A., Elliott, M. N., Bogart, L. M., Kanouse, D. E., Vestal, K. D., Klein, D. J., et al. (2013). Cost of Talking Parents, Healthy Teens: A worksite-based intervention to promote parent–adolescent sexual health communication. *Journal of Adolescent Health, 53,* 595–601.

Lagus, K. A., Bernat, D. H., Bearinger, L. H., Resnick, M. D., & Eisenberg, M. E. (2011). Parental perspectives on sources of sex information for young people. *Journal of Adolescent Health, 49,* 87–89.

Lammers, C., Ireland, M., Resnick, M., & Blum, R. (2000). Influences on adolescents' decision to postpone onset of sexual intercourse: A survival analysis of virginity among youths aged 13 to 18 years. *Journal of Adolescent Health, 26,* 42–48.

Landor, A. M., & Simons, L. G. (2014). Why virginity pledges succeed or fail: The moderating effect of religious commitment versus religious participation. *Journal of Child and Family Studies, 23,* 1102–1113.

Langley, C. (2016). Father knows best: Paternal presence and sexual debut in African-American adolescents living in poverty. *Family Process, 55,* 155–170.

Langley, C., Barbee, A. P., Antle, B., Christensen, D., Archuleta, A., Sar, B. K., et al. (2015). Enhancement of Reducing the Risk for the 21st century: Improvement to a curriculum developed to prevent teen pregnancy and STI transmission. *American Journal of Sexuality Education, 10,* 40–69.

Lansford, J. E. (2009). Parental divorce and children's adjustment. *Perspectives in Psychological Science, 4,* 140–152.

Lansford, J. E., Dodge, K. A., Fontaine, R. G., Bates, J. E., & Pettit, G. S. (2014). Peer rejection, affiliation with deviant peers, delinquency, and risky sexual behavior. *Journal of Youth and Adolescence, 43,* 1742–1751.

Lansford, J. E., Yu, T., Erath, S. A., Pettit, G. S., Bates, J. E., & Dodge, K. (2010). Developmental precursors of number of sexual partners from ages 16 to 22. *Journal of Research on Adolescence, 20,* 651–677.

Lantos, H., Bajos, N., & Moreau, C. (2016). Determinants and correlates of preventive behaviors at first sex with a first partner and second partner: Analysis of the FECOND study. *Journal of Adolescent Health, 58,* 644–651.

Laqueur, T. W. (2003). *Solitary sex: A cultural history of masturbation.* New York: Zone Books.

Larsson, I., & Svedin, C. G. (2002). Sexual experiences in childhood: Young adults' recollections. *Archives of Sexual Behavior, 31,* 263–273.

Lau, M., Lin, H., & Flores, G. (2015). Clusters of factors identify a high prevalence of pregnancy involvement among US adolescent males. *Maternal and Child Health Journal, 19,* 1713–1723.

Lau, M., Lin, H., & Flores, G. (2016). Factors associated with being pleased with a female partner pregnancy among sexually active U.S. adolescent males. *American Journal of Men's Health, 10,* 192–206.

Lau, M., Markham, C., Lin, H., Flores, G., & Chacko, M. R. (2009). Dating and sexual attitudes in Asian-American adolescents. *Journal of Adolescent Research, 24,* 91–113.

Laumann, E. O., Gagnon, J. H., Michael, R. T., & Michaels, S. (1994). *The social organization of sexuality.* Chicago: University of Chicago Press.

Leadbeater, B. J. R. (2014). *Growing up fast: Re-visioning adolescent mothers' transitions to young adulthood.* New York: Psychology Press.

Lee, S. Y., Lee, H. J., Kim, T. K., Lee, S. G., & Park, E. C. (2015). Sexually transmitted infections and first sexual intercourse age in adolescents: The nationwide retrospective cross-sectional study. *Journal of Sexual Medicine, 12,* 2313–2323.

Legate, N., Ryan, R. M., & Weinstein, N. (2012). Is coming out always a "good thing"?: Exploring the relations of autonomy support, outness, and wellness for lesbian, gay, and bisexual individuals. *Social Psychological and Personality Science, 3,* 145–152.

Lehmiller, J. J., VanderDrift, L. E., & Kelly, J. R. (2014). Sexual communication, satisfaction, and condom use behavior in friends with benefits and romantic partners. *Journal of Sex Research, 51,* 74–85.

Lehr, S. T., Demi, A. S., Diiorio, C., & Facteau, J. (2005). Predictors of father–son communication about sexuality. *Journal of Sex Research, 42,* 119–129.

Lehrer, J. A., Pantell, R., Tebb, K., & Shafer, M. A. (2007). Forgone health care among U.S. adolescents: Associations between risk characteristics and confidentiality concern. *Journal of Adolescent Health, 40,* 218–226.

Lehti, V., Sourander, A., Klomek, A., Niemelä, S., Sillanmäki, L., Piha, J., et al. (2011). Childhood bullying as a predictor for becoming a teenage mother in Finland. *European Child and Adolescent Psychiatry, 20,* 49–55.

Leitenberg, H., Detzer, M. J., & Srebnik, D. (1993). Gender differences in masturbation and the relation of masturbation experience in preadolescence and/or early adolescence to sexual behavior and sexual adjustment in young adulthood. *Archives of Sexual Behavior, 22,* 87–98.

Leitenberg, H., Greenwald, E., & Tarran, M. J. (1989). The relation between sexual activity among children during preadolescence and/or early adolescence and sexual behavior and sexual adjustment in young adulthood. *Archives of Sexual Behavior, 18,* 299–313.

Leplatte, D., Rosenblum K. L., Stanton, E., Miller, N., & Muzik, M. (2012). Mental health in primary care for adolescent parents. *Mental Health in Family Medicine, 9,* 39–45.

Levine, J. (2002). *Harmful to minors: The perils of protecting children from sex.* New York: Da Capo Press.

Levinson, R. A., Jaccard, J., & Beamer, L. (1995). Older adolescents' engagement in casual sex: Impact of risk perception and psychosocial motivations. *Journal of Youth and Adolescence, 24,* 349–364.

Lewin, A., Mitchell, S. J., Burrell, L., Beers, L. S., & Duggan, A. K. (2011). Patterns and predictors of involvement among fathers of children born to adolescent mothers. *Journal of Family Social Work, 14,* 335–353.

Lewin, A., Mitchell, S. J., Waters, D., Hodgkinson, S., Southammakosane, C., & Gilmore, J. (2015). The protective effects of father involvement for infants of teen mothers with depressive symptoms. *Maternal Child Health Journal, 19,* 1016–1023.

Lewis, M. A., Granato, H., Blayney, J. A., Lostutter, T. W., & Kilmer, J. R. (2012). Predictors of hooking up sexual behaviors and emotional reactions among U.S. college students. *Archives of Sexual Behavior, 41,* 1219–1229.

Lewis, R., & Marston, C. (2016). Oral sex, young people, and gendered narratives of reciprocity. *Journal of Sex Research, 53,* 776–787.

Li, G., & Hines, M. (2016). In search of emerging same-sex sexuality: Romantic attractions at age 13 years. *Archives of Sexual Behavior, 45,* 1839–1849.

Li, G., Kung, K. T. F., & Hines, M. (2017). Childhood gender-typed behavior and adolescent sexual orientation: A longitudinal population-based study. *Developmental Psychology, 53,* 764–777.

Lien, L., Haavet, O. R., & Dalgard, F. (2010). Do mental health and behavioural problems of early menarche persist into late adolescence?: A three year follow-up study among adolescent girls in Oslo, Norway. *Social Science and Medicine, 71,* 529–533.

Lightfoot, M. (2012). HIV prevention for adolescents: Where do we go from here? *American Psychologist, 67,* 661–671.

Lin, A. J., & Santelli, J. S. (2008). The accuracy of condom information in three selected abstinence-only education curricula. *Sexuality Research and Social Policy, 5,* 56–70.

Lindberg, L. D., Jones, R., & Santelli, J. S. (2008). Noncoital sexual activities among adolescents. *Journal of Adolescent Health, 43,* 231–238.

Lindberg, L. D., Maddow-Zimet, I., & Boonstra, H. (2016). Changes in adolescents' receipt of sex education, 2006–2013. *Journal of Adolescent Health, 58,* 621–627.

Lindberg, L., Santelli, J., & Desai, S. (2016). Understanding the recent decline in adolescent fertility in the United States, 2007–2013. *Journal of Adolescent Health, 58,* S100–S101.

Lipman, E. L., Georgiades, K., & Boyle, M. H. (2011). Young adult outcomes of children born to teen mothers: Effects of being born during their teen or later years. *Journal of the American Academy of Child and Adolescent Psychiatry, 50,* 232–241.

Livingston, J. A., Testa, M., Windle, M., & Bay-Cheng, L. Y. (2015). Sexual risk at first coitus: Does alcohol make a difference? *Journal of Adolescence, 43,* 148–158.

Löfgren-Mårtenson, L., & Månsson, S. A. (2010). Lust, love, and life: A qualitative study of Swedish adolescents' perceptions and experiences with pornography. *Journal of Sex Research, 47,* 568–579.

Long-Middleton, E. R., Burke, P. J., Lawrence, C. A. C., Blanchard, L. B., Amudala, N. H., & Rankin, S. H. (2013). Understanding motivations for abstinence among adolescent young women: Insights into effective sexual risk reduction strategies. *Journal of Pediatric Health Care, 27,* 342–350.

Longmore, M. A., Eng, A. L., Giordano, P. C., & Manning, W. D. (2009). Parenting and adolescents' sexual initiation. *Journal of Marriage and Family, 71,* 969–982.

Longmore, M. A., Manning, W. D., & Giordano, P. C. (2001). Preadolescent parenting strategies and teens' dating and sexual initiation: A longitudinal analysis. *Journal of Marriage and Family, 63,* 322–335.

Lopez Sanchez, F., Del Campo, A., & Guijo, V. (2002). Pre-pubertal sexuality. *Sexologies, 11,* 49–58.

Lucassen, M. F. G., Clark, T. C., Denny, S. J., Fleming, T. M., Rossen, F. V., Sheridan, J., et al. (2015). What has changed from 2001 to 2012 for sexual minority youth in New Zealand? *Journal of Paediatrics and Child Health, 51,* 410–418.

Luker, K. (1996). *Dubious conceptions: The politics of teenage pregnancy.* Cambridge, MA: Harvard University Press.

Luker, K. (2007). *When sex goes to school: Warring views on sex—and sex education—since the sixties.* New York: Norton.

Lyons, H., Giordano, P. C., Manning, W. D., & Longmore, M. A. (2011). Identity, peer relationships, and adolescent girls' sexual behavior: An exploration of the contemporary double standard. *Journal of Sex Research, 48,* 437–449.

Lyons, H., Manning, W., Giordano, P., & Longmore, M. (2013). Predictors of heterosexual casual sex among young adults. *Archives of Sexual Behavior, 42,* 585–593.

Lyons, H. A., Manning, W. D., Longmore, M. A., & Giordano, P. C. (2014). Young adult casual sexual behavior: Life-course-specific motivations and consequences. *Sociological Perspectives, 57,* 79–101.

Lyons, H. A., Manning, W. D., Longmore, M. A., & Giordano, P. C. (2015). Gender and casual sexual activity from adolescence to emerging adulthood: Social and life course correlates. *Journal of Sex Research, 52,* 543–557.

Macapagal, K., Coventry, R., Arbeit, M. R., Fisher, C. B., & Mustanski, B. (2017). "I won't out myself just to do a survey": Sexual and gender minority adolescents' perspectives on the risks and benefits of sex research. *Archives of Sexual Behavior, 46,* 1393–1409.

Maguen, S., & Armistead, L. (2006). Abstinence among female adolescents: Do parents matter above and beyond the influence of peers? *American Journal of Orthopsychiatry, 76,* 260–264.

Malabarey, O. T., Balayla, J., Klam, S. L., Shrim, A., & Abenhaim, H. A. (2012).

Pregnancies in young adolescent mothers: A population-based study on 37 million births. *Journal of Pediatric and Adolescent Gynecology, 25,* 98–102.

Malacane, M., & Beckmeyer, J. J. (2016). A review of parent-based barriers to parent–adolescent communication about sex and sexuality: Implications for sex and family educators. *American Journal of Sexuality Education, 11,* 27–40.

Malacane, M., & Martins, N. (2017). Sexual socialization messages in television programming produced for adolescents. *Mass Communication and Society, 20,* 23–46.

Manago, A. M., Ward, L. M., & Aldana, A. (2015). The sexual experience of Latino young adults in college and their perceptions of values about sex communicated by their parents and friends. *Emerging Adulthood, 3,* 14–23.

Maness, S. B., Buhi, E. R., Daley, E. M., Baldwin, J. A., & Kromrey, J. D. (2016). Social determinants of health and adolescent pregnancy: An analysis from the National Longitudinal Study of Adolescent to Adult Health. *Journal of Adolescent Health, 58,* 636–643.

Manlove, J. (1997). Early motherhood in an intergenerational perspective: The experiences of a British cohort. *Journal of Marriage and Family, 59,* 263–279.

Manlove, J., Logan, C., Ikramullah, E., & Holcombe, E. (2008). Factors associated with multiple partner fertility among fathers. *Journal of Marriage and Family, 70,* 536–548.

Manlove, J., Wildsmith, E., Ikramullah, E., Terry-Humen, E., & Schelar, E. (2012). Family environments and the relationship context of first adolescent sex: Correlates of first sex in a casual versus steady relationship. *Social Science Research, 41,* 861–875.

Manning, W. D., Giordano, P. C., & Longmore, M. A. (2006). Hooking up: The relationship contexts of "nonrelationship" sex. *Journal of Adolescent Research, 21,* 459–483.

Manning, W. D., Longmore, M. A., & Giordano, P. C. (2000). The relationship context of contraceptive use at first intercourse. *Family Planning Perspectives, 32,* 104–110.

Maravilla, J. C., Betts, K. S., Abajobir, A. A., Cruz, C. C., & Alati, R. (2016). The role of community health workers in preventing adolescent repeat pregnancies and births. *Journal of Adolescent Health, 59,* 378–390.

Marceau, K., Ram, N., Houts, R. M., Grimm, K. J., & Susman, E. J. (2011). Individual differences in boys' and girls' timing and tempo of puberty: Modeling development with nonlinear growth models. *Developmental Psychology, 47,* 1389–1409.

Marin, B. V. O., Kirby, D. B., Hudes, E. S., Coyle, K. K., & Gómez, C. A. (2006). Boyfriends, girlfriends and teenagers' risk of sexual involvement. *Perspectives on Sexual and Reproductive Health, 38,* 76–83.

Markham, C. M., Lormand, D., Gloppen, K. M., Peskin, M. F., Flores, B., Low, B., et al. (2010). Connectedness as a predictor of sexual and reproductive health outcomes for youth. *Journal of Adolescent Health, 46,* S23–S41.

Marks, M. J., & Fraley, R. C. (2005). The sexual double standard: Fact or fiction? *Sex Roles, 52,* 175–186.

Marques, S. S., Lin, J. S., Starling, M. S., Daquiz, A. G., Goldfarb, E. S., Garcia, K. C. R., et al. (2015). Sexuality education websites for adolescents: A framework-based content analysis. *Journal of Health Communication, 20,* 1310–1319.

Marshal, M. P., Friedman, M. S., Stall, R., King, K. M., Miles, J., Gold, M. A., et al. (2008). Sexual orientation and adolescent substance use: A meta-analysis and methodological review. *Addiction, 103,* 546–556.

Marsiglio, W., & Roy, K. (2013). Fathers' nurturance of children over the life course. In G. W. Peterson & K. R. Bush (Eds.), *Handbook of marriage and the family* (3rd ed., pp. 353–376). New York: Springer.

Marston, C., & King, E. (2006). Factors that shape young people's sexual behavior: A systematic review. *Lancet, 368,* 1581–1586.

Martin, A., Brazil, A., & Brooks-Gunn, J. (2012). The socioemotional outcomes of young children of teenage mothers by paternal coresidence. *Journal of Family Issues, 34,* 1217–1237.

Martin, J. A., Hamilton, B. E., Osterman, M. J., Curtin, S. C., & Mathews, T. J. (2015, January 15). *Births: Final data for 2013.* Hyattsville, MD: National Center for

Health Statistics. Retrieved July 24, 2016, from *www.cdc.gov/nchs/data/nvsr/nvsr64/nvsr64_01.pdf*.

Martin, K. A. (1996). *Puberty, sexuality, and the self: Boys and girls at adolescence.* New York: Routledge.

Martinez, G., Copen, C. E., & Abma, J. C. (2011). Teenagers in the United States: Sexual activity, contraceptive use, and childbearing, 2006–2010 National Survey of Family Growth. *Vital Health Statistics, 23,* 1–35.

Martino, S. C., Elliott, M. N., Collins, R. L., Kanouse, D. E., & Berry, S. H. (2008). Virginity pledges among the willing: Delays in first intercourse and consistency of condom use. *Journal of Adolescent Health, 43,* 341–348.

Martino, S. C., Elliott, M. N., Corona, R., Kanouse, D. E., & Schuster, M. A. (2008). Beyond the "big talk": The roles of breadth and repetition in parent–adolescent communication about sexual topics. *Pediatrics, 121,* e612–e618.

Martin-Storey, A., & August, E. G. (2016). Harassment due to gender nonconformity mediates the association between sexual minority identity and depressive symptoms. *Journal of Sex Research, 53,* 85–97.

Martos, A. J., Nezhad, S., & Meyer, I. H. (2015). Variations in sexual identity milestones among lesbians, gay men, and bisexuals. *Sexual Research and Social Policy, 12,* 24–33.

Mason-Jones, A. J., Crisp, C., Momberg, M., Koech, J., De Koker, P., & Mathews, C. (2012). A systematic review of the role of school-based healthcare in adolescent sexual, reproductive, and mental health. *Systematic Reviews, 1,* 49. Retrieved July 27, 2016, from *http://systematicreviewsjournal.biomedcentral.com/articles/10.1186/2046-4053-1-49*.

Maticka-Tyndale, E., & Barnett, J. P. (2010). Peer-let interventions to reduce HIV risk of youth: A review. *Evaluation and Program Planning, 33,* 98–112.

Matson, P. A., Chung, S. E., & Ellen, J. M. (2014). Perceived neighborhood partner availability, partner selection, and risk for sexually transmitted infections within a cohort of adolescent females. *Journal of Adolescent Health, 55,* 122–127.

Mattebo, M., Larsson, M., Tydén, T., & Häggström-Nordin, E. (2013). Professionals' perceptions of the effect of pornography on Swedish adolescents. *Public Health Nursing, 31,* 196–205.

Mattebo, M., Tydén, T., Häggström-Nordin, E., Nilsson, K. W., & Larsson, M. (2013). Pornography consumption, sexual experiences, lifestyles, and self-rated health among male adolescents in Sweden. *Journal of Developmental and Behavioral Pediatrics, 34,* 460–468.

Maxwell, C. (2006). Context and "contextualization" in sex and relationships education. *Health Education, 106,* 437–449.

Maxwell, C., & Chase, E. (2008). Peer pressure: Beyond rhetoric to reality. *Sex Education, 8,* 303–314.

Mayer, K. H., Garofalo, R., & Makadon, H. J. (2014). Promoting the successful development of sexual and gender minority youths. *American Journal of Public Health, 104,* 976–981.

Mayeux, L., Sandstrom, M. J., & Cillessen, A. H. N. (2008). Is being popular a risky proposition? *Journal of Research on Adolescence, 18,* 49–74.

Mazur, A., Halpern, C., & Udry, J. R. (1994). Dominant looking male teenagers copulate earlier. *Ethology and Sociobiology, 15,* 87–94.

McFarland, K., & Williams, D. J. (2016). Macro sex-negativity to micro implications: My personal experience with absent (abstinence) sex education. *Journal of Positive Sexuality, 2,* 5–10.

McHale, S. M., Bissell, J., & Kim, J. Y. (2009). Sibling relationship, family, and genetic factors in sibling similarity in sexual risk. *Journal of Family Psychology, 23,* 562–572.

McLanahan S., & Sandefur, G. (1994). *Growing up with a single parent: What hurts, what helps.* Cambridge, MA: Harvard University Press.

McMichael, C. (2013). Unplanned but not unwanted?: Teen pregnancy and parenthood among young people with refugee backgrounds. *Journal of Youth Studies, 16,* 663–678.

McNeely, C., Shew, M. L., Beuhring, T., Sieving, R., Miller, B. C., & Blum, R. W. (2002). Mothers' influence on the timing of first sex among 14- and 15-year-olds. *Journal of Adolescent Health, 31,* 256–265.

McRee, A. L., Reiter, P. L, Gottlieb, S. L., & Brewer, N. T. (2011). Mother–daughter communication about HPV vaccine. *Journal of Adolescent Health, 48,* 314–317.

Meade, C. S., Kershaw, T. S., & Ickovics, J. R. (2008). The intergenerational cycle of teenage motherhood: An ecological approach. *Health Psychology, 27,* 419–429.

Meier, A. M. (2007). Adolescent first sex and subsequent mental health. *American Journal of Sociology, 112,* 1811–1847.

Meier, A., & Allen G. (2009). Romantic relationships from adolescence to young adulthood: Evidence from the National Longitudinal Study of Adolescent Health. *Sociological Quarterly, 50,* 308–335.

Mendle, J., & Ferrero, J. (2012). Detrimental psychological outcomes associated with pubertal timing in adolescent boys. *Developmental Review, 32,* 49–66.

Mendle, J., Ferrero, J., Moore, S. R., & Harden, K. P. (2013). Depression and adolescent sexual activity in romantic and nonromantic relational contexts: A genetically-informative sibling comparison. *Journal of Abnormal Psychology, 122,* 51–63.

Mendle, J., Harden, K. P., Turkheimer, E., Van Hulle, C. A., D'Onofrio, B. M., Brooks-Gunn, J., et al. (2009). Associations between father absence and age of first sexual intercourse. *Child Development, 80,* 1463–1480.

Mendle, J., Turkheimer, E., & Emery, R. E. (2007). Detrimental psychological outcomes associated with early pubertal timing in adolescent girls. *Developmental Review, 27,* 151–171.

Mereish, E. H., Goldbach, J. T., Burgess, C., & DiBello, A. M. (2017). Sexual orientation, minority stress, social norms, and substance use among racially diverse adolescents. *Drug and Alcohol Dependence, 178,* 49–56.

Merghati-Khoei, E., Abolghasemi, N., & Smith, T. G. (2014). "Children are sexually innocent": Iranian parents' understanding of children's sexuality. *Archives of Sexual Behavior, 43,* 587–595.

Merianos, A. L., Rosen, B. L., King, K. A., Vidourek, R. A., & Fehr, S. K. (2015). The association of early substance use with lifetime/past year contraction of sexually transmitted diseases: A national study. *American Journal of Sexuality Education, 10,* 158–176.

Merrick, E. N. (1995). Adolescent childbearing as a career "choice": Perspective from an ecological context. *Journal of Counseling and Development, 73,* 288–295.

Mesch, G. S. (2009). Social bonds and Internet pornographic exposure among adolescents. *Journal of Adolescence, 32,* 601–618.

Meyer, I. H. (2003). Prejudice, social stress, and mental health in lesbian, gay, and bisexual populations: Conceptual issues and research evidence. *Psychological Bulletin, 129,* 674–697.

Michael, K. (2016). Sexual behavior and risk-taking among adolescents: Gender, socioeconomic status, sexual status, and longitudinal analysis. *Megamot, 50,* 117–152.

Michaud, P. A., Suris, J. C., & Deppen, A. (2006). Gender-related psychological and behavioural correlates of pubertal timing in a national sample of Swiss adolescents. *Molecular and Cellular Endocrinology, 254–255,* 172–178.

Miller, B. C., Benson, B., & Galbraith, K. A. (2001). Family relationships and adolescent pregnancy risk: A research synthesis. *Developmental Review, 21,* 1–38.

Milrod, C. (2014). How young is too young: Ethical concerns in genital surgery of the transgender MTF adolescent. *Journal of Sexual Medicine, 11,* 338–346.

Minguez, M., Santelli, J. S., Gibson, E., Orr, M., & Samant, S. (2015). Reproductive health impact of a school health center. *Journal of Adolescent Health, 56,* 338–344.

Mirzazadeh, A., Biggs, M. A., Viitanen, A., Horvath, H., Wang, L. Y., Dunville, R., et al. (2018). Do school-based programs prevent HIV and other sexually transmitted infections in adolescents?: A systematic review and meta-analysis. *Prevention Science, 19,* 490–506.

Mitchell, K. J., Finkelhor, D., Jones, L. M., & Wolak, J. (2012). Prevalence and characteristics of youth sexting: A national study. *Pediatrics, 129,* 13–20.

Mitchell, K. J., Ybarra, M. L., & Korchmaros, J. D. (2014). Sexual harassment among adolescents of different sexual orientations and gender identities. *Child Abuse and Neglect, 38,* 280–295.

Moffitt, T. E. (2005). The new look of behavioral genetics in developmental psychopathology: Gene–environment interplay in antisocial behaviors. *Psychological Bulletin, 131,* 533–554.

Moffitt, T. E., Arseneault, L., Belsky, D., Dickson, N., Hancox, R. J., Harrington, H. L., et al. (2010). A gradient of childhood self-control predicts health, wealth, and public safety. *Proceedings of the National Academy of Sciences of the USA, 108,* 2693–2698.

Moffitt, T. E., Poulton, R., & Caspi, A. (2013). Lifelong impact of early self-control. *American Scientist, 101,* 352–359.

Mohammadyari, G. (2014). The relationship between parental style and attitude to premarital sex among students: A case study in Iran. *International Journal of Psychology and Behavioral Research, 3,* 24–28.

Moilanen, K. L. (2015). Predictors of latent growth in sexual risk taking in late adolescence and early adulthood. *Journal of Sex Research, 52,* 83–97.

Moilanen, K. L., Crockett, L. J., Raffaelli, M., & Jones, B. L. (2010). Trajectories of sexual risk from mid-adolescence to early adulthood. *Journal of Research on Adolescence, 20,* 114–139.

Mollborn, S. (2007). Making the best of a bad situation: Material resources and teenage parenthood. *Journal of Marriage and the Family, 69,* 92–104.

Mollborn, S. (2010). Predictors and consequences of adolescents' norms against teenage pregnancy. *Sociological Quarterly, 51,* 303–328.

Mollborn, S., & Jacobs, J. (2015). "I'll be there for you": Teen parents' coparenting relationships. *Journal of Marriage and Family, 77,* 373–387.

Mollborn, S., & Lovegrove, P. J. (2011). How teenage fathers matter for children: Evidence from the ECLS-B. *Journal of Family Issues, 32,* 3–30.

Monahan, K. C., & Lee, J. M. (2008). Adolescent sexual activity: Links between relational context and depressive symptoms. *Journal of Youth and Adolescence, 37,* 917–927.

Monto, M. A., & Carey, A. G. (2014). A new standard of sexual behavior?: Are claims associated with the "hookup culture" supported by General Social Survey data? *Journal of Sex Research, 51,* 605–615.

Moore, S. R., Harden, K. P., & Mendle, J. (2014). Pubertal timing and adolescent sexual behavior in girls. *Developmental Psychology, 50,* 1734–1745.

Moran, J. P. (2000). *Teaching sex: The shaping of adolescence in the 20th century.* Cambridge, MA: Harvard University Press.

Moreno, M. A., Brockman, L. N., Wasserheit, J. N., & Christakis, D. A. (2012). A pilot evaluation of older adolescents' sexual reference displays on Facebook. *Journal of Sex Research, 49,* 390–399.

Morrison-Beedy, D., Xia, Y., & Passmore, D. (2013). Sexual risk factors for partner age discordance in adolescent girls and their male partners. *Journal of Clinical Nursing, 22,* 3289–3299.

Moser, C., Kleinplatz, P. J., Zuccarini, D., & Reiner, W. G. (2004). Situating unusual child and adolescent sexual behavior in context. *Child and Adolescent Psychiatric Clinics, 13,* 569–589.

Mueller, A. S., James, W., Abrutyn, S., & Levin, M. L. (2015). Suicide ideation and bullying among US adolescents: Examining the intersections of sexual orientation, gender, and race/ethnicity. *American Journal of Public Health, 105,* 980–985.

Mustanski, B., Birkett, M., Greene, G. J., Rosario, M., Bostwick, W., & Everett, B. G. (2014). The association between sexual orientation identity and behavior across race/ethnicity, sex, and age in a probability sample of high school students. *American Journal of Public Health, 104,* 237–244.

Mustanski, B., DuBois, L. Z., Prescott, T. L., & Ybarra, M. L. (2014). A mixed-methods study of condom use and decision making among adolescent gay and bisexual males. *AIDS and Behavior, 18,* 1955–1969.

Mustanski, B., & Liu, R. T. (2013). A longitudinal study of predictors of suicide attempts among lesbian, gay, bisexual, and transgender youth. *Archives of Sexual Behavior, 42,* 437–448.

Mustanski, B., Newcomb, M. E., & Clerkin,

E. M. (2011). Relationship characteristics and sexual risk-taking in young men who have sex with men. *Health Psychology, 30,* 597–605.

Mustanski, B. S., Garofalo, R., & Emerson, E. M. (2010). Mental health disorders, psychological distress, and suicidality in a diverse sample of lesbian, gay, bisexual, and transgender youths. *American Journal of Public Health, 100,* 2426–2432.

Myers, K., & Geist, C. (2015, April). *Why wait?: Gender, race, and class as predictors of teens' attitudes towards pregnancy.* Paper presented at the annual meeting of the Population Association of America, San Diego, CA. Retrieved July 24, 2016, from *http://paa2015.princeton. edu/uploads/151018.*

Nack, A. (2000). Damaged goods: Women managing the stigma of STDs. *Deviant Behavior, 21,* 95–121.

Nagamatsu, M., Yamawaki, N., Sato, T., Nakagawa, A., & Saito, H. (2013). Factors influencing attitudes toward sexual activity among early adolescents in Japan. *Journal of Early Adolescence, 33,* 267–288.

Napper, L. E., Kenney, S. R., & LaBrie, J. W. (2015). The longitudinal relationships among injunctive norms and hooking up attitudes and behavior. *Journal of Sex Research, 52,* 499–506.

National Campaign to Prevent Teen and Unplanned Pregnancy. (2013). *Counting it up: The public costs of teen childbearing.* Washington, DC: Author. Retrieved September 21, 2016, from *http://thenationalcampaign.org/ why-it-matters/public-cost.*

National Campaign to Prevent Teen and Unplanned Pregnancy. (2016). *National and state data.* Washington, DC: Author. Retrieved November 2, 2016, from *https:// thenationalcampaign.org/data/landing.*

NBC News/People Magazine. (2005). Nearly 3 in 10 young teens "sexually active." Retrieved July 10, 2016, from *www.nbcnews. com/id/6839072/print/1/displaymode/1098.*

Negriff, S., & Susman, E. J. (2011). Pubertal timing, depression, and externalizing problems: A framework, review, and examination of gender differences. *Journal of Research on Adolescence, 21,* 717–746.

Nelson, R. J. (2011). *An introduction to behavioral endocrinology* (4th ed.). Sunderland, MA: Sinauer.

Newcomb, M. E., Birkett, M., Corliss, H. L., & Mustanski, B. (2014). Sexual orientation, gender, and racial differences in illicit drug use in a sample of US high school students. *American Journal of Public Health, 104,* 304–310.

Newcomb, M. E., & Mustanski, B. (2016). Developmental change in the effects of sexual partner and relationship characteristics on sexual risk behavior in young men who have sex with men. *AIDS and Behavior, 20,* 1284–1294.

Newcomb, M. E., Ryan, D. T., Garofalo, R., & Mustanski, B. (2014). The effects of sexual partnership and relationship characteristics on three sexual risk variables in young men who have sex with men. *Archives of Sexual Behavior, 43,* 61–72.

Newcomer, S. F., & Udry, J. R. (1985). Oral sex in an adolescent population. *Archives of Sexual Behavior, 14,* 41–46.

Newton, D. C., & McCabe, M. (2008). Sexually transmitted infections: Impact on individuals and their relationships. *Journal of Health Psychology, 13,* 864–869.

NHS Bristol. (2009). Parent attitudes to teenage health, pregnancy and sex and relationships education (MSS Research Project No. MR 4689). Retrieved July 11, 2016, from *www.4ypbristol.co.uk/professionals_supportparents.*

Noar, S. M. (2011). Computer technology-based interventions in HIV prevention: State of the evidence and future directions for research. *AIDS Care, 23,* 525–533.

Noar, S. M., Black, H. G., & Pierce, L. B. (2009). Efficacy of computer technology-based HIV prevention interventions: A meta-analysis. *AIDS, 23,* 107–115.

Noar, S. M., Carlyle, K., & Cole, C. (2006). Why communication is crucial: Meta-analysis of the relationship between safer sexual communication and condom use. *Journal of Health Communication, 11,* 365–390.

Noar, S. M., Pierce, L. B., & Black, H. G. (2010). Can computer-mediated interventions change theoretical mediators of safer sex?: A meta-analysis. *Human Communication Research, 36,* 261–297.

Nogueira Avelar e Silva, R., van de Bongardt, D., Baams, L., & Raat, H. (2018). Bidirectional associations between adolescents' sexual behaviors and psychological well-being. *Journal of Adolescent Health, 62,* 63–71.

Noll, J. G., & Shenk, C. E. (2013). Teen birth rates in sexually abused and neglected females. *Pediatrics, 131,* 1181–1187.

Noll, J. G., Trickett, P. K., Long, J. D., Negriff, S., Susman, E. J., Shalev, I., et al. (2017). Childhood sexual abuse and early timing of puberty. *Journal of Adolescent Health, 60,* 65–71.

Noller, P., & Callan, V. J. (1991). *The adolescent in the family.* London: Routledge.

Norris, A. E., Pettigrew, J., Miller-Day, M., Hecht, M. L., Hutchison, J., & Campoe, K. (2015). Resisting pressure from peers to engage in sexual behavior: What communication strategies do early adolescent Latino girls use? *Journal of Early Adolescence, 35,* 562–580.

Novak, D. P., & Karlsson, R. B. (2005). Gender differed factors affecting male condom use. A population-based study of 18-year-old Swedish adolescents. *International Journal of Adolescent Medicine and Health, 17,* 379–390.

Nsuami, M. J., Sanders, L. S., & Taylor, S. N. (2010). Knowledge of sexually transmitted infections among high school students. *American Journal of Health Education, 41,* 206–217.

Obama's Father's Day Speech. (2008, June 23). *Huffington Post.*

Ocasio, M. A., Feaster, D. J., & Prado, G. (2016). Substance use and sexual risk behavior in sexual minority Hispanic adolescents. *Journal of Adolescent Health, 59,* 599–601.

O'Hara, R. E., Gibbons, F. X., Gerrard, M., Li, Z., & Sargent, J. D. (2012). Greater exposure to sexual content in popular movies predicts earlier sexual debut and increased sexual risk taking. *Psychological Science, 23,* 984–993.

Okami, P., Olmstead, R., & Abramson, P. R. (1997). Sexual experiences in early childhood: 18-year longitudinal data from the UCLA Family Lifestyles Project. *Journal of Sex Research, 34,* 339–347.

Okazaki, S. (2002). Influences of culture on Asian-Americans' sexuality. *Journal of Sex Research, 39,* 34–41.

Oliveira-Campos, M., Giatti, L., Malta, D., & Barreto, S. M. (2013). Contextual factors associated with sexual behavior among Brazilian adolescents. *Annals of Epidemiology, 23,* 629–635.

Oman, R. F., Vesely, S. K., Aspy, C. B., Tolma, E. L., Gavin, L., Bensyl, D. M., et al. (2013). A longitudinal study of youth assets, neighborhood conditions, and youth sexual behaviors. *Journal of Adolescent Health, 52,* 779–785.

Ompad, D. C., Strathdee, S. A., Celentano, D. D., Latkin, C., Poduska, J. M., Kellam, S. G., et al. (2006). Predictors of early initiation of vaginal and oral sex among urban young adults in Baltimore, Maryland. *Archives of Sexual Behavior, 35,* 53–65.

Orgilés, M., Carratalá, E., & Espada, J. P. (2015). Perceived quality of the parental relationship and divorce effects on sexual behaviour in Spanish adolescents. *Psychology, Health and Medicine, 20,* 8–17.

Ostovich, J. M., & Sabini, J. (2005). Timing of puberty and sexuality in men and women. *Archives of Sexual Behavior, 34,* 197–206.

O'Sullivan, L. F., Cheng, M. M., Harris, K. M., & Brooks-Gunn, J. (2007). I wanna hold your hand: The progression of social, romantic and sexual events in adolescent relationships. *Perspectives on Sexual and Reproductive Health, 39,* 100–107.

O'Sullivan, L. F., & Meyer-Bahlburg, H. F. L. (2003). African-American and Latina inner-city girls' reports of romantic and sexual development. *Journal of Social and Personal Relationships, 20,* 221–238.

O'Sullivan, L. F., Meyer-Bahlburg, H. F. L., & Watkins, B. X. (2001). Mother–daughter communication about sex among urban African American and Latino families. *Journal of Adolescent Research, 16,* 269–292.

Oswalt, S. B., Cameron, K. A., & Koob, J. J. (2005). Sexual regret in college students. *Archives of Sexual Behavior, 34,* 663–669.

Ott, M. A., Katschke, A., Tu, W., & Fortenberry, J. D. (2011). Longitudinal associations among relationship factors, partner change, and sexually transmitted infection acquisition in adolescent women. *Sexually Transmitted Diseases, 38,* 153–157.

Ott, M. Q., Corliss, H. L., Wypij, D., Rosario, M., & Austin, S. B. (2011). Stability and change in self-reported sexual orientation identity in young people: Application of mobility metrics. *Archives of Sexual Behavior, 40,* 519–532.

Oudekerk, B. A., Allen, J. P., Hafen, C. A., Hessel, E. T., Szwedo, D. E., & Spilker, A. (2014). Maternal and paternal psychological control as moderators of the link between peer attitudes and adolescents' risky sexual behavior. *Journal of Early Adolescence, 34,* 413–435.

Oudekerk, B. A., Guarnera, L. A., & Reppucci, N. D. (2014). Older opposite-sex romantic partners, sexual risk, and victimization in adolescence. *Child Abuse and Neglect, 38,* 1238–1248.

Outlaw, A. Y., Phillips, G., II, Hightow-Weidman, L. B., Fields, S. D., Hidalgo, J., Halpern-Felsher, B., et al. (2011). Age of MSM sexual debut and risk factors: Results from a multisite study of racial/ethnic minority YMSM living with HIV. *AIDS Patient Care and STDs, 25,* S23–S29.

Owen, J., & Fincham, F. D. (2011). Young adults' emotional reactions after hooking up encounters. *Archives of Sexual Behavior, 40,* 321–330.

Owen, J., Fincham, F. D., & Moore, J. (2011). Short-term prospective study of hooking up among college students. *Archives of Sexual Behavior, 40,* 331–341.

Owen, J., Quirk, K., & Fincham, F. (2014). Toward a more complete understanding of reactions to hooking up among college women. *Journal of Sex and Marital Therapy, 40,* 396–409.

Owen, J. J., Rhoades, G. K., Stanley, S. M., & Fincham, F. D. (2010). "Hooking up" among college students: Demographic and psychosocial correlates. *Archives of Sexual Behavior, 39,* 653–663.

Owens, E. W., Behun, R. J., Manning, J. C., & Reid, R. C. (2012). The impact of Internet pornography on adolescents: A review of the research. *Sexual Addiction and Compulsivity, 19,* 99–122.

Padilla-Walker, L. M., & Carlo, G. (2007). Personal values as a mediator between parent and peer expectations and adolescent behaviors. *Journal of Family Psychology, 21,* 538–541.

Palmer, M. J., Clarke, L., Ploubidis, G. B., Mercer, C. H., Johnson, A. M., Copas, A. J., et al. (2017). Is "sexual competence" at first heterosexual intercourse associated with subsequent sexual health status? *Journal of Sex Research, 54,* 91–104.

Paradise, J. E., Cote, J., Minsky, S., Lourenco, A., & Howland, J. (2001). Personal values and sexual decision-making among virginal and sexually experienced urban adolescent girls. *Journal of Adolescent Health, 28,* 404–409.

Pardun, C. J., L'Engle, K. L., & Brown, J. D. (2005). Linking exposure to outcomes: Early adolescents' consumption of sexual content in six media. *Mass Communication and Society, 8,* 75–91.

Park, B. K., & Calamaro, C. (2013). A systematic review of social networking sites: Innovative platforms for health research targeting adolescents and young adults. *Journal of Nursing Scholarship, 45,* 256–264.

Parkes, A., Henderson, M., Wight, D., & Nixon, C. (2011). Is parenting associated with teenagers' early sexual risk-taking, autonomy and relationship with sexual partners? *Perspectives on Sexual and Reproductive Health, 43,* 30–40.

Patchen, L., Letourneau, K., & Berggren, E. (2013). Evaluation of an integrated services program to prevent subsequent pregnancy and birth among urban teen mothers. *Social Work in Health Care, 52,* 642–655.

Paton, D., & Wright, L. (2017). The effect of spending cuts on teen pregnancy. *Journal of Health Economics, 54,* 135–146.

Paul, E. L., McManus, B., & Hayes, A. (2000). "Hookups": Characteristics and correlates of college students' spontaneous and anonymous sexual experiences. *Journal of Sex Research, 37,* 76–88.

Paul, J. P., Catania, J., Pollack, L., Moskowitz, J., Canchola, J., Mills, T., et al. (2002). Suicide attempts among gay and bisexual men: Lifetime prevalence and antecedents. *American Journal of Public Health, 92,* 1338–1345.

Pears, K. C., Pierce, S. L., Kim, H. K., Capaldi, D. M., & Owen, L. D. (2005). The timing of entry into fatherhood in young, at-risk men. *Journal of Marriage and Family, 67,* 429–447.

Pelucchi, C., Esposito, S., Galeone, C., Semino,

M., Sabatini, C., Picciolli, I., et al. (2010). Knowledge of human papillomavirus infection and its prevention among adolescents and parents in the greater Milan area, northern Italy. *BMC Public Health, 10,* 378.

Peplau, L. A., Cochran, S. D., & Mays, V. M. (1997). A national survey of the intimate relationships of African American lesbians and gay men: A look at commitment, satisfaction, sexual behavior, and HIV disease. In B. Greene (Ed.), *Psychological perspectives on lesbian and gay issues: Vol. 3. Ethnic and cultural diversity among lesbians and gay men* (pp. 11–38). Thousand Oaks, CA: SAGE.

Peris, T. S., & Emery, R. E. (2004). A prospective study of the consequences of marital disruption for adolescents: Predisruption family dynamics and postdisruption adolescent adjustment. *Journal of Clinical Child and Adolescent Psychology, 33,* 694–704.

Perkins, A. B., Becker, J. V., Tehee, M., & Mackelprang, E. (2014). Sexting behaviors among college students: Cause for concern? *International Journal of Sexual Health, 26,* 79–92.

Perrin, K. K., & DeJoy, S. B. (2003). Abstinence-only education: How we got here and where we're going. *Journal of Public Health Policy, 24,* 445–459.

Peskin, H. (1973). Influence of the developmental schedule of puberty on learning and ego functioning. *Journal of Youth and Adolescence, 2,* 273–290.

Peskin, M. F., Shegog, R., Markham, C. M., Thiel, M., Baumler, E. R., Addy, R. C., et al. (2015). Efficacy of It's Your Game-Tech: A computer-based sexual health education program for middle school youth. *Journal of Adolescent Health, 56,* 515–521.

Peter, J., & Valkenburg, P. M. (2006a). Adolescents' exposure to sexually explicit online material and recreational attitudes toward sex. *Journal of Communication, 56,* 639–660.

Peter, J., & Valkenburg, P. M. (2006b). Adolescents' exposure to sexually explicit material on the Internet. *Communication Research, 33,* 178–204.

Peter, J., & Valkenburg, P. M. (2010). Processes underlying the effects of adolescents' use of sexually explicit Internet material: The role of perceived realism. *Communication Research, 37,* 375–399.

Peter, J., & Valkenburg, P. M. (2016). Adolescents and pornography: A review of 20 years of research. *Journal of Sex Research, 53,* 509–531.

Petersen, J. L., & Hyde, J. S. (2010). A meta-analytic review of research on gender differences in sexuality. *Psychological Bulletin, 136,* 21–38.

Pew Research Center. (2013, June). A survey of LGBT Americans: Attitudes, experiences and values in changing times. Retrieved February 21, 2015, from *www.pewsocialtrends.org/2013/06/13/chapter-3-the-coming-out-experience.*

Picot, J., Shepherd, J., Kavanagh, J., Cooper, K., Harden, A., Barnett-Page, E., et al. (2012). Behavioural interventions for the prevention of sexually transmitted infections in young people aged 13–19 years: A systematic review. *Health Education Research, 27,* 495–512.

Pierce, R. V. (1875). *The people's common sense medical adviser in plain English.* Buffalo, NY: World's Dispensary Printing Office and Bindery.

Pilgrim, N. A., Ahmed, S., Gray, R. H., Sekasanvu, J., Lutalo, T., Nalugoda, F., et al. (2014). Family structure effects on early sexual debut among adolescent girls in Rakai, Uganda. *Vulnerable Children and Youth Studies, 9,* 193–205.

Pingel, E. S., Bauermeister, J. A., Elkington, K. S., Fergus, S., Caldwell, C. H., & Zimmerman, M. A. (2012). Condom use trajectories in adolescence and the transition to adulthood: The role of mother and father support. *Journal of Research on Adolescence, 22,* 350–366.

Pinto, N., & Moleiro, C. (2015). Gender trajectories: Transsexual people coming to terms with their gender identities. *Professional Psychology: Research and Practice, 46,* 12–20.

Pistella, C. L. Y., & Bonati, F. A. (1999). Adolescent women's recommendations for enhanced parent–adolescent communication about sexual behavior. *Child and Adolescent Social Work Journal, 16,* 305–315.

Pluhar, E., Jennings, T., & Diiorio, C. (2006).

Getting an early start: Communication about sexuality among mothers and children 6–10 years old. *Journal of HIV/AIDS Prevention in Children and Youth, 7,* 7–35.

Pogarsky, G., Thornberry, T. P., & Lizotte, A. J. (2006). Developmental outcomes for children of young mothers. *Journal of Marriage and Family, 68,* 332–344.

Ponzetti, J. J., Jr. (Ed.). (2016). *Evidence-based approaches to sexuality education: A global perspective.* New York: Routledge.

Potard, C., Courtois, R., & Rusch, E. (2008). The influence of peers on risky sexual behaviour during adolescence. *European Journal of Contraception and Reproductive Health Care, 13,* 264–270.

Poteat, V. P., Russell, S. T., & Dewaele, A. (2017). Sexual health risk behavior disparities among male and female adolescents using identity and behavior indicators of sexual orientation. *Archives of Sexual Behavior.*

Price, J., Patterson, R., Regnerus, M., & Walley, J. (2016). How much more XXX is generation X consuming?: Evidence of changing attitudes and behaviors related to pornography since 1973. *Journal of Sex Research, 53,* 12–20.

Priebe, G., & Svedin, C. G. (2013). Operationalization of three dimensions of sexual orientation in a national survey of late adolescents. *Journal of Sex Research, 50,* 727–738.

Primack, B. A., Gold, M. A., Schwarz, E. B., & Dalton, M. A. (2008). Degrading and non-degrading sex in popular music: A content analysis. *Public Health Reports, 123,* 593–600.

Prinstein, M. J., Choukas-Bradley, S. C., Helms, S. W., Brechwald, W. A., & Rancourt, D. (2011). High peer popularity longitudinally predicts adolescent health risk behavior, or does it?: An examination of linear and quadratic associations. *Journal of Pediatric Psychology, 36,* 980–990.

Prinstein, M. J., Meade, C. S., & Cohen, G. L. (2003). Adolescent oral sex, peer popularity, and perceptions of best friends' sexual behavior. *Journal of Pediatric Psychology, 28,* 243–249.

Prinstein, M. J., & Wang, S. S. (2005). False consensus and adolescent peer contagion: Examining discrepancies between perceptions and actual reported levels of friends' deviant and health risk behaviors. *Journal of Abnormal Child Psychology, 33,* 293–306.

Pronin, E., & Kugler, M. B. (2010). People believe they have more free will than others. *Proceedings of the National Academy of Sciences of the USA, 107,* 22469–22474.

Protogerou, C., & Johnson, B. T. (2014). Factors underlying the success of behavioral HIV-prevention interventions for adolescents: A meta-review. *AIDS and Behavior, 18,* 1847–1863.

Puckett, J. A., Horne, S. G., Surace, F., Carter, A., Noffsinger-Frazier, N., Shulman, J., et al. (2017). Predictors of sexual minority youth's reported suicide attempts and mental health. *Journal of Homosexuality, 64,* 697–715.

Quinlan, R. J. (2003). Father absence, parental care, and female reproductive development. *Evolution and Human Behavior, 24,* 376–390.

Raatikainen, K., Heiskanen, N., Verkasalo, P. K., & Heinonen, S. (2006). Good outcome of teenage pregnancies in high-quality maternity care. *European Journal of Public Health, 16,* 157–161.

Rachlin, H., Raineri, A., & Cross, D. (1991). Subjective probability and delay. *Journal of the Experimental Analysis of Behavior, 55,* 233–244.

Raeburn, P. (2014). *Do fathers matter?: What science is telling us about the parent we've overlooked.* New York: Farrar, Straus & Giroux.

Ragsdale, K., Bersamin, M. M., Schwartz, B. L., Zamboanga, B. L., Kerrick, M. R., & Grube, J. W. (2014). Development of sexual expectancies among adolescents: Contributions by parents, peers and the media. *Journal of Sex Research, 51,* 551–560.

Rahimi-Naghani, S., Merghati-Khoei, E., Shahbazi, M., Khalajabadi Farahani, F., Motamedi, M., Salehi, M., et al. (2016). Sexual and reproductive health knowledge among men and women aged 15 to 49 years in metropolitan Tehran. *Journal of Sex Research, 53,* 1153–1164.

Raiford, J. L., Seth, P., & DiClemente, R. J. (2013). What girls won't do for love: Human immunodeficiency virus/sexually transmitted infections risk among young

African-American women driven by a relationship imperative. *Journal of Adolescent Health, 52,* 566–571.

Raine, T. R., Gard, J. C., Boyer, C. B., Haider, S., Brown, B. A., Hernandez, F. A. R., et al. (2010). Contraceptive decision-making in sexual relationships: Young men's experiences, attitudes and values. *Culture, Health and Sexuality, 12,* 373–386.

R-Almendarez, R., & Wilson, A. D. (2013). The effect of gender and ethnicity on the sexual behaviors of adolescents. *Family Journal: Counseling and Therapy for Couples and Families, 21,* 104–111.

Ralph, L. J., Berglas, N. F., Schwartz, S. L., & Brindis, C. D. (2011). Finding teens in TheirSpace: Using social networking sites to connect youth to sexual health services. *Sexuality Research and Social Policy, 8,* 38–49.

Ramiro, M. T., Teva, I., Bermúdez, M. P., & Buela-Casal, G. (2013). Social support, self-esteem and depression: Relationship with risk for sexually transmitted infections/HIV transmission. *International Journal of Clinical and Health Psychology, 13,* 181–188.

Ramsey, G. V. (1943). The sex information of younger boys. *American Journal of Orthopsychiatry, 13,* 347–352.

Ream, G. L., & Savin-Williams, R. C. (2005). Reciprocal associations between adolescent sexual activity and quality of youth–parent interactions. *Journal of Family Psychology, 19,* 171–179.

Reece, M., Herbenick, D., Schick, V., Sanders, S. A., Dodge, B., & Fortenberry, J. D. (2010). Condom use rates in a national probability sample of males and females ages 14 to 94 in the United States. *Journal of Sexual Medicine, 7,* 266–276.

Regnerus, M. D. (2007). *Forbidden fruit: Sex & religion in the lives of American teenagers.* New York: Oxford University Press.

Regnerus, M. D., & Luchies, L. B. (2006). The parent–child relationship and opportunities for adolescents' first sex. *Journal of Family Issues, 27,* 159–183.

Regnerus, M., & Uecker, J. (2011). *Premarital sex in America: How young Americans meet, mate, and think about marrying.* New York: Oxford University Press.

Reich, W. (1986). *The sexual revolution: Toward a self-regulating character structure.* New York: Farrar, Straus, & Giroux.

Reisner, S. L., Conron, K. J., Tardiff, L. A., Jarvi, S., Gordon, A. R., & Austin, S. B. (2014). Monitoring the health of transgender and other gender minority populations: Validity of natal sex and gender identity survey items in a U.S. national cohort of young adults. *BMC Public Health, 14,* 1–19.

Reisner, S. L., Greytak, E. A., Parsons, J. T., & Ybarra, M. L. (2015). Gender minority social stress in adolescence: Disparities in adolescent bullying and substance use by gender identity. *Journal of Sex Research, 52,* 243–256.

Reitz, E., van de Bongardt, D., Baams, L., Doornwaard, S., Dubas, J., van Aken, M., et al. (2015). Project STARS (Studies on Trajectories of Adolescent Relationships and Sexuality): A longitudinal, multi-domain study on sexual development of Dutch adolescents. *European Journal of Developmental Psychology, 12,* 613–626.

Remafedi, G., Resnick, M., Blum, R., & Harris, L. (1992). Demography of sexual orientation in adolescents. *Pediatrics, 89,* 714–721.

Reyna, V. F., & Mills, B. A. (2014). Theoretically motivated interventions for reducing sexual risk taking in adolescence: A randomized controlled experiment applying fuzzy-trace theory. *Journal of Experimental Psychology: General, 143,* 1627–1648.

Rhee, S. H., & Waldman, I. D. (2002). Genetic and environmental influences on antisocial behavior: A meta-analysis of twin and adoption studies. *Psychological Bulletin, 128,* 490–529.

Rhule, D. M., McMahon, R. J., Spieker, S. J., & Munson, J. A. (2006). Positive adjustment and associated protective factors in children of adolescent mothers. *Journal of Child and Family Studies, 15,* 231–251.

Rice, E., Gibbs, J., Winetrobe, H., Rhoades, H., Plant, A., Montoya, J., et al. (2014). Sexting and sexual behavior among middle school students. *Pediatrics, 134,* e21–e28.

Rice, E., Rhoades, H., Winetrobe, H., Sanchez, M., Montoya, J., Plant, A., et al. (2012). Sexually explicit cell phone messaging associated with sexual risk among adolescents. *Pediatrics, 130,* 667–673.

Rideout, V. J. (2007, June). *Parents, children and media: A Kaiser Family Foundation survey.* Menlo Park, CA: Henry J. Kaiser Family Foundation. Retrieved July 11, 2016, from *https://kaiserfamilyfoundation.files.wordpress.com/2013/01/7638.pdf.*

Rideout, V. J., Foehr, U. G., & Roberts, D. F. (2010, January). *Generation M²: Media in the lives of 8- to 18-year-olds.* Menlo Park, CA: Henry J. Kaiser Family Foundation. Retrieved July 11, 2016, from *http://files.eric.ed.gov/fulltext/ED527859.pdf.*

Rink, E., Tricker, R., & Harvey, S. M. (2007). Onset of sexual intercourse among female adolescents: The influence of perceptions, depression, and ecological factors. *Journal of Adolescent Health, 41,* 398–406.

Ritchwood, T. D., Ford, H., DeCoster, J., Sutton, M., & Lochman, J. E. (2015). Risky sexual behavior and substance use among adolescents: A meta-analysis. *Children and Youth Services Review, 52,* 74–88.

Robbins, C. L., Schick, V., Reece, M., Herbenick, D., Sanders, S. A., Dodge, B., et al. (2011). Prevalence, frequency, and associations of masturbation with partnered sexual behaviors among US adolescents. *Archives of Pediatric and Adolescent Medicine, 165,* 1087–1093.

Roberto, A. J., Carlyle, K. E., Zimmerman, R. S., Abner, E. L., Cupp, P. K., & Hansen, G. L. (2008). The short-term effects of a computer-based pregnancy, STD, and HIV prevention program. *Communication Quarterly, 56,* 29–48.

Roberts, M. E., Gibbons, F. X., Gerrard, M., Weng, C. Y., Murry, V. M., Simons, L. G., et al. (2012). From racial discrimination to risky sex: Prospective relations involving peers and parents. *Developmental Psychology, 48,* 89–102.

Robillard, A. (2012). Music videos and sexual risk in African American adolescent girls: Gender, power and the need for media literacy. *American Journal of Health Education, 43,* 93–103.

Robinson, J. P., & Espelage, D. L. (2011). Inequities in educational and psychological outcomes between LGBTQ and straight students in middle and high school. *Educational Researcher, 40,* 315–330.

Robinson, J. P., Espelage, D. L., & Rivers, I. (2013). Developmental trends in peer victimization and emotional distress in LGB and heterosexual youth. *Pediatrics, 131,* 423–430.

Rocca, C. H., Doherty, I., Padian, N. S., Hubbard, A. E., & Minnis, A. M. (2010). Pregnancy intentions and teenage pregnancy among Latinas: A mediation analysis. *Perspectives on Sexual and Reproductive Health, 42,* 186–196.

Roche, K. M., & Leventhal, T. (2009). Beyond neighborhood poverty: Family management, neighborhood disorder, and adolescents' early sexual onset. *Journal of Family Psychology, 23,* 819–827.

Rogers, A. A., Ha, T., Stormshak, E. A., & Dishion, T. J. (2015). Quality of parent-adolescent conversations about sex and adolescent sexual behavior: An observational study. *Journal of Adolescent Health, 57,* 174–178.

Rohrbach, L. A., Berglas, N. F., Jerman, P., Angulo-Olaiz, F., Chou, C. P., & Constantine, N. A. (2015). A rights-based sexuality education curriculum for adolescents: 1-year outcomes from a cluster-randomized trial. *Journal of Adolescent Health, 57,* 399–406.

Romero, L., Pazol, K., Warner, L., Cox, S., Kroelinger, C., Besera, G., et al. (2016, April 29). Reduced disparities in birth rates among teens aged 15–19 years: United States, 2006–2007 and 2013–2014. *Morbidity and Mortality Weekly Report, 65.* Washington, DC: U.S. Department of Health and Human Services, Centers for Disease Control and Prevention. Retrieved September 21, 2016, from *www.cdc.gov/mmwr/volumes/65/wr/mm6516a1.htm.*

Romo, L. F., Lefkowitz, E. S., Sigman, M., & Au, T. K. (2002). A longitudinal study of maternal messages about dating and sexuality and their influence on Latino adolescents. *Journal of Adolescent Health, 31,* 59–69.

Ronis, S. T., & O'Sullivan, L. F. (2011). A longitudinal analysis of predictors of male and female adolescents' transitions to intimate sexual behavior. *Journal of Adolescent Health, 49,* 321–323.

Rosario, M., Corliss, H. L., Everett, B. G., Reisner, S. L., Austin, B., & Buchting, F.

O., et al. (2014). Mediation by peer violence victimization of sexual orientation disparities in cancer-related tobacco, alcohol, and sexual risk behaviors: Pooled youth risk behavior surveys. *American Journal of Public Health, 104,* 245–254.

Rosario, M., Hunter, J., Maguen, S., Gwadz, M., & Smith, R. (2001). The coming-out process and its adaptational and health-related associations among gay, lesbian, and bisexual youths: Stipulation and exploration of a model. *American Journal of Community Psychology, 29,* 133–160.

Rosario, M., Schrimshaw, E. W., & Hunter, J. (2004). Ethnic/racial differences in the coming-out process of lesbian, gay, and bisexual youths: A comparison of sexual identity development over time. *Cultural Diversity and Ethnic Minority Psychology, 10,* 215–228.

Rose, E., DiClemente, R. J., Wingood, G. M., Sales, J. M., Latham, T. P., Crosby, R. A., et al. (2009). The validity of teens' and young adults' self-reported condom use. *Archives of Pediatrics and Adolescent Medicine, 163,* 61–64.

Rosenbaum, J. E. (2009). Patient teenagers?: A comparison of the sexual behavior of virginity pledgers and matched nonpledgers. *Pediatrics, 123,* e110–e120.

Rosenthal, D. A., & Feldman, S. S. (1999). The importance of importance: Adolescents' perceptions of parental communication about sexuality. *Journal of Adolescence, 22,* 835–851.

Rosenthal, D. A., Feldman, S. S., & Edwards, D. (1998). Mum's the word: Mothers' perspectives on communication about sexuality with adolescents. *Journal of Adolescence, 21,* 727–743.

Rosin, H. (2012, September). Boys on the side. *The Atlantic.* Retrieved July 10, 2016, from *www.theatlantic.com/magazine/archive/2012/09/boys-on-the-side/309062.*

Rosin, H. (2014, November). Why kids sext. *The Atlantic.* Retrieved July 11, 2016, from *www.theatlantic.com/magazine/archive/2014/11/why-kids-sext/380798.*

Rossi, E., Poulin, F., & Boislard, M. A. (2017). Trajectories of annual number of sexual partners from adolescence to emerging adulthood: Individual and family predictors.

Journal of Youth and Adolescence, 46, 995–1008.

Rothman, E. F., Sullivan, M., Keyes, S., & Boehmer, U. (2012). Parents' supportive reactions to sexual orientation disclosure associated with better health: Results from a population-based survey of LGB adults in Massachusetts. *Journal of Homosexuality, 59,* 186–200.

Rouvier, M., Campero, L., Walker, D., & Caballero, M. (2011). Factors that influence communication about sexuality between parents and adolescents in the cultural context of Mexican families. *Sex Education, 11,* 175–191.

Rowe, D. C. (2002). On genetic variation in menarche and age at first sexual intercourse: A critique of the Belsky–Draper hypothesis. *Evolution and Human Behavior, 23,* 365–372.

Ruditis, P. (2005). *Rainbow party.* New York: Simon Plus.

Ruedinger, E., & Cox, J. E. (2012). Adolescent childbearing: Consequences and interventions. *Current Opinion in Pediatrics, 24,* 446–452.

Russell, S. T., & Fish, J. N. (2016). Mental health in lesbian, gay, bisexual, and transgender (LGBT) youth. *Annual Review of Clinical Psychology, 12,* 465–487.

Russell, S. T., Seif, H., & Truong, N. L. (2001). School outcomes of sexual minority youth in the United States: Evidence from a national study. *Journal of Adolescence, 24,* 111–127.

Russell, S. T., & Toomey, R. B. (2012). Men's sexual orientation and suicide: Evidence for U.S. adolescent-specific risk. *Social Science and Medicine, 74,* 523–529.

Ryan, R. M. (2015). Nonresident fatherhood and adolescent sexual behavior: A comparison of siblings approach. *Developmental Psychology, 51,* 211–223.

Ryan, S., Franzetta, K., Manlove, J., & Holcombe, E. (2007). Adolescents' discussions about contraception or STDs with partners before first sex. *Perspectives on Sexual and Reproductive Health, 39,* 149–157.

Saewyc, E. M. (2011). Research on adolescent sexual orientation: Development, health disparities, stigma, and resilience. *Journal of Research on Adolescence, 21,* 256–272.

Saewyc, E. M., Bauer, G. R., Skay, C. L., Bearinger, L. H., Resnick, M. D., Reis, E., et al. (2004). Measuring sexual orientation in adolescent health surveys: Evaluation of eight school-based surveys. *Journal of Adolescent Health, 35,* 345, e1–e15.

Saftner, M. A., Martyn, K. K., & Lori, J. R. (2011). Sexually active adolescent women: Assessing family and peer relationships using event history calendars. *Journal of School Nursing, 27,* 225–236.

Sakaluk, J. K., & Milhausen, R. R. (2012). Factors influencing university students explicit and implicit sexual double standards. *Journal of Sex Research, 49,* 464–476.

Salam, R. A., Faqqah, A., Sajjad, N., Lassi, Z. S., Das, J. K., Kaufman, M., et al. (2016). Improving adolescent sexual and reproductive health: A systematic review of potential interventions. *Journal of Adolescent Health, 59,* S11–S28.

Salazar, L. F., DiClemente, R. J., Wingood, G. M., Crosby, R. A., Harrington, K., Davies, S., et al. (2004). Self-concept and adolescents' refusal of unprotected sex: A test of mediating mechanisms among African American girls. *Prevention Science, 5,* 137–149.

Salazar, L. F., Head, S., Crosby, R. A., DiClemente, R. J., Sales, J. M., Wingood, G. M., et al. (2011). Personal and social influences regarding oral sex among African American female adolescents. *Journal of Women's Health, 20,* 161–167.

Sales, J., Brown, J. L., DiClemente, R. J., Davis, T. L., Kottke, M. J., & Rose, E. S. (2012). Age differences in STDs, sexual behaviors, and correlates of risky sex among sexually experienced adolescent African-American females. *Journal of Pediatric Psychology, 37,* 33–42.

Saliares, E., Wilkerson, J. M., Sieving, R. E., & Brady, S. S. (2017). Sexually experienced adolescents' thoughts about sexual pleasure. *Journal of Sex Research, 54,* 604–618.

Samarova, V., Shilo, G., & Diamond, G. M. (2014). Changes in youths' perceived parental acceptance of their sexual minority status over time. *Journal of Research on Adolescence, 24,* 681–688.

Samkange-Zeeb, F. N., Spallek, L., & Zeeb, H. (2011). Awareness and knowledge of sexually transmitted diseases (STDs) among school-going adolescents in Europe: A systematic review of published literature. *BMC Public Health, 11,* 727.

Sandberg-Thoma, S. E., & Duch, C. M. K. (2014). Casual sexual relationships and mental health in adolescence and emerging adulthood. *Journal of Sex Research, 51,* 121–130.

Sandfort, T. G., & Cohen-Kettenis, P. T. (2000). Sexual behavior in Dutch and Belgian children as observed by their mothers. *Journal of the Psychology and Human Sexuality, 12,* 105–115.

Santa Maria, D., Markham, C., Bluethmann, S., & Mullen, P. D. (2015). Parent-based adolescent sexual health interventions and effect on communication outcomes: A systematic review and meta-analyses. *Perspectives on Sexual and Reproductive Health, 47,* 37–50.

Santelli, J. S., Lindberg, L. D., Finer, L. B., & Singh, S. (2007). Explaining recent declines in adolescent pregnancy in the United States: The contribution of abstinence and improved contraceptive use. *American Journal of Public Health, 97,* 150–156.

Santelli, J. S., Nystrom, R. J., Brindis, C., Juszczak, L., Klein, J. D., Bearss, N., et al. (2003). Reproductive health in school-based health centers: Findings from the 1998–99 census of school-based health centers. *Journal of Adolescent Health, 32,* 443–451.

Santelli, J., Ott, M. A., Lyon, M., Rogers, J., Summers, D., & Schleifer, R. (2006). Abstinence and abstinence-only education: A review of U.S. policies and programs. *Journal of Adolescent Health, 38,* 72–81.

Santelli, J. S., Sandfort, T., & Orr, M. (2008). Transnational comparisons of adolescent contraceptive use: What can we learn from these comparisons? *Archives of Pediatrics and Adolescent Medicine, 162,* 92–94.

Santelli, J. S., Sharma, V., & Viner, R. (2013). Inequality, national wealth, economic development and global trends in teenage birth rates, 1990–2010. *Journal of Adolescent Health, 53,* S4–S5.

Saraswathi, T. S., & Pai, S. (1997). Socialization in the Indian context. In H. S. R. Kao & D.

Sinha (Eds.), *Asian perspectives on psychology* (pp. 74–92). Thousand Oaks, CA: SAGE.

Sasaki, S., Ozaki, K., Yamagata, S., Takahashi, Y., Shikishima, C., Kornacki, T., et al. (2016). Genetic and environmental influences on traits of gender identity disorder: A study of Japanese twins across developmental stages. *Archives of Sexual Behavior, 45,* 1681–1695.

Satterwhite, C. L., Torrone, E., Meites, E., Dunne, E. F., Mahajan, R., Ocfemia, M. C. B., et al. (2013). Sexually transmitted infections among US women and men: Prevalence and incidence estimates, 2008. *Sexually Transmitted Diseases, 40,* 187–193.

Savin-Williams, R. C. (1994). Dating those you can't love and loving those you can't date. In R. Montemayor, G. R. Adams, & T. P. Gullotta (Eds.), *Personal relationships during adolescence* (pp. 196–215). Thousand Oaks, CA: SAGE.

Savin-Williams, R. C. (1998a). The disclosure to families of same-sex attractions by lesbian, gay, and bisexual youths. *Journal of Research on Adolescence, 8,* 49–68.

Savin-Williams, R. C. (1998b). " . . . And then I became gay": Young men's stories. New York: Routledge.

Savin-Williams, R. C. (2005). *The new gay teenager.* Cambridge, MA: Harvard University Press.

Savin-Williams, R. C. (2011). Identity development among sexual-minority youth. In S. J. Schwartz, K. Luyckx, & V. L. Vignoles (Eds.), *Handbook of identity theory and research* (pp. 671–689). New York: Springer.

Savin-Williams, R. C. (2014). An exploratory study of the categorical versus spectrum nature of sexual orientation. *Journal of Sex Research, 51,* 446–453.

Savin-Williams, R. C., & Diamond, L. M. (2000). Sexual identity trajectories among sexual-minority youths: Gender comparisons. *Archives of Sexual Behavior, 29,* 607–627.

Savin-Williams, R. C., Joyner, K., & Rieger, G. (2012). Prevalence and stability of self-reported sexual orientation identity during young adulthood. *Archives of Sexual Behavior, 41,* 103–110.

Savin-Williams, R. C., & Ream, G. L. (2003). Suicide attempts among sexual minority male youth. *Journal of Clinical Child and Adolescent Psychology, 32,* 509–522.

Savolainen, J., Mason, W. A., Hughes, L. A., Ebeling, H., Hurtig, T. M., & Taanila, A. M. (2015). Pubertal development and sexual intercourse among adolescent girls: An examination of direct, mediated, and spurious pathways. *Youth and Society, 47,* 520–538.

Schalet, A. T. (2011). Beyond abstinence and risk: A new paradigm for adolescent sexual health. *Women's Health Issues, 21*(Suppl. 3), S5–S7.

Scharf, M., & Mayseless, O. (2008). Late adolescent girls' relationships with parents and romantic partner: The distinct role of mothers and fathers. *Journal of Adolescence, 31,* 837–855.

Schmid, A., Leonard, N. R., Ritchie, A. S., & Gwadz, M. V. (2015). Assertive communication in condom negotiation: Insights from late adolescent couples' subjective ratings of self and partner. *Journal of Adolescent Health, 57,* 94–99.

Schmidt, S. C., Wandersman, A., & Hills, K. J. (2015). Evidence-based sexuality education programs in schools: Do they align with the National Sexuality Education standards? *American Journal of Sexuality Education, 10,* 177–195.

Schmiedeberg, C., Huyer-May, B., Castiglioni, L., & Johnson, M. D. (2017). The more or the better?: How sex contributes to life satisfaction. *Archives of Sexual Behavior, 46,* 465–473.

Scholl, T. O., Hediger, M. L., & Ances, I. G. (1990). Maternal growth during pregnancy and decreased infant birth weight. *American Journal of Clinical Nutrition, 51,* 790–793.

Schuster, M. A., Corona, R., Elliott, M. N., Kanouse, D. E., Eastman, K. L., Zhou, A. J., et al. (2008). Evaluation of Talking Parents, Healthy Teens, a new worksite based parenting program to promote parent–adolescent communication about sexual health: Randomized controlled trial. *BMJ, 337,* a308.

Scott, M. E., Steward-Streng, N. R., Manlove, J., & Moore, K. A. (2012, June). *The characteristics and circumstances of teen fathers: At the birth of their first child and beyond* (Research Brief No. 2012-19, 1-6). Washington, DC: Child Trends. Retrieved July 24, 2016, from *www.*

childtrends.org/wp-content/uploads/2013/03/ Child_Trends-2012_06_01_RB_TeenFathers. pdf.

Scott-Sheldon, L. A. J., Carey, K. B., Cunningham, K., Johnson, B. T., & Carey, M. P. (2016). Alcohol use predicts sexual decision-making: A systematic review and meta-analysis of the experimental literature. *AIDS Behavior, 20,* S19–S39.

Scott-Sheldon, L. A. J., Huedo-Medina, T. B., Warren, M. R., Johnson, B. T., & Carey, M. P. (2011). Efficacy of behavioral interventions to increase condom use and reduce sexually transmitted infections: A meta-analysis, 1991–2010. *Journal of Acquired Immune Deficiency Syndromes, 58,* 489–498.

Secor-Turner, M., Sieving, R. E., Eisenberg, M. E., & Skay, C. (2011). Associations between sexually experienced adolescents' sources of information about sex and sexual risk outcomes. *Sex Education, 11,* 489–500.

Sedgh, G., Finer, L. B., Bankole, A., Eilers, M. A., & Singh, S. (2015). Adolescent pregnancy, birth, and abortion rates across countries: Levels and recent trends. *Journal of Adolescent Health, 56,* 223–230.

Selkie, E. M., Benson, M., & Moreno, M. (2011). Adolescents' views regarding uses of social networking websites and text messaging for adolescent sexual health education. *American Journal of Health Education, 42,* 205–212.

Seth, P., Patel, S. N., Sales, J. M., DiClemente, R. J., Wingood, G. M., & Rose, E. S. (2011). The impact of depressive symptomatology on risky sexual behavior and sexual communication among African American female adolescents. *Psychology, Health and Medicine, 16,* 346–356.

Seth, P., Raiji, P. T., DiClemente, R. J., Wingood, G. M., & Rose, E. (2009). Psychological distress as a correlate of a biologically confirmed STI, risky sexual practices, self-efficacy and communication with male sex partners in African-American female adolescents. *Archives of Pediatric Adolescent Medicine, 156,* 599–606.

Ševčíková, A., Simon, L., Daneback, K., & Kvapilik, T. (2015). Bothersome exposure to online sexual content among adolescent girls. *Youth and Society, 47,* 486–501.

Sexuality and U. (2016). Statistics on oral sex experience among Canadian teenagers. Retrieved July 10, 2016, from *www.sexualityandu.ca/sexual-health/statistics1/statistics-on-oral-sex-experience-among-canadian-teenagers.*

Shackleton, N., Jamal, F., Viner, R. M., Dickson, K., Patton, G., & Bonell, C. (2016). School-based interventions going beyond health education to promote adolescent health: Systematic review of reviews. *Journal of Adolescent Health, 58,* 382–396.

Shearer, A., Herres, J., Kodish, T., Squitieri, H., James, K., Russon, J., et al. (2016). Differences in mental health symptoms across lesbian, gay, bisexual, and questioning youth in primary care settings. *Journal of Adolescent Health, 59,* 38–43.

Shepherd, L. M., Sly, K. F., & Girard, J. M. (2017). Comparison of comprehensive and abstinence-only sexuality education in young African American adolescents. *Journal of Adolescence, 61,* 50–63.

Shields, J. P., Cohen, R., Glassman, J. R., Whitaker, K., Franks, H., & Bertolini, I. (2013). Estimating population size and demographic characteristics of lesbian, gay, bisexual, and transgender youth in middle school. *Journal of Adolescent Health, 52,* 248–250.

Shilo, G., & Mor, Z. (2014). The impact of minority stressors on the mental and physical health of lesbian, gay, and bisexual youths and young adults. *Health Social Work, 39,* 161–171.

Shilo, G., & Mor, Z. (2015). Sexual activity and condom use among Israeli adolescents. *Journal of Sexual Medicine, 12,* 1732–1736.

Shilo, G., & Savaya, R. (2012). Mental health of lesbian, gay, and bisexual youth and young adults: Differential effects of age, gender, religiosity, and sexual orientation. *Journal of Research on Adolescence, 22,* 310–325.

Shulman, S., Seiffge-Krenke, I., & Walsh, S. D. (2017). Is sexual activity during adolescence good for future romantic relationships? *Journal of Youth and Adolescence, 46,* 1867–1877.

Sidze, E. M., Elungata'a, P., Maina, B. W., & Mutua, M. M. (2015). Does the quality of parent–child connectedness matter for adolescents' sexual behaviors in Nairobi informal settlements? *Archives of Sexual Behavior, 44,* 631–638.

SIECUS. (2009, October). SIECUS fact sheet: Comprehensive sex education. Retrieved April 22, 2018, from *www.siecus.org/index. cfm?fuseaction=Page.ViewPage&PageID=1193*.

Sieving, R. E., Eisenberg, M. E., Pettingell, S., & Skay, C. (2006). Friends' influence on adolescents' first sexual intercourse. *Perspectives on Sexual and Reproductive Health, 38,* 13–19.

Sieving, R. E., McMorris, B. J., Beckman, K. J., Pettingell, S. L., Secor-Turner, M., Kugler, K., et al. (2011). Prime Time: 12-month sexual health outcomes of a clinic-based intervention to prevent pregnancy risk behaviors. *Journal of Adolescent Health, 49,* 172–179.

Sieving, R. E., McRee, A. L., McMorris, B. J., Beckman, K. J., Pettingell, S. L., Bearinger, L. H., et al. (2013). Prime Time: Sexual health outcomes at 24 months for a clinic-linked intervention to prevent pregnancy risk behaviors. *JAMA Pediatrics, 167,* 333–340.

Silk, J., & Romero, D. (2014). The role of parents and families in teen pregnancy prevention: An analysis of programs and policies. *Journal of Family Issues, 35,* 1339–1362.

Silva, M. (2002). The effectiveness of school-based sex education programs in the promotion of abstinent behavior: A meta-analysis. *Health Education Research, 17,* 471–481.

Silventoinen, K., Haukka, J., Dunkel, L., Tynelius, P., & Rasmussen, F. (2008). Genetics of pubertal timing and its associations with relative weight in childhood and adult height: The Swedish young male twins study. *Pediatrics, 121,* e885–e891.

Silverstein, L. B., & Auerbach, C. F. (1999). Deconstructing the essential father. *American Psychologist, 54,* 397–407.

Simon, L., & Daneback, K. (2013). Adolescents' use of the Internet for sex education: A thematic and critical review of the literature. *International Journal of Sexual Health, 25,* 305–319.

Simons, L., Schrager, S. M., Clark, L. F., Belzer, M., & Olson, J. (2013). Parental support and mental health among transgender adolescents. *Journal of Adolescent Health, 53,* 791–793.

Simons, L. G., Sutton, T. E., Simons, R. L., Gibbons, F. X., & Murry, V. M. (2016). Mechanisms that link parenting practices to adolescents' risky sexual behavior: A test of six competing theories. *Journal of Youth and Adolescence, 45,* 255–270.

Singh, D., & Young, R. K. (1995). Body weight, waist-to-hip ratio, breasts, and hips: Role in judgments of female attractiveness and desirability for relationships. *Ethology and Sociobiology, 16,* 483–507.

Sipsma, H., Biello, K. B., Cole-Lewis, H., & Kershaw, T. (2010). Like father, like son: The intergenerational cycle of adolescent fatherhood. *American Journal of Public Health, 100,* 517–524.

Sipsma, H. L., Ickovics, J. R., Lewis, J. B., Ethier, K. A., & Kershaw, T. S. (2011). Adolescent pregnancy desired and pregnancy incidence. *Women's Health Issues, 21,* 110–116.

Sly, D. F., Riehman, K., Wu, C., Eberstein, I., Quadagno D., & Kistner, J. (1995). Early childhood differentials in mother–child AIDS-information interaction. *AIDS Education and Prevention, 7,* 337–354.

Smahel, D., Brown, B. B., & Blinka, L. (2012). Associations between online friendship and Internet addiction among adolescents and emerging adults. *Developmental Psychology, 48,* 381–388.

Smiler, A. P., Frankel, L. B. W., & Savin-Williams, R. C. (2011). From kissing to coitus?: Sex-of-partner differences in the sexual milestone achievement of young men. *Journal of Adolescence, 34,* 727–735.

Smiler, A. P., Ward, M., Caruthers, A., & Merriwether, A. (2005). Pleasure, empowerment, and love: Factors associated with a positive first coitus. *Sexuality Research and Social Policy, 2,* 41–55.

Smith, A. M., Rosenthal, D. A., & Reichler, H. (1996). High schoolers masturbatory practices: Their relationship to sexual intercourse and personal characteristics. *Psychological Reports, 79,* 499–509.

Smith, M., Gertz, E., Alvarez, S., & Lurie, P. (2006). The content and accessibility of sex education information on the Internet. *Health Education and Behavior, 27,* 684–694.

Snapp, S., Ryu, E., & Kerr, J. (2015). The upside to hooking up: College students' positive hookup experiences. *International Journal of Sexual Health, 27,* 43–56.

Sneed, C. D., Tan, H. P., & Meyer, J. C. (2015). The influence of parental communication and perception of peers on adolescent sexual behavior. *Journal of Health Communication, 20,* 888–892.

Social Security Act. (2018, February). Title V, Section 510(b)(2)(A-H). Separate program for abstinence education. Retrieved April 22, 2018, from *www.ssa.gov/OP_Home/ssact/title05/0510.htm.*

Solebello, N., & Elliott, S. (2011). "We want them to be as heterosexual as possible": Fathers talk about their teen children's sexuality. *Gender and Society, 25,* 293–315.

Somers, C. L., & Paulson, S. E. (2000). Students' perceptions of parent–adolescent closeness and communication about sexuality: Relations with sexual knowledge, attitudes, and behaviors. *Journal of Adolescence, 23,* 629–644.

Song, A. V., & Halpern-Felsher, B. L. (2011). Predictive relationship between adolescent oral and vaginal sex. *Archives of Pediatrics and Adolescent Medicine, 165,* 243–249.

Spack, N. P., Edwards-Leeper, L., Feldman, H. A., Leibowitz, S., Mandel, F., Diamond, D. A., et al. (2012). Children and adolescents with gender identity disorder referred to a pediatric medical center. *Pediatrics, 129,* 418–425.

Spitalnick, J. S., DiClemente, R. J., Wingood, G. M., Crosby, R. A., Milhausen, R. R., Sales, J. M., et al. (2007). Brief report: Sexual sensation seeking and its relationship to risky sexual behavior among African-American adolescent females. *Journal of Adolescence, 30,* 165–173.

Sprecher, S. (2014). Evidence of change in men's versus women's emotional reactions to first sexual intercourse: A 23-year study in a human sexuality course at a Midwestern university. *Journal of Sex Research, 51,* 466–472.

Sprecher, S., Harris, G., & Meyers, A. (2008). Perceptions of sources of sex education and targets of sex communication: Sociodemographic and cohort effects. *Journal of Sex Research, 45,* 17–26.

Sprecher, S., & Regan, P. C. (1996). College virgins: How men and women perceive their sexual status. *Journal of Sex Research, 33,* 3–15.

Sprecher, S., & Treger, S. (2015). Virgin college students' reasons for and reactions to their abstinence from sex: Results from a 23-year study at a Midwestern U.S. university. *Journal of Sex Research, 52,* 936–948.

Sprecher, S., Treger, S., & Sakaluk, J. K. (2013). Premarital sexual standards and sociosexuality: Gender, ethnicity, and cohort differences. *Archives of Sexual Behavior, 42,* 1395–1405.

Stark, L., Tan, T. M., Muldoon, K. A., King, D., Lamin, D. F. M., Lilley, S., et al. (2016). Family structure and sexual and reproductive health outcomes among adolescents in rural Sierra Leone. *Global Public Health, 11,* 309–321.

Stattin, H., Kerr, M., & Skoog, T. (2011). Early pubertal timing and girls' problem behavior: Integrating two hypotheses. *Journal of Youth and Adolescence, 40,* 1271–1287.

Steele, J. (1999). Teenage sexuality and media practice: Factoring in the influences of family, friends, and school. *Journal of Sex Research, 36,* 331–341.

Steensma, T. D., Kreukels, B. P. C., de Vries, A. L. C., & Cohen-Kettenis, P. T. (2013). Gender identity development in adolescence. *Hormones and Behavior, 64,* 288–297.

Steinberg, L. (2008). A social neuroscience perspective on adolescent risk-taking. *Developmental Review, 28,* 78–106.

Stepp, L. S. (1999, July 8). Parents are alarmed by an unsettling new fad in middle schools: Oral sex. *Washington Post.* Retrieved July 10, 2016, from *www.washingtonpost.com/archive/politics/1999/07/08/parents-are-alarmed-by-an-unsettling-new-fad-in-middle-schools-oral-sex/4130d1ef-5e0f-4078-99ec-faa75fe294c5.*

Sternberg, R. J. (2004). A triangular theory of love. In H. T. Reis & C. E. Rusbult (Eds.), *Close relationships* (pp. 258–276). New York: Psychology Press.

Stillman, S. (2016, March 14). The list: When juveniles are found guilty of sexual misconduct, the sex-offender registry can be a life sentence. *New Yorker.* Retrieved August 26, 2016, from *www.newyorker.com/magazine/2016/03/14/when-kids-are-accused-of-sex-crimes.*

Stinson, R. D. (2010). Hooking up in young adulthood: A review of factors influencing the sexual behavior of college students. *Journal of College Student Psychotherapy, 24,* 98–115.

Stone, D. M., Luo, F., Lippy, C., & McIntosh, W. L. (2015). The role of social connectedness and sexual orientation in the prevention of youth suicide ideation and attempts among sexually active adolescents. *Suicide and Life-Threatening Behavior, 45,* 415–430.

Stone, D. M., Luo, F., Ouyang, L., Lippy, C., Hertz, M. F., & Crosby, A. E. (2014). Sexual orientation and suicide ideation, plans, attempts, and medically serious attempts: Evidence from local youth risk behavior surveys, 2001–2009. *American Journal of Public Health, 104,* 262–271.

Stone, N., Hatherall, B., Ingham, R., & McEachran, J. (2006). Oral sex and condom use among young people in the United Kingdom. *Perspectives on Sexual and Reproductive Health, 38,* 6–12.

Strassberg, D. S., McKinnon, R. K., Sustaita, M. A., & Rullo, J. (2013). Sexting by high school students: An exploratory and descriptive study. *Archives of Sexual Behavior, 42,* 15–21.

Strassberg, D. S., Rullo, J. E., & Mackaronis, J. E. (2014). The sending and receiving of sexually explicit cell phone photos ("sexting") while in high school: One college's students' retrospective reports. *Computers in Human Behavior, 41,* 177–183.

Strohschein, L. (2012). Parental divorce and child mental health: Accounting for pre-disruption differences. *Journal of Divorce and Remarriage, 53,* 489–502.

Strokoff, J., Owen, J., & Fincham, F. D. (2015). Diverse reactions to hooking up among U.S. university students. *Archives of Sexual Behavior, 44,* 935–943.

Strunk, J. A. (2008). The effect of school-based health clinics on teenage pregnancy and parenting outcomes: An integrated literature review. *Journal of School Nursing, 24,* 13–20.

Sturgeon, S. W. (2008, November). *The relationship between family structure and adolescent sexual activity.* Washington, DC: Heritage Foundation. Retrieved July 10, 2016, from *www.familyfacts.org.*

Suleiman, A. B., & Deardorff, J. (2015). Multiple dimensions of peer influence in adolescent romantic and sexual relationships: A descriptive, qualitative perspective. *Archives of Sexual Behavior, 44,* 765–775.

Suleiman, A. B., Galván, A., Harden, K. P., & Dahl, R. E. (2017). Becoming a sexual being: The "elephant in the room" of adolescent brain development. *Developmental Cognitive Neuroscience, 25,* 209–220.

Sullivan, K., Clark, J., Castrucci, B., Samsel, R., Fonseca, V., & Garcia, I. (2011). Continuing education mitigates the negative consequences of adolescent childbearing. *Maternal Child Health Journal, 15,* 360–366.

Sullivan, P. S., Salazar, L., Buchbinder, S., & Sanchez, T. H. (2009). Estimating the proportion of HIV transmissions from main sex partners among men who have sex with men in five US cities. *AIDS, 23,* 1153–1162.

Susman, E. J., & Rogol, A. (2004). Puberty and psychological development. In R. L. Lerner & L. Steinberg (Eds.), *Handbook of adolescent psychology* (2nd ed., pp. 15–44). New York: Wiley.

Sutton, M. Y., Lasswell, S. M., Lanier, Y., & Miller, K. S. (2014). Impact of parent–child communication interventions on sex behaviors and cognitive outcomes for black/African-American and Hispanic/Latino youth: A systematic review, 1988–2012. *Journal of Adolescent Health, 54,* 369–384.

Suwarni, L., Ismail, D., Prabandari, Y. S., & Adiyanti, M. G. (2015). Perceived parental monitoring on adolescence premarital sexual behavior in Pontianak City, Indonesia. *International Journal of Public Health Science, 4,* 211–219.

Suzuki, L. K., & Calzo, J. P. (2004). The search for peer advice in cyberspace: An examination of online teen bulletin boards about health and sexuality. *Applied Developmental Psychology, 25,* 685–698.

Svedin, C. G., Åkerman, I., & Priebe, G. (2011). Frequent users of pornography: A population based epidemiological study of Swedish male adolescents. *Journal of Adolescence, 34,* 779–788.

Swain, C. R., Ackerman, L. K., & Acherman, M. A. (2006). The influence of individual characteristics and contraceptive beliefs on parent–teen sexual communications: A structural model. *Journal of Adolescent Health, 38,* 753.e9–753.e18.

Swartzendruber, A., Zenilman, J. M., Niccolai, L. M., Kershaw, T. S., Brown, J. L., DiClemente, R. J., et al. (2013). It takes 2: Partner attributes associated with sexually transmitted infections among adolescents. *Sexually Transmitted Diseases, 40,* 372–378.

Tabatabaie, A. (2015). Childhood and adolescent sexuality, Islam, and problematics of sex education: A call for re-examination. *Sex Education, 15,* 276–288.

Talley, A. E., Hughes, T. L., Aranda, F., Birkett, M., & Marshal, M. P. (2014). Exploring alcohol-use behaviors among heterosexual and sexual minority adolescents: Intersections with sex, age, and race/ethnicity. *American Journal of Public Health, 104,* 295–303.

Taylor, K. (2013, July 12). Sex on campus: She can play that game, too. *New York Times.* Retrieved July 10, 2016, from *www.nytimes.com/2013/07/14/fashion/sex-on-campus-she-can-play-that-game-too.html?pagewanted=all&_r=0.*

Taylor, L. D. (2005). Effects of visual and verbal sexual television content and perceived realism on attitudes and beliefs. *Journal of Sex Research, 42,* 130–137.

Temple, J. R., & Choi, H. (2014). Longitudinal association between teen sexting and sexual behavior. *Pediatrics, 134,* e1287–e1292.

ter Bogt, T. F. M., Engels, R. C. M. E., Bogers, S., & Kloosterman, M. (2010). "Shake it baby, shake it": Media preferences, sexual attitudes and gender stereotypes among adolescents. *Sex Roles, 63,* 844–859.

Thomas, J. C., & Sampson, L. A. (2005). High rates of incarceration as a social force associated with community rates of sexually transmitted infection. *Journal of Infectious Diseases, 191*(Suppl. 1), S55–S60.

Thomson, E., & McLanahan, S. S. (2012). Reflections on "Family structure and child well-being: Economic resources vs. parental socialization." *Social Forces, 91,* 45–53.

Thornburg, H. D. (1981). Adolescent sources of information on sex. *Journal of School Health, 51,* 274–277.

Timmermans, M., van Lier, P. A. C., & Koot, H. M. (2008). Which forms of child/adolescent externalizing behaviors account for late adolescent risky sexual behavior and substance use? *Journal of Child Psychology and Psychiatry, 49,* 386–394.

Tither, J. M., & Ellis, B. J. (2008). Impact of fathers on daughters' age of menarche: A genetically and environmentally controlled sibling study. *Developmental Psychology, 44,* 1409–1420.

Tolli, M. V. (2012). Effectiveness of peer education interventions for HIV prevention, adolescent pregnancy prevention and sexual health promotion for young people: A systematic review of European studies. *Health Education Research, 27,* 904–913.

Tolman, D. L. (2005). *Dilemmas of desire: Teenage girls talk about sexuality.* Cambridge, MA: Harvard University Press.

Tolman, D. L. (2012). Female adolescents, sexual empowerment and desire: A missing discourse of gender inequity. *Sex Roles, 66,* 746–757.

Tolman, D. L., & McClelland, S. I. (2011). Normative sexuality development in adolescence: A decade in review, 2000–2009. *Journal of Research on Adolescence, 21,* 242–255.

Tomić, I., Burić, J., & Štulhofer, A. (in press). Associations between Croatian adolescents' use of sexually explicit material and sexual behavior: Does parental monitoring play a role? *Archives of Sexual Behavior.*

Tortolero, S. R., Markham, C. M., Peskin, M. F., Shegog, R., Addy, R. C., Escobar-Chaves, L., et al. (2010). It's your game: Keep it real. Delaying sexual behavior with an effective middle school program. *Journal of Adolescent Health, 46,* 169–179.

Townsend, J. M., & Wasserman, T. H. (2011). Sexual hookups among college students: Sex differences in emotional reactions. *Archives of Sexual Behavior, 40,* 1173–1181.

Trenholm, C., Devancy, B., Fortson, K., Quay, L., Wheeler, J., & Clark, M. (2007). *Impacts of four Title V, Section 510 abstinence education programs.* Washington, DC: Mathematica Policy Research. Retrieved July 27, 2016, from *http://files.eric.ed.gov/fulltext/ED496286.pdf.*

Troiden, R. R. (1989). The formation of homosexual identities. *Journal of Homosexuality, 17,* 43–73.

Tschann, J. M., & Adler, N. E. (1997). Sexual self-acceptance, communication with partner, and contraceptive use among adolescent females: A longitudinal study. *Journal of Research on Adolescence, 7,* 413–430.

Tsitsika, A., Critselis, E., Kormas, G., Konstantoulaki, E., Constantopoulos, E., & Kafetzis, D. (2009). Adolescent pornographic Internet site use: A multivariate regression analysis of the predictive factors of use and psychosocial implications. *CyberPsychology and Behavior, 12,* 545–550.

Tubman, J. G., Windle, M., & Windle, R. C. (1996). The onset and cross-temporal patterning of sexual intercourse in middle adolescence: Prospective relations with behavioral and emotional problems. *Child Development, 67,* 327–343.

Tucker, J. S., Ewing, B. A., Espelage, D. L., Green, H. D., Jr., de la Haye, K., & Pollard, M. S. (2016). Longitudinal associations of homophobic name-calling victimization with psychological distress and alcohol use during adolescence. *Journal of Adolescent Health, 59,* 110–115.

Turnbull, T., van Wersch, A., & van Schaik, P. (2008). A review of parental involvement in sex education: The role for effective communication in British families. *Health Education Journal, 67,* 182–195.

Twenge, J. M., Sherman, R. A., & Wells, B. E. (2016). Changes in American adults' reported same-sex sexual experiences and attitudes, 1973–2014. *Archives of Sexual Behavior, 45,* 1713–1730.

Udry, J. R. (1990). Hormonal and social determinants of adolescent sexual initiation. In J. Bancroft & J. M. Reinisch (Eds.), *Adolescence and puberty* (pp. 70–87). New York: Oxford University Press.

Udry, J. R., Billy, J. O. G., Morris, N. M., Groff, T. R., & Raj, M. H. (1985). Serum androgenic hormones motivate sexual behavior in adolescent boys. *Fertility and Sterility, 43,* 90–94.

Udry, J. R., & Campbell, B. C. (1994). Getting started on sexual behavior. In A. S. Rossi (Ed.), *Sexuality across the life course* (pp. 187–208). Chicago: University of Chicago Press.

Udry, J. R., Talbert, L. M., & Morris, N. M. (1986). Biosocial foundations for adolescent female sexuality. *Demography, 23,* 217–228.

Uecker, J. E., Angotti, N., & Regnerus, M. D. (2008). Going most of the way: "Technical virginity" among American adolescents. *Social Science Research, 37,* 1200–1215.

Ueno, K. (2005). Sexual orientation and psychological distress in adolescence: Examining interpersonal stressors and social support processes. *Social Psychological Quarterly, 68,* 258–277.

Underhill, K., Montgomery, P., & Operario, D. (2007). Sexual abstinence only programmes to prevent HIV infection in high income countries: Systematic review. *British Medical Journal, 335,* 248–252.

Ungar, M. T. (2000). The myth of peer pressure. *Adolescence, 35,* 167–180.

United Nations Population Fund. (2013). Motherhood in childhood: Facing the challenge of adolescent pregnancy (United Nations report). Retrieved July 24, 2016, from *www.unfpa.org/sites/default/files/pub-pdf/EN-SWOP2013-final.pdf.*

Upchurch, D. M., Aneshensel, C. S., Sucoff, C. A., & Levy-Storms, L. (1999). Neighborhood and family contexts of adolescent sexual activity. *Journal of Marriage and the Family, 61,* 920–933.

Upchurch, D. M., Mason, W. M., Kusonuki, Y., & Kriechbaum, M. J. (2004). Social and behavioral determinants of self-reported STD among adolescents. *Perspectives on Sexual and Reproductive Health, 36,* 276–287.

Urošević, S., Collins, P., Muetzel, R., Lim, K., & Luciana, M. (2012). Longitudinal changes in behavioral approach system sensitivity and brain structures involved in reward processing during adolescence. *Developmental Psychology, 48,* 1488–1500.

U.S. Census Bureau. (2017, September). Median household income (Current Population Reports, 2017). Retrieved September 25, 2017, from *www.census.gov/data/tables/time-series/demo/income-poverty/cps-finc/finc-03.html.*

U.S. Department of Health and Human Services. (2010). *Healthy People 2010.*

Washington, DC: U.S. Government Printing Office. Retrieved July 10, 2016, from *https://bookstore.gpo.gov/products/sku/017-001-00579-7*.

van Beusekom, G., Baams, L., Bos, H. M. W., Overbeek, G., & Sandfort, T. G. M. (2016). Gender nonconformity, homophobic peer victimization, and mental health: How same-sex attraction and biological sex matter. *Journal of Sex Research, 53,* 98–108.

van de Bongardt, D., de Graaf, H., Reitz, E., & Deković, M. (2014). Parents as moderators of longitudinal associations between sexual peer norms and Dutch adolescents' sexual initiation and intention. *Journal of Adolescent Health, 55,* 388–393.

van de Bongardt, D., Reitz, E., & Deković, M. (2016). Indirect over-time relations between parenting and adolescents' sexual behaviors and emotions through global self-esteem. *Journal of Sex Research, 53,* 273–285.

van de Bongardt, D., Reitz, E., Sandfort, T., & Deković, M. (2015). A meta-analysis of the relations between three types of peer norms and adolescent sexual behavior. *Personality and Social Psychology Review, 19,* 203–234.

van Gelder, M. M. H. J., Reefhuis, J., Herron, A. M., Williams, M. L., & Roeleveld, N. (2011). Reproductive health characteristics of marijuana and cocaine users: Results from the 2002 National Survey of Family Growth. *Perspectives on Sexual and Reproductive Health, 43,* 164–172.

van Oosten, J. M. F., Peter, J., & Boot, I. (2015). Exploring associations between exposure to sexy online self-presentations and adolescents' sexual attitudes and behavior. *Journal of Youth and Adolescence, 44,* 1078–1091.

van Oosten, J. M. F., Peter, J., & Vandenbosch, L. (2017). Adolescents' sexual media use and willingness to engage in casual sex: Differential relations and underlying processes. *Human Communication Research, 43,* 127–147.

Vandenbosch, L., & Eggermont, S. (2013). Sexually explicit websites and sexual initiation: Reciprocal relationships and the moderating role of pubertal status. *Journal of Research on Adolescence, 23,* 621–634.

Vandenbosch, L., Vervloessem, D., & Eggermont, S. (2013). "I might get your heart racing in my skin-tight jeans": Sexualization on music entertainment television. *Communication Studies, 64,* 178–194.

Vannier, S. A., & Byers, E. S. (2013). A qualitative study of university students' perceptions of oral sex, intercourse, and intimacy. *Archives of Sexual Behavior, 42,* 1573–1581.

Vannier, S. A., & O'Sullivan, L. F. (2012). Who gives and who gets: Why, when, and with whom young people engage in oral sex. *Journal of Youth and Adolescence, 41,* 572–582.

Vasilenko, S. A. (2017). Age-varying associations between nonmarital sexual behavior and depressive symptoms across adolescence and young adulthood. *Developmental Psychology, 53,* 366–378.

Vasilenko, S. A., Kugler, K. C., Butera, N. M., & Lanza, S. T. (2015). Patterns of adolescent sexual behavior predicting young adult sexually transmitted infections: A latent class analysis approach. *Archives of Sexual Behavior, 44,* 705–715.

Vasilenko, S. A., Kugler, K. C., & Rice, C. E. (2016). Timing of first sexual intercourse and young adult health outcomes. *Journal of Adolescent Health, 59,* 291–297.

Vasilenko, S. A., Lefkowitz, E. S., & Maggs, J. L. (2012). Short-term positive and negative consequences of sex based on daily reports among college students. *Journal of Sex Research, 49,* 558–569.

Vasilenko, S. A., Lefkowitz, E. S., & Welsh, D. P. (2014). Is sexual behavior healthy for adolescents?: A conceptual framework for research on adolescent sexual behavior and physical, mental, and social health. *New Directions for Child and Adolescent Development, 144,* 3–19.

Vasilenko, S. A., Maas, M. K., & Lefkowitz, E. S. (2015). "It felt good but weird at the same time": Emerging adults' first experiences of six different sexual behaviors. *Journal of Adolescent Research, 30,* 586–606.

Vaughan, B., Trussell, J., Kost, K., Singh, S., & Jones, R. (2008). Discontinuation and resumption of contraceptive use: Results from the 2002 National Survey of Family Growth. *Contraception, 78,* 271–283.

Veale, J. R., Watson, R. J., Peter, T., & Saewyc, E. M. (2017). Mental health disparities among Canadian transgender youth. *Journal of Adolescent Health, 60,* 44–49.

Vespa, J., Lewis, J. M., & Kreider, R. M. (2013, August). *America's families and living arrangements: 2012* (Current Population Reports, No. P20-570). Washington, DC: U.S. Census Bureau. Retrieved December 3, 2016, from *www.census.gov/prod/2013pubs/p20-570.pdf.*

Villarruel, A. M., Loveland-Cherry, C. J., & Ronis, D. (2010). Testing the efficacy of a computer-based parent–adolescent sexual communication intervention for Latino parents. *Family Relations, 59,* 533–543.

Voisin, D. R., Hotton, A. L., Tan, K., & DiClemente, R. (2013). A longitudinal examination of risk and protective factors associated with drug use and unsafe sex among young African American females. *Children and Youth Services Review, 35,* 1440–1446.

Voisin, D. R., Tan, K., & DiClemente, R. J. (2013). A longitudinal examination of the relationship between sexual sensation seeking and STI-related risk factors among African American females. *AIDS Education and Prevention, 25,* 124–134.

Voisin, D. R., Tan, K., Salazar, L. F., Crosby, R., & DiClemente, R. J. (2012). Correlates of sexually transmitted infection prevention knowledge among African American girls. *Journal of Adolescent Health, 51,* 197–199.

Voisin, D. R., Tan, K., Tack, A. C., Wade, D., & DiClemente, R. (2012). Examining parental monitoring as a pathway from community violence exposure to drug use, risky sex, and recidivism among detained youth. *Journal of Social Service Research, 38,* 699–711.

von Sadovszky, V., Draudt, B., & Boch, S. (2014). A systematic review of reviews of behavioral interventions to promote condom use. *Worldviews on Evidence-Based Nursing, 11,* 107–117.

Vrangalova, Z. (2015a). Hooking up and psychological well-being in college students: Short-term prospective links across different hookup definitions. *Journal of Sex Research, 52,* 485–498.

Vrangalova, Z. (2015b). Does casual sex harm college students' well-being?: A longitudinal investigation of the role of motivation. *Archives of Sexual Behavior, 44,* 945–959.

Vrangalova, Z., & Savin-Williams, R. C. (2011). Adolescent sexuality and positive well-being: A group-norms approach. *Journal of Youth and Adolescence, 40,* 931–944.

Waldfogel, J., Craigie, T. A., & Brooks-Gunn, J. (2010). Fragile families and child wellbeing. *Future of Children, 20,* 87–112.

Wallerstein, J. S., Lewis, J. M., & Blakeslee, S. (2001). *The unexpected legacy of divorce: The 25 year landmark study.* New York: Hyperion.

Wallien, M. S. C., & Cohen-Kettenis, P. T. (2008). Psychosexual outcome of gender-dysphoric children. *Journal of the American Academy of Child and Adolescent Psychiatry, 47,* 1413–1423.

Walper, S., & Wendt, E. V. (2015). Adolescents' relationships with mother and father and their links to the quality of romantic relationships: A classification approach. *European Journal of Developmental Psychology, 12,* 516–532.

Wang, B., Stanton, B., Deveaux, L., & Lunn, S. (2015). Dynamic relationships between parental monitoring, peer risk involvement and sexual risk behavior among Bahamian mid-adolescents. *International Perspectives on Sexual and Reproductive Health, 41,* 89–98.

Wang, N. (2016). Parent–adolescent communication about sexuality in Chinese families. *Journal of Family Communication, 16,* 229–246.

Ward, L. M. (2016). Media and sexualization: State of empirical research, 1995–2015. *Journal of Sex Research, 53,* 560–577.

Warner, T. D. (2018). Adolescent sexual risk taking: The distribution of youth behaviors and perceived peer attitudes across neighborhood contexts. *Journal of Adolescent Health, 62,* 226–233.

Warner, T. D., Giordano, P. C., Manning W. D., & Longmore, M. A. (2011). Everybody's doin' it (right?): Neighborhood norms and sexual activity in adolescence. *Social Science Research, 40,* 1676–1690.

Wasserman, A. M., Crockett, L. J., & Hoffman, L. (2017). Reward seeking and cognitive control: Using the dual systems model to predict adolescent sexual behavior. *Journal of Research on Adolescence, 27,* 907–913.

Watson, A. F., & McKee, A. (2013). Masturbation and the media. *Sexuality and Culture, 17,* 449–475.

Waylen, A., & Wolke, D. (2004). Sex 'n' drugs

'n' rock 'n' roll: The meaning and social consequences of pubertal timing. *European Journal of Endocrinology, 151*(Suppl. 3), U151–U159.

Weber, J. B. (2012). Becoming teen fathers: Stories of teen pregnancy, responsibility, and masculinity. *Gender and Society, 26,* 900–921.

Weber, M., Quiring, O., & Daschmann, G. (2012). Peers, parents and pornography: Exploring adolescents' exposure to sexually explicit material and its developmental correlates. *Sexuality and Culture, 16,* 408–427.

Weed, S. E., & Lickona, T. (2014). Abstinence education in context: History, evidence, premises, and comparison to comprehensive sexuality education. In M. C. Kenny (Ed.), *Sex education: Attitude of adolescents, cultural differences and school's challenges* (pp. 27–69). Hauppauge, NY: Nova Science.

Wei, E. H., Loeber, R., & Stouthamer-Loeber, M. (2002). How many of the offspring born to teenage fathers are produced by repeat serious delinquents? *Criminal Behaviour and Mental Health, 12,* 83–98.

Weigel, M. (2016). *Labor of love: The invention of dating.* New York: Farrar, Straus & Giroux.

Whitaker, K., Shapiro, V. B., & Shields, J. P. (2016). School-based protective factors related to suicide for lesbian, gay, and bisexual adolescents. *Journal of Adolescent Health, 58,* 63–68.

White, C. N., & Warner, L. A. (2015). Influence of family and school-level factors on age of sexual initiation. *Journal of Adolescent Health, 56,* 231–237.

Wickrama, T., Merten, M. J., & Wickrama, K. A. S. (2012). Early socioeconomic disadvantage and young adult sexual health. *American Journal of Health Behavior, 36,* 834–848.

Widman, L., Choukas-Bradley, S., Helms, S. W., Golin, C. E., & Prinstein, M. J. (2014). Sexual communication between early adolescents and their dating partners, parents, and best friends. *Journal of Sex Research, 51,* 731–741.

Widman, L., Choukas-Bradley, S., Helms, S. W., & Prinstein, M. J. (2016). Adolescent susceptibility to peer influence in sexual situations. *Journal of Adolescent Health, 58,* 323–329.

Widman, L., Choukas-Bradley, S., Noar, S. M., Nesi, J., & Garrett, K. (2016). Parent–adolescent sexual communication and adolescent safer sex behavior: A meta-analysis. *Journal of the American Medical Association Pediatrics, 170,* 52–61.

Widman, L., Noar, S. M., Choukas-Bradley, S., & Francis, D. B. (2014). Adolescent sexual health communication and condom use: A meta-analysis. *Health Psychology, 33,* 1113–1124.

Wight, D., & Fullerton, D. (2013). A review of interventions with parents to promote the sexual health of their children. *Journal of Adolescent Health, 52,* 4–27.

Wight, D., Williamson, L., & Henderson, M. (2006). Parental influences on young people's sexual behavior: A longitudinal analysis. *Journal of Adolescence, 29,* 473–494.

Williams, S., & Thompson, M. P. (2013). Examining the prospective effects of making a virginity pledge among males across their 4 years of college. *Journal of American College Health, 61,* 114–120.

Willoughby, B. J., Carroll, J. S., & Busby, D. M. (2014). Differing relationship outcomes when sex happens before, on, or after first dates. *Journal of Sex Research, 51,* 52–61.

Wilson, E. K., Dalberth, B. T., Koo, H. P., & Gard, C. (2010). Parents' perspectives on talking to preteenage children about sex. *Perspectives on Sexual and Reproductive Health, 42,* 56–63.

Wilson, P. M. (1986). Black culture and sexuality. In L. Lister (Ed.), *Human sexuality, ethno-culture, and social work* (pp. 29–46). Binghamton, NY: Haworth Press.

Wilson, W. J. (2012). *The truly disadvantaged: The inner city, the underclass, and public policy* (2nd ed.). Chicago: University of Chicago Press.

Wingood, G. M., DiClemente, R. J., Harrington, K., Davies, S., Hook, E. W., & Oh, M. K. (2001). Exposure to X-rated movies and adolescents' sexual and contraceptive-related attitudes and behaviors. *Pediatrics, 107,* 1116–1119.

Winter, T., Karvonen, S., & Rose, R. J. (2014). Associations between sexual abstinence ideals, religiosity, and alcohol abstinence: A longitudinal study of Finnish twins. *Journal of Sex Research, 51,* 197–207.

Wolak, J., Finkelhor, D., & Mitchell, K. J. (2012). How often are teens arrested for sexting?: Data from a national sample of police cases. *Pediatrics, 129,* 4–12.

Wolak, J., Mitchell, K., & Finkelhor, D. (2007). Unwanted and wanted exposure to online pornography in a national sample of youth Internet users. *Pediatrics, 119,* 247–257.

Wolfers, M., de Zwart, O., & Kok, G. (2011). Adolescents in the Netherlands underestimate risk for sexually transmitted infections and deny the need for sexually transmitted infection testing. *AIDS Patient Care and STDs, 25,* 311–319.

Wong, M. L., Chan, R. K. W., Koh, D., Tan, H. H., Lim, F. S., Emmanuel, S., & Bishop, G. (2009). Premarital sexual intercourse among adolescents in an Asian country: Multilevel ecological factors. *Pediatrics, 124,* e44–e52.

Wood, H., Sasaki, S., Bradley, S. J., Singh, D., Fantus, S., Owen-Anderson, A., et al. (2013). Patterns of referral to a gender identity service for children and adolescents (1976–2011): Age, sex ratio, and sexual orientation. *Journal of Sex and Marital Therapy, 39,* 1–6.

Wood, J. R., McKay, A., Komarnicky, T., & Milhausen, R. R. (2016). Was it good for you too?: An analysis of gender differences in oral sex practices and pleasure ratings among heterosexual Canadian university students. *Canadian Journal of Human Sexuality, 25,* 21–29.

Woodward, L. J., & Fergusson, D. M. (1999). Early conduct problems and later risk of teenage pregnancy in girls. *Developmental Psychopathology, 11,* 127–141.

Woodward, L., Fergusson, D. M., & Horwood, L. J. (2001). Risk factors and life processes associated with teenage pregnancy: Results of a prospective study from birth to 20 years. *Journal of Marriage and the Family, 63,* 1170–1184.

Wright, P. J. (2011). Mass media effects on youth sexual behavior: Assessing the claim for causality. In C. T. Salmon (Ed.), *Communication Yearbook 35* (pp. 343–386). New York: Routledge.

Wright, P. J., Malamuth, N. M., & Donnerstein, E. (2012). Research on sex in the media: What do we know about effects on children and adolescents? In D. G. Singer & J. L. Singer (Eds.), *Handbook of children and the media* (pp. 273–302). Thousand Oaks, CA: SAGE.

Wright, P. J., Randall, A. K., & Arroyo, A. (2013). Father–daughter communication about sex moderates the association between exposure to MTV's *16 and Pregnant/Teen Mom* and female students' pregnancy-risk behavior. *Sexuality and Culture, 17,* 50–66.

Xie, H., Cairns, B. D., & Cairns, R. B. (2001). Predicting teen motherhood and teen fatherhood: Individual characteristics and peer affiliations. *Social Development, 10,* 488–511.

Yasmin, G., Kumar, A. T., & Parihar, B. (2014). Teenage pregnancy: Its impact on maternal and fetal outcome. *International Journal of Scientific Study, 1,* 9–13.

Ybarra, M., & Mitchell, K. (2007). How risky are social networking sites?: A comparison of places online where youth sexual solicitation and harassment occurs. *Pediatrics, 121,* e350–e357.

Ybarra, M. L., & Mitchell, K. J. (2014). "Sexting" and its relation to sexual activity and sexual risk behavior in a national survey of adolescents. *Journal of Adolescent Health, 55,* 757–764.

Ybarra, M. L., Mitchell, K. J., & Kosciw, J. (2015). The relation between suicidal ideation and bullying victimization in a national sample of transgender and non-transgender adolescents. In P. Goldblum, D. L. Espelage, J. Chu, & B. Bongar (Eds.), *Youth suicide and bullying: Challenges and strategies for prevention and intervention* (pp. 121–133). New York: Oxford University Press.

Ybarra, M. L., Rosario, M., Saewyc, E., & Goodenow, C. (2016). Sexual behaviors and partner characteristics by sexual identity among adolescent girls. *Journal of Adolescent Health, 58,* 310–316.

Ybarra, M. L., Strasburger, V. C., & Mitchell, K. J. (2014). Sexual media exposure, sexual behavior, and sexual violence victimization in adolescence. *Clinical Pediatrics, 53,* 1239–1247.

Young, A. M., & d'Arcy, H. (2005). Older boyfriends of adolescent girls: The cause or a sign of the problem? *Journal of Adolescent Health, 36,* 410–419.

Young, M. D., Deardorff, J., Ozer, E., & Lahiff, M. (2011). Sexual abuse in childhood and adolescence and the risk of early pregnancy among women ages 18–22. *Journal of Adolescent Health, 49,* 287–293.

Zhang, J., Jemmott, J. B., & Jemmott, L. A. (2015). Mediation and moderation of an efficacious theory-based abstinence-only intervention for African American adolescents. *Health Psychology, 34,* 1175–1184.

Zhao, Y., Montoro, R., Igartua, K., & Thombs, B. D. (2010). Suicidal ideation and attempt among adolescents reporting "unsure" sexual identity or heterosexual identity plus same-sex attraction or behavior: Forgotten groups? *Journal of the American Academy of Child and Adolescent Psychiatry, 49,* 104–113.

Zimmer-Gembeck, M. J., & Collins, W. A. (2008). Gender, mature appearance, alcohol use, and dating as correlates of sexual partner accumulation from ages 16–26 years. *Journal of Adolescent Health, 42,* 564–572.

Zimmer-Gembeck, M. J., & Helfand, M. (2008). Ten years of longitudinal research on U.S. adolescent sexual behavior: Developmental correlates of sexual intercourse, and the importance of age, gender, and ethnic background. *Developmental Review, 28,* 153–224.

Zimmer-Gembeck, M. J., Siebenbruner, J., & Collins, W. A. (2004). A prospective study of intraindividual and peer influences on adolescents' heterosexual romantic and sexual behavior. *Archives of Sexual Behavior, 33,* 381–394.

Ziol-Guest, K. M., & Dunifon, R. E. (2014). Complex living arrangements and child health: Examining family structure linkages with children's health outcomes. *Family Relations, 63,* 424–437.

Zito, R. C., & De Coster, S. (2016). Family structure, maternal dating, and sexual debut: Extending the conceptualization of instability. *Journal of Youth and Adolescence, 45,* 1003–1019.

Zucker, K. J. (2010). The DSM diagnostic criteria for gender identity disorder in children. *Archives of Sexual Behavior, 39,* 477–498.

Zucker, K. J., Bradley, S. J., Owen-Anderson, A., Kibblewhite, S. J., & Cantor, J. M. (2008). Is gender identity disorder in adolescents coming out of the closet? *Journal of Sex and Marital Therapy, 34,* 287–290.

Zuckerman, M. (1994). *Behavioral expressions and biosocial bases of sensation seeking.* Cambridge, UK: Cambridge University Press.

Author Index

Subject Index

Note. *f* after a page number indicates a figure.